# The Two Psychiatries

# The Two Psychiatries:
## The Transformation of Psychiatric Work in Saskatchewan, 1905-1984

**Harley D. Dickinson**

Canadian Plains Research Center
University of Regina
1989

**Canadian Cataloguing in Publication Data**

Dickinson, Harley D., 1951–
The two psychiatries : the transformation of psychiatric work in Saskatchewan, 1905–1984

(Canadian plains studies, ISSN 0317–6290 ; 15)
Includes bibliographical references and index.
ISBN: 0–88977–048–4

1. Psychiatry — Saskatchewan — History. 2. Social psychiatry — Saskatchewan — History. I. University of Regina. Canadian Plains Research Center. II. Title. III. Series

RC448.S32D53 616.89'0097124 C89–098066–7

*For*
*Jane, John and Sarah*

# Contents

# Figures

# Tables

# Abbreviations

ACCL: All Canadian Congress of Labour
BSW: Bachelor of Social Work
CAP: Canadian Assistance Plan
CCF: Co-operative Commonwealth Federation
CCL: Canadian Congress of Labour
CMHA: Canadian Mental Health Association
CMP: Capitalist Mode of Production
CPN: Community Psychiatric Nurse
DPH: Department of Public Health
DPW: Department of Public Works
ECT: Electro-Convulsive Therapy
EDP: Electronic Data Processing
FP: Forces of Production
GSA: Government Services Association
MCIC: Medical Care Insurance Commission
MLA: Member of the Legislative Assembly
MSW: Master of Social Work
NCMH: National Committee for Mental Hygiene
NDP: New Democratic Party
NWT: North-West Territories
PAPC: Prince Albert Psychiatric Centre
PSB: Psychiatric Services Branch
PSC: Public Service Commission
PSS: Psychological Society of Saskatchewan

| | |
|---|---|
| PSW: | Psychiatric Social Worker |
| RN: | Registered Nurse |
| RPN: | Registered Psychiatric Nurse |
| SAB: | Saskatchewan Archives Board |
| SCPS: | Saskatchewan College of Physicians and Surgeons |
| SHNB: | Saskatchewan Hospital North Battleford |
| SWH: | Saskatchewan Hospital Weyburn |
| SPNA: | Saskatchewan Psychiatric Nurses Association |
| SRNA: | Saskatchewan Registered Nurses Association |
| SRP: | Social Relations of Production |
| SW: | Social Worker |
| TLC: | Trades and Labour Congress |
| UCSC: | United Civil Servants of Canada |
| YPC: | Yorkton Psychiatric Centre |

# Preface

This book is an analysis of the nature and organization of psychiatric work in Saskatchewan. It focusses on the forces that contributed to the formation and transformation of psychiatry, considered as a form of work, throughout this century. As such, this study is a contribution to the development of a sociology of psychiatry. The development of a distinct sociology of psychiatry was suggested by Schatzman and Strauss in the early 1970s, both for its own sake and as a preliminary for the development of an adequate sociology of mental disorder or mental illness. They claimed that an understanding of mental disorders required an understanding of the social practices which resulted in the diagnosis and treatment of those disorders.

The analysis presented here shows there has been a major transformation in the nature and organization of psychiatric practice in this century. I argue that psychiatry, especially since World War II, is characterized by an institutional bifurcation. On the one hand, we have seen the development of a medically dominated, private sector psychiatric services system wherein treatment, generally in the form of psychotropic drugs, is provided on an out-patient basis by general practitioners or psychiatrists working on a fee-for-service basis. If in-patient treatment is required it is most often provided in psychiatric wards, or even general wards, of general hospitals. On the other hand, we have also seen the development and expansion of a public sector psychiatric services system wherein diagnosis and treatment is provided by non-medical mental health professions, such as social workers, psychologists and community psychiatric nurses, usually working for a salary within a mental health clinic setting. These are the "two psychiatries" referred to in the title.

Within these two psychiatries we find substantial differences in terms of who does what, to whom, where and with what consequences. Although I do not provide a comprehensive examination of all the differences in this study, the observation of these differences supports Schatzman and Strauss's claim that the development of a sociology of mental disorder or mental illness first requires the development of a sociology of psychiatry.

It is important to note that the instituional bifurcation identified in this study serves to link the sociology of psychiatry to a much broader sociological project — the sociology of social reproduction. That is, the transformation in the nature and organization of psychiatry suggests that there has been a transformation in the nature and organization of social reproduction processes in general. Social reproduction refers to the ways, and the extent to which, individuals are constituted as social agents and active subjects who are available, willing and able to perform socially determined roles and functions. Recent estimates indicate that in Canada as many as one person in three will receive some form of treatment within the official mental health services systems. This may or may not indicate higher rates of prevalence or incidence of mental disorders than in the past. What it does clearly indicate, however, is a revolution in the form and content of at least certain aspects of the social reproduction processes of modern societies. More specifically it suggests that people are increasingly turning to scientifically trained experts for assistance with their problems in living. The professionally dominated processes of scientized reproduction are, as this study indicates, also subjected to attempts to increase the efficiency and reduce the costs of service delivery. That is, the processes of social reproduction increasingly are being rationalized. The consequences of the rationalization of reproduction for service recipients remain to be analyzed.

The consequences of this rationalization for the nature and organization of service provider's work, however, have been at least partly analyzed in the present study.

This study, which was originally a doctoral dissertation undertaken at the University of Lancaster, England, was made possible because of access I was granted to a unique and valuable data source.

Nine of the former ministers of public health for Saskatchewan granted me permission to use their restricted access archive materials. Thus, I had access to restricted files stored by the Saskatchewan Archives Board (SAB) covering the entire 1944-76 period. Most of these files had never before been used for research purposes. Use of these records required written permission from each of the former ministers, which was granted in all but two cases.

Although a number of studies have used archival materials, including case notes and personal files, ministerial documents are largely an untapped data source.

It was decided to concentrate on the records of former provincial ministers of public health since they were ultimately responsible for the provision of psychiatric services in the province, and thus any documents, records or reports relating to the organization of psychiatry as work, rather than as treatment, would be in their files. Saskatchewan law states that government department records be transferred to SAB when a government changes and it was anticipated that these files would be a rich source of data. They included copies of correspondence, memos, reports and briefs which came directly from the minister's office, as well as a full range of documents from individuals, government departments, and occupational and other groups interested in the development of psychiatric services. In a few cases there were even copies of letters written, but not sent, as well as written accounts of telephone conversations wherein important discussions concerning management strategy or tactics were summarized.

The documentation amounts to a detailed record of factors considered in the development and management of the provincial psychiatric system. It is particularly valuable as sociological data because it constitutes a record of these developments as a product of various social practices.

The richness of the data raised the question of presentation. The temptation with this type of qualitative data is to quote the material at length, in order to make as much as possible available to the reader. Doing this, however, invariably results in a longer manuscript. The alternative, which is to paraphrase and précis the material, allows for a more concise presentation, but obscures the richness of the data. Throughout the book I have attempted to strike a balance between these alternatives.

Other sources of data were also used. These included: (1) personal interviews with former Saskatchewan ministers of public health, including T.C. Douglas. I also interviewed psychiatrists, social workers, psychologists, psychiatric nurses and others involved in, or knowledgeable about, the development of psychiatry in the province; (2) personal files containing unpublished documents, reports, papers and minutes of meetings; (3) unrestricted access archival materials; and (4) various secondary sources, such as published articles, books and reports. Of particular use were the Annual Reports of the Saskatchewan Department of Public Health, the Public Accounts of the Province of Saskatchewan, and the Annual Reports of the Saskatchewan Medical Care Insurance Commission. Much of the empirical data presented as tables and graphs is derived from these sources. In combination, these data sources provided the basis for the account of the transformation of psychiatric work presented here.

The book consists of seven chapters and an appendix. Chapter One introduces the focus of analysis and the approach to be used. Chapters Two through Six constitute an account of the development of community psychiatry in Saskatchewan between 1914 and 1980. Chapter Two examines the nature and organization of mental hospital work, and various attempts to transform insanity into mental illness in the 1914-44 period. Chapter Three continues with an analysis of the transformation of the mental hospital labour process up to 1963. It focusses on the creation of the occupation of psychiatric nursing and the transformation of mental hospital work from a custodial to a therapeutic labour process. It also examines the relationship of this process to the development of community psychiatry and the medicalization of psychiatric work. Chapter Four focusses on the development of the community psychiatric labour process, the emergence of the community psychiatric division of labour and the transformation of the principal locus of psychiatric work. It is suggested that the development of this division of labour cannot best be understood in terms of the deskilling of psychiatric work. Chapter Five looks at the depopulation of the mental hospitals in relationship to the medicalization of psychiatric work and the expansion of community psychiatry. Throughout the 1963-71 period covered by this chapter there is evidence of the systematic deskilling of psychiatric work. Chapter Six, the last substantive chapter, continues with an examination of the community psychiatric labour process and its relationship to what I see as an incipient de-medicalization of community psychiatric work. Chapter Seven provides the conclusions to the book. The appendix outlines the principal concepts and techniques of a theory of the labour process.

# Acknowledgements

I am greatly indebted to a large number of people for their assistance at different stages of this project.

I would like to thank the former Saskatchewan ministers of public health, J.W. Erb, W.G. Davies, A.E. Blakeney, D.G. Steuart, G.B. Grant, W. Smishek, W. Robbins, and the late T.C. Douglas and T.J. Bentley, who granted me access to restricted archival materials. I must also thank the people interviewed for sharing their time and knowledge, W.G. Davies, J.W. Erb, M.J. Katz, W. Ford, F. Coburn, T. Greenough, G. Rutherford, P. Griffiths, H. Stallwick, I. MacDonald, the late T.C. Douglas, and D. Bennett of Maudsley Hospital, London, England.

I would also like to thank Kent Silzer and Wayne Fritz for their invaluable assistance and many fruitful leads, as well as others at Psychiatric Services Branch, Regina, who provided me with much useful information. I also appreciate the kind cooperation of the staff of the Saskatchewan Archives Board at both the Regina and Saskatoon offices.

This monograph was first prepared as a doctoral dissertation at the University of Lancaster, England. I would like to give special thanks to Drs. Keith Soothill and Larry Ray, who were my Ph.D. supervisors. My doctoral studies were funded by the Social Sciences and Humanities Research Council in the form of a doctoral fellowship. I gratefully acknowledge that support.

I would also like to thank Mark Stobbe, Glenn Andre, Dexter Slugoski, Eric Kempthorne, and Anita Wong.

My many friends and colleagues in the Department of Sociology and in the College of Arts and Science, University of Saskatchewan, have provided both intellectual and institutional support which I greatly appreciate.

Mr. Gordon Arnott, of Arnott, Kelley, O'Connor & Associates, Ltd. of Regina kindly provided me with the original architectural drawing for the Psychiatric Centre in Yorkton.

I am grateful to Gillian Wadsworth Minifie and Brian Mlazgar of the Canadian Plains Research Center, University of Regina, for their experience and editorial skills.

Many thanks to my parents for their support. Above and beyond all others, however, it was Jane who supported, encouraged and assisted me throughout — thanks!

# Permissions

Permissions to quote from the following previously published materials are gratefully acknowledged:

Chapter 1, note 7, p. 309. Reprinted with permission of Croom Helm, London, from "The Futures of Professionalization" by Eliot Friedson in *Health and the Division of Labour*, ed. Margaret Stacey et al., 1977.

Chapter 1, notes 26, 28-33, pp. 310-311. Copyright 1979 by Andrew T. Scull, 1979. Reproduced by permission of Allen Lane The Penguin Press, from *Museums of Madness: The Social Organization of Insanity in Nineteenth-Century England.*

Chapter 1, note 37, p. 311. Reproduced with permission of Routledge from I.K. Zola, "Medicine as Social Control," in *The Sociological Review* 20 (1972): 487.

Chapter 3, note 136, p. 328. Copyright 1985 Merrill Publishing Co., Columbus, Ohio. Reproduced from *Deviance and Medicalization: From Badness to Sickness* by Peter Conrad and Joseph W. Schneider.

Chapter 4, note 18, p. 329. Reproduced with permission of the Minister of Supply and Services Canada from *Trends in Psychiatric Care* by D.G. McKerracher, 1966.

Chapter 4, note 36, p. 329. Reprinted with permission of the Canadian Hospital Association from J.D. McMillan, "Community Mental Health," in *The Canadian Hospital* 34 (May 1957): 41-42.

Chapter 5, note 3, p. 333. Reprinted with permission of the Minister of Supply and Services Canada from *Trends in Psychiatric Care* by D.G. McKerracher, 1966.

Chapter 5, notes 58, 59 and 61, p. 336. Reprinted with permission of the Minister of Supply and Services Canada from Helen K. Mussallem, *Nursing Education in Canada*, 1966.

Appendix, notes 1 and 5, p. 351, note 33, p. 353, notes 36, 51 and 52, p. 354. Reproduced by permission of Penguin Books, Ltd. from *Capital, A Critique of Political Economy Volume 1* by Karl Marx, 1976.

Appendix, note 2, p. 351. Copyright 1974 by Harry Braverman. Reprinted by permission of Monthly Review Foundation.

Appendix, note 6, p. 352. Copyright 1973 by the AAAS.

Appendix, note 8, p. 352. Copyright 1973 by Monthly Review Inc. Reprinted by permission of Monthly Review Foundation.

Appendix, note 13, p. 352. Copyright 1976 by Monthly Review Inc. Reprinted by permission of Monthly Review Foundation.

# Chapter One

# The Sociology of Psychiatric Work

This book examines aspects of the development of community psychiatry in terms of a transformation in the nature and organization of psychiatric work. In general, it examines various conditions and processes associated with the historical medicalization and incipient de-medicalization of public sector psychiatry in Saskatchewan. More specifically, it examines the hypothesis that development of the occupational division of labour associated with community psychiatry is based upon the de-skilling of psychiatric work.

The focus on psychiatric practice as work was suggested almost twenty years ago by Schatzman and Strauss. Noting that most of the relevant sociological literature at the time constituted a sociology in and for, not about, psychiatry, they proposed a research programme for the sociology of psychiatry. The programme consisted of five models which provided a framework for the examination of the process of professional role-creation and negotiation in various work locales, and various socio-cultural and political processes external to, but influential in, workplace interactions. Having adopted this focus, they claimed they then had "little interest in certain standard problems — for example, in studies of prevalence and incidence — since the search for mental disturbance is not viewed as independent of the 'production' of it."[1]

This is not to say a sociological analysis of mental illness is not fruitful. I agree with Robertson that "sociology can make a distinctive contribution to an understanding of the causes of mental disorder."[2] The sociology of mental disorders, however, is analytically distinct from the sociology of psychiatry, and the two cannot properly be conflated. For this reason, the extensive body of sociological literature which has contributed to an understanding of the etiology and epidemiology of mental illness is not examined here.[3] By analyzing the rise and development of community psychiatry in terms of the transformation of psychiatric work, I hope to make a contribution to the sociology of psychiatry.

Analyzing community psychiatry in terms of the transformation of psychiatric work entails more than an analysis of the changing nature of psychiatrists' work. As Kahn has pointed out, besides the medically trained psychiatrist,

> the practitioner of community psychiatry may also be a social worker, a psychologist, a nurse, or a member of a related profession who has had a degree of clinical training and who has been prepared for the role.[4]

Community psychiatry is conceptualized as a labour process which in part consists of a particular occupational division of labour. Therefore, an understanding of the rise and development of community psychiatry necessitates an understanding of the rise and development of the community psychiatric division of labour, including the non-medical occupational groups. It also necessitates an analysis of the institutional context within which community psychiatric work is performed, as well as the relationship between the institutional context and the occupational division of labour. In other words, it involves attempting to determine why the principal locus of psychiatric work shifted from the mental hospital to the community, and what the relationship was between this transition and the development of the community psychiatric occupational division of labour.

The usual approach of the sociology of psychiatry has been to analyze psychiatric work, and the historical change of psychiatric work, in terms of the processes of professionalization. Thus Schatzman and Strauss, and others working within the interactionist tradition, analyze the various struggles in which different professions engage as they attempt to negotiate a workplace role that will give them power and autonomy. Bucher and Stelling, for example, observe:

> What one sees in many organizations is the struggle of different groups for varying degrees of professional recognition, with differential success in different locales. The reward for success is autonomy and influence: the group is accorded the competence to define problems, determine solutions, and monitor the functioning of the system.[5]

Similarly, Andrew Scull analyzes the rise of the asylum and the medicalization of insanity in nineteenth-century England as part of a process associated with the professionalization of mental hospital medical superintendents' work. Thus the main focus for these studies is professions and/or the process of professionalization. Freidson points out, however, that there are certain conceptual and empirical problems endemic to the concepts of profession and professionalization, and suggests a new research programme. The balance of this chapter includes a brief exposition of Freidson's critique of the sociology of professions and his programmatic recommendations. Also included is a critical examination of the work of Andrew Scull and the derivative work of Diana Ralph, in terms of their contribution to the analysis of community psychiatry.

## Freidson and the Sociology of Professions

Freidson has noted that, with few exceptions,[6] the literature of the sociology of professions has been characterized by "a remarkable unanimity."[7] Specifically, it is agreed that professions exist as a type of occupation with special importance to the effective and humane functioning of modern society, that they have been growing in number and importance throughout this century, and that they will continue to increase in both number and importance into the next century.[8]

With regard to these assessments and predictions, however, he concludes "we are left in limbo . . . for they do not provide us with the intellectual tools by which we can connect them to concrete occupations."[9] In addition, a closer examination of the literature indicates that the unanimity may be more apparent than real. This is because the concept of profession is used in different ways by different authors. Freidson identifies four distinct uses.

The least practical usage for sociological purposes is as an ideological claim. Various occupational groups lay claim to the title "professional" in an attempt to substantiate their demands for increased status, pay or power. By claiming to be professions, many insist that such rewards are their due. Although the use of the concept as an ideological claim might be an effective bargaining tool, it has no utility for sociological analysis.

Another usage, which he calls the "market-related labour" approach, is based on the difference between "professional" and "amateur." The operative distinction is whether one is paid for one's work. On the basis of this distinction, it is argued that the number of professions is expanding because increasing numbers of people are being drawn into the paid labour force. This observation is interesting in light of Marx's conceptualization of capital accumulation as multiplication of the proletariat;[10] a process referred to as proletarianization. Thus, using the "market-related labour" approach, professionalization and proletarianization, usually understood as opposites, refer to the same process. This approach is the least sophisticated variant of the "professionalization of everyone" thesis critically examined by Wilensky.[11]

The attribute approach is probably most common. This approach posits that an occupation is a profession if it is characterized by certain traits. Although the attributes vary from profession to profession, some of the most common include years of formal education, skill, service orientation, an esoteric theory, collegial body and self-regulation.

Habenstein has shown that the structural-functionalist approach, which addresses the question of what unique roles or functions professions serve for society, is a sophisticated variant of the attribute approach.[12] This is because the question itself is based on the assumption that professions have a "constellation of characteristics" which allow them to serve some unique function. This should be demonstrated, however, rather than assumed.

Freidson notes it is often argued by those using the attribute approach that professions also constitute a distinct class. This, however, often obscures important differences between occupations and the institutions in which they work. Thus he observes that "A particular kind of work . . . can be organized as a profession at one point in history and not at another, and in one nation and not in another."[13] Similarly, Bucher and Stelling, working within the interactionist tradition, note that "Occupational label is no necessary indicator of professional status; the status of people of particular occupational titles can vary markedly in different formal organizations."[14] Psychiatrists, for example, can be independent private practitioners, salaried employees of private and public corporations, managers of various facilities or research scientists deriving their income from grants. Although all are psychiatrists, the differences in the nature and organization of their work, and consequently their specific workplace and career interests, outweigh the similarities common training may generate. A good example of this is the relationship between public and private sector psychiatrists in Saskatchewan throughout the 1960s and 1970s.

Defining class membership on the basis of common attributes, rather than in relational terms, also limits one's ability to analyze the differences between occupations within different work settings. As Freidson states, the concept of class is inappropriate for analyzing the nature and organization of work at the concrete level. He claims that a better understanding of

> the division of labour and . . . the crucial differences *among* occupations . . . requires . . . an emphasis on

> the degree to which they, as occupations rather than classes, have gained the organized power to control themselves the terms, conditions and content of their work in the settings where they perform their work.[15]

This, which is in essence the fourth way the concept of profession is used, is referred to as the occupational monopoly and dominance approach, and is used by the interactionists in the analysis of specific occupational struggles for workplace power and autonomy. Although the reward for successful negotiation is supposedly professional recognition, the interactionist approach does not permit specification of "the conditions under which a group succeeds or fails in the achievement of professional status."[16]

The explanatory limitations of the interactionist approach are further highlighted by Schatzman and Bucher. Following an account of a division of labour in a state mental hospital, they observe that different occupational groups "Undoubtedly . . . meet with variable success in negotiating their claims"[17] for professional status. This is followed by the somewhat vacuous conclusion that

> the modern scene . . . will offer more negotiation among professionals, particularly as working situations become increasingly complex and interprofessional in structure.[18]

Certain sociologically interesting questions remain unasked, such as what leads to, and what the nature of the changing division of labour is, and why some occupational groups are successful and others are not. The interactionist approach remains a method in search of a theory.

In order to avoid these problems Freidson suggests that there are three elements to be considered in the definition of a profession: (1) the form of occupational organization, which provides (2) a labour market monopoly, and (3) autonomy within an occupational division of labour.[19] Although this is conceptually superior to the attribute approach, it is still beset with empirical difficulties. For example, there is no evidence that a form of occupational organization exists which can, in general, generate a labour market monopoly and workplace autonomy. As the interactionists have demonstrated, occupational status and power are contingent upon context. In addition, labour market monopoly is no guarantee of workplace autonomy. A good example of this is the case of psychiatric nurses in Saskatchewan. Although they had a legislative monopoly of on-ward mental hospital work after 1948, they were completely dominated by medical superintendants and physicians within the mental hospital division of labour.

If a profession cannot be identified by a particular form of occupational organization or a labour market monopoly, one is left with the criterion of workplace autonomy. As Freidson puts it, given an occupational organization and a labour market monopoly, a profession is an occupation with "a place in the division of labour that is free of the authority of others over their work."[20] If this is taken at face value, however, no occupation working within the context of an employment relation could be a profession, since the work of all employees is subject to employer authority. This observation corresponds to the professionalization-bureaucratization dichotomy found in some literature of the sociology of professions.[21] Even if one does not adopt this hardline, however, there are problems with using workplace autonomy as definitive of professions. If autonomy and control are contingent and variable between and within occupations, as the interactionists have demonstrated, how is one to use these criteria to distinguish a profession from a non-profession? How much power and autonomy within the workplace is needed to accord an occupation professional status? Which aspects of an occupation's work must be subject to self-direction and control?

The problem is, of course, that no matter what answer is given, it can always be criticized for being arbitrary. This lends credence to Habenstein's contention that the concept of profession has little analytical utility. It also concurs with Freidson that "the analysis of the organization of control over work, and its consequences for work, workers, organizations and society"[22] is more sociologically important than attempting to determine if an occupation is, or is not, a profession.

In terms of giving theoretical coherence to the sociology of professions, Freidson also suggests that a focus on the organization of control over work will facilitate "the critical use of at least some of the perspectives and analytical tools developed by Marxist theory."[23] His comment suggests the possible utility of a Marxist theory of the labour process for understanding the changing nature and organization of psychiatric work associated with the development of community psychiatry. One of the objectives of this book is to address that question. For an extended discussion of labour process theory in this regard see the Appendix.

## Andrew Scull and the Rise and Fall of the Asylum

Andrew Scull has made a major contribution to the development of a sociology of psychiatry. Prior to Scull's work, much of the literature concerned with the history of psychiatry consisted of cataloguing how ideas about the insane changed over time, and/or discovering modern psychiatric ideas in the writings of previous epochs.[24] Works of this type have usually been written by psychiatrists with few sociological aspirations. As a consequence, the mechanism of social change is often located in some idealized march of medical science. Within this model, medical knowledge of insanity progresses from ignorance to enlightenment, and psychiatric practice from barbarous punishment to benevolent treatment, notwithstanding the fact that many medical treatments were (and may still be) barbarous.[25] Scull claims the nineteenth-century medicalization of insanity cannot be explained in terms of the march of science. He observes, for example, that "as an ideological prop for the professional claims of psychiatry, this claim has obvious merits; as an historical analysis of the process itself it has none."[26]

The work of Thomas Szasz[27] is an interesting inversion of the march of medicine approach. Although Szasz is himself a medically trained psychiatrist, he presents an account of the development of modern medical psychiatry as the machinations of a malevolent and imperialistic profession. Rather than psychiatric treatment being viewed as the apogee of humanism and modern medical science, it is presented as a sophisticated form of oppression perpetrated through a gigantic fraud. Like the march of medicine approach, the anti-psychiatry of Szasz has little explanatory value. It does, however, have obvious merits as an ideology for those non-medical occupational groups struggling against the medical domination of the community psychiatric division of labour.

In *Museums of Madness* Scull sets out to explain what the march of medicine authors take for granted or use as explanation. Thus he asks how insanity was transformed into mental illness; why the asylum emerged as the principal locus of psychiatric work in the nineteenth century; what its relation was to the professionalization of psychiatry; and why these changes took the form they did. These are all important sociological questions, and Scull's answers are a major contribution to the historical sociology of psychiatry. However, his analysis is characterized by a number of weaknesses.

My critique of Scull has two objectives. The first is to show that in an attempt to prove asylum-based psychiatric work had been successfully professionalized and medicalized by the early part of the twentieth century, a number of disparate occupational practices are conflated. Thus he ignores a number of subsequent developments characteristic of psychiatric work in the twentieth century. The second is to demonstrate that his decarceration thesis is one-sided, and incapable of adequately accounting for the nature and form of community-based alternatives to mental hospitals which have developed since World War II.

Scull provides an explanation of the rise of the asylum in terms of the medicalization of insanity and the professionalization of asylum doctors' work in the nineteenth century. He has correctly observed that

> At the close of the century . . . the professional status of the asylum doctors remained distinctly questionable. Conspicuously mired in the status of salaried employees . . . they shared with similarly situated groups like workhouse doctors and public health officers at best a tenuous hold on social respectability and but a paltry measure of the autonomy usually

> granted to those engaged in professional work. Since then, however, practitioners of psychological medicine have, with somewhat more success, laid claim to these standard accoutrements of professional status.[28]

By the conceptual sleight of hand of transforming asylum doctors into practitioners of psychological medicine, Scull concludes that asylum doctors have subsequently achieved professional status, a conclusion which is important for his later analysis of the twentieth-century decarceration movement. How was this professional status supposedly achieved?

First, Scull argues that the asylum itself, as the material base from which the drive for professional status took place, was of strategic importance. This was because the asylum "assured [psychiatry's] cognitive monopoly and guaranteed a (captive) market for its services."[29] Given these two advantages, he then argues that

> psychiatry needed only to develop a plausible esoteric theory and a course of professional training to transmit it, in order to persuade the public of its expertise and thus to secure its independence from outside scrutiny and interference in its line of work.[30]

Leaving aside his use of the attribute approach to professionalization and the dubious claim that professional independence from outside scrutiny can be secured by the development of a plausible esoteric theory and course of training, let us examine the argument upon which this claim is based. Scull has suggested that psychoanalytic theory, or Freudian ideas, fulfilled the function of a plausible esoteric theory, and that the transmission of these through a course of training were critical to the attainment of workplace autonomy, "notwithstanding the obvious impracticality of applying them in an asylum context."[31] However, surely a plausible esoteric theory that cannot be practically applied in the workplace is unlikely to "persuade the public of its [psychiatry's] expertise and thus . . . secure its independence." Yet this is precisely what Scull has claimed. How did Freudian ideas achieve this? Apparently "by encouraging the development of the whole new realm of office practice, coping with upper class neurotics,"[32] and thereby allowing psychiatry at once

> to dilute the ill-effects of overly close association with the poor, the stigmatized, and the unwanted; and to establish among the elite its credentials as a doubly worthy enterprise.[33]

This seems to have been the objective of his earlier conceptual transformation of asylum doctors into practitioners of psychological medicine. By transforming asylum doctors, medically trained private practice psychiatrists and psychoanalysts into one profession — practitioners of psychological medicine — Scull can then conclude that asylum doctors had achieved professional autonomy and independence from outside scrutiny and control.

This conflation is, however, analytically and historically illegitimate. Analytically, it must be recognized that asylum doctors working within the asylums, and medically trained private practice psychiatrists and psychoanalysts working within the "whole new realm of office practice," do not constitute a unified profession. It would appear evident, even in terms of Scull's account, that the physician working with psychotics in the asylum and the psychoanalyst working with upper-class neurotics in an office setting are not doing the same type of work. They are, in fact, engaged in quite distinct labour processes, characterized by specific social forces and relations of production.

Historically it is illegitimate because psychoanalytic theory was developed by Freud as a psychological alternative to the neurological theory of insanity embraced by medically trained psychiatrists. Freud, however, did not believe there was anything in the nature of psychoanalytic theory which would preclude its use in psychiatric practice. In his introductory lectures, given around the turn of the century, he claimed that it was not psychiatry but psychiatrists who opposed psychoanalysis.[34] In light of this, the fact that Freudian ideas were enthusiastically embraced by American psychiatrists in the interwar years needs to be explained. Although Ray has made some suggestions regarding the basis of the unlikely marriage of psychoanalysis and psychiatry, a complete analysis has yet to be done.[35]

In addition, it cannot be assumed, as Scull does, that the adoption of psychoanalytical theory,

> having secured psychiatry's position *vis-à-vis* the insane . . . provided the basis for the profession's subsequent efforts to engulf other forms of deviance, and reduce these to a medical paradigm.[36]

Thus, Scull's analysis of the professionalization of psychiatry and medicalization of madness is subsequently presented as an example of a more general tendency towards the medicalization of deviance. In an influential paper entitled "Medicine as an Institution of Social Control," first published in 1972, Zola clearly stated this medicalization of deviance thesis: "medicine is becoming a major institution of social control, nudging aside if not incorporating, the more traditional institutions of religion and law."[37] This is echoed by Scull in the conclusion of *Museums of Madness*.[38]

This medicalization of deviance thesis implicitly informs Scull's analysis of the post-World War II decarceration movement. Decarceration is usually defined as "a state-sponsored effort to de-institutionalize deviant populations [which] has become a central element in the social control practices of advanced capitalist societies,"[39] although at times other meanings are attached to the term.

When Scull wishes to argue that decarceration is simply the abandonment of various problem populations, especially the mentally ill, it refers solely to a process of depopulating the mental hospitals. When he talks about deviant populations other than the mentally ill, such as the criminal, it refers to a policy of developing various facilities designed to divert people from the traditional institutions of social control.[40]

Based upon the argument that the main features of the social control apparatuses in England and America, "prior to the adoption of a policy of de-institutionalization," were "progressive institutionalization, bureaucratization, and professionalization," Scull purports to provide an explanation of the apparent reversal of these trends in terms of "the complex dialectical interplay between transformations in the social control apparatus . . . and changes in the wider social system."[41]

This takes the form of an argument that the principal impetus for decarceration is the control of state expenditures. Even on this issue, however, Scull tends to be somewhat confused. On the one hand, following Gough, he argues that the "problem" of rapid increases in state expenditures following World War II is "undoubtedly exacerbated in the case of state services by the absence of competitive pressures to reduce costs."[42] Contradictorily, he states the principal cause and explanation of decarceration is to be found in pervasive and intense cost-cutting pressures:

> Once the drive for the control of soaring costs is seen as the factor underlaying the move towards decarceration . . . this change which formerly appeared either fortuitous or inexplicable becomes readily comprehensible.[43]

What remains incomprehensible is how a policy of decarceration can be caused by pressures to reduce state expenditures if, as he claims, the provision of state services is characterized by an absence of pressure to reduce costs. Even more problematic for Scull's account is the fact that, in many cases, total costs are not reduced. This can only be explained by Scull in terms of state bureaucrats misleading both government officials and academic researchers by "statistical juggling and administrative sleight of hand."[44] One wonders, however, just who is performing this juggling, and why. Unfortunately, Scull avoids these questions.

Other problems exist with Scull's account. Perhaps the most significant is that the cost-cutting argument, despite Scull's assertions to the contrary, does not account for the characteristic form assumed by the diverse community-based alternatives to the mental hospital. The assertion that "it is the pervasiveness and intensity of these [cost-cutting] pressures . . . which account for most of the characteristic features of the new system of community 'care and treatment' "[45] can only be accepted as true if one accepts the assumption that decarceration entails the replacement of institution-based care and treatment with nothing — the abandonment of problem populations to the "sewers of human misery."[46]

Although Scull notes that the decarceration process can be, and has been, slowed down and even reversed by union struggles and other sources of political opposition,[47] he dismisses these as being of marginal importance. By so doing, he is able to revert to a simple economic reductionism.[48]

Although economic motives may underlie the depopulation of the mental hospitals, this does not explain the form taken by the many community-based alternatives. Of particular concern is the fact that this economism provides no explanation of the particular occupational division of labour associated with the rise of community psychiatry. Similarly, it cannot explain the myriad facilities developed as alternatives to the mental hospitals, and within which community psychiatric work occurs.

It has been argued that two factors have resulted in Scull conflating the complex and varied processes of decarceration into "a single, unitary phenomenon."[49] The first is the view that decarceration is the product of pressures to reduce state expenditures. The second is the assumption that most forms of deviance have been effectively medicalized. This second assumption allows Scull to conflate deviants, be they mentally ill, criminals or juvenile deliquents, into a more or less homogeneous "problem population" which is engulfed or discharged by various social control apparatuses depending on what is considered to be most cost effective at the time.

The view that complete and unproblematic medical control of the "mentally ill" had been achieved by the end of the nineteenth century or early part of the twentieth century is not uncommon. Jones has pointed out, however, that the Lunacy Act of 1890, passed following the death of Lord Shaftesbury, transformed control of the definition of insanity into a legal matter.[50] Although state-supported asylums were managed by medically trained superintendents, control of the initial definition and disposition of the insane had become a legal prerogative. Shaftesbury, who piloted the British Lunacy Act of 1845 through Parliament, was a great champion of the medicalization of insanity. He was firmly committed to the ideology that the cure for mental illness lay in early treatment. "In fact," as Skultans has noted, "the importance attributed to early treatment explains Shaftesbury's opposition to the introduction of more comprehensive safeguards for the liberty of the subject."[51] Shaftesbury and other proponents of the medical model of mental illness

> regarded the legalization of insanity as representing a threat to the early treatment of mental illness. Thus it was only after his death that the Lunacy Consolidation Bill ('the triumph of legalism') could become law in 1890.[52]

Following passage of this act, medical control of the definition of mental illness was at best partial. The situation was similar in North America at that time. The first decades of this century were thus characterized by various attempts to transform insanity into mental illness. This process, especially as it occurred in Saskatchewan, is examined in Chapter Two.

Scull's failure to recognize and account for the tenuous and shifting nature of occupational control of the definition and treatment of the insane in the twentieth century, coupled with a simplistic economic reductionism, has resulted in significant inadequacies both in his account of decarceration and, more importantly, in his (almost complete lack of) analysis of the various community-based alternatives to the mental hospitals which have developed since World War II.

Under the pressure of similar criticisms,[53] Scull has recently reconsidered his views, at least in regard to criminal populations. He insists, however, that he remains

> convinced that for the subpopulations of deviants with whom *Decarceration* was primarily concerned, the mentally ill, this is essentially an accurate representation.[54]

It is my intention to demonstrate that community psychiatry is not a policy of non-intervention and that Scull is incorrect in insisting that it is.

Others have made similar observations. Diana Ralph, for example, in a book highly derivative of Scull's work, states that although *Decarceration*

> is an excellent exposition of the deinstitutionalizing aspect of community psychiatry, it virtually ignores the

> much larger problem of the geometrical expansion in the number of non-psychotic people who get processed through the community psychiatric programs.[55]

In order to correct this deficiency, Ralph takes a particular theme which runs through Scull's work, that "the attempt to manage an increasing proportion of the 'deviant' within the community [is] a response to the changing exigencies of domestic pacification and control"[56] and transforms it into a mono-causal explanation of community psychiatry. She calls this the labour theory of community psychiatry.

As conceptualized by Ralph, community psychiatry is "a nationalized form of industrial psychology" which, motivated by "management's fears of labour militancy on the one hand, and worker and potential worker breakdown on the other," was developed by "the capitalist class and its state" to control both actual and potential labour unrest. Ralph, outlining the implications of her theory, has stated that community psychiatry serves two major functions. Firstly it is intended

> to increase worker tolerance to ever more alienated and pressured work, and to reduce their (and their families') resistance against these alienating situations. Secondarily it serves to pacify displaced workers and potential workers such as housewives, adolescents, and minorities, without rendering them permanently unemployable.[57]

The reliance on a functionalist explanation and a crude conflict model of capitalist society weakens Ralph's analysis. In particular, difficulties exist in demonstrating the causal connections (if any) between the development of community psychiatry and labour unrest. This is especially problematic given the fact that in North America community psychiatry was first developed on a large scale in the non-industrial province of Saskatchewan as a result of the policies of a government avowedly committed to the eradiction of capitalism. These facts hardly provide support for the labour theory of community psychiatry. In addition, it is not clear from Ralph's analysis why community psychiatry assumed the specific institutional form it did, or why it is characterized by a particular occupational division of labour.

Ralph has made a contribution to the analysis of community psychiatry, however, by questioning the assumption of complete and unproblematic medicalization of community psychiatric work. Having drawn attention to the fact that community psychiatry cannot be understood as a simple extension of asylum psychiatry into non-asylum settings, Ralph incorrectly dismisses medical psychiatry as being of secondary significance in shaping the development of community psychiatry. At times she even seems to assume that community psychiatry corresponds to the complete demedicalization of community psychiatric work. Part of the problem is that she assumes community psychiatry must have developed from either public clinical psychiatry or industrial psychology. Within this dichotomy there is no possibility of analyzing community psychiatry as the convergence of a number of interrelated processes, or to see it as having developed from some other distinct, but related, base.

I perceive community psychiatry as a particular manifestation of the public health movement, and this viewpoint is generally accepted. Yolles, for example, maintains that the origin of community psychiatry lies in "the adoption of public health practice to mental health service."[58]

Public health practice, which is based upon an ideological commitment to prevention, usually takes the form of (1) direct intervention into the environment (community), (2) early treatment of incipient disorders, and (3) the mobilization of community resources in an attempt to achieve the first two objectives. The most vigorous advocates of this approach to mental illness throughout the first half of this century were the proponents of the mental hygiene movement. In North America the mental hygienists were organized as the National Committee for Mental Hygiene (NCMH). The membership of the NCMH, until 1950, consisted largely of medically trained physicians, academics, prominent business figures and politicians. In order to facilitate the application of public health principles to psychiatric practice, the NCMH, which had close funding arrangements with the Rockefeller Foundation, engaged in three interrelated activities: (1) propagandizing; (2) political lobbying; and (3) establishing demonstration projects.

The propaganda was an attempt to convince skeptics that mental illness was a disease that could be prevented. The political lobbying was directed towards securing the passage of legislation intended to reform the asylum system and to ensure medical control of the treatment of mental illness. The demonstration projects consisted of training and employing various categories of non-medical labour power to provide follow-up services to discharged mental patients, the objective of which was to convince legislators that hospitalization rates and inmate population levels could effectively and economically be reduced. Although these demonstration projects did, in some cases, entail the training and employment of psychologists, they also consisted of the training and employment of psychiatric social workers and psychiatric nurses. Therefore, Ralph's reduction of community psychiatry to a nationalized version of industrial psychology seems analytically unwarranted and historically incorrect. It is also somewhat surprising, given her observation that post-World War II psychiatry has been characterized by a shift "from an individual clinical model of treatment to a mass public health conception of its mandate."[59]

Neither Scull nor Ralph specifically analyzes community psychiatry as a form of work. This, however, is the principal focus of this book, a focus drawn from the interactionist branch of the sociology of professions, particularly that segment involved in developing a sociology of psychiatry. Based on a critique of the sociology of professions approach, Freidson has suggested it might be sociologically fruitful to replace the analysis of professionalization with an analysis of the organization and control over work, a change which he suggests might also permit the critical use of certain concepts and analytical tools. This comment raised the question of the potential utility of a theory of the labour process in understanding the rise and development of community psychiatry. This book addresses that question.

# Chapter Two

# Psychiatry and Psychiatric Work in Saskatchewan, 1905-1944

This chapter has two objectives: first the examination of various attempts to medicalize mental illness, and second a description of the nature and organization of mental hospital work in the pre-1944 period. The object of examining pre-war mental hospital work is to provide the context within which the subsequent transformation of psychiatric work associated with the development of community psychiatry in Saskatchewan can be understood.

Saskatchewan did not exist as a province prior to 1905. Before that time, what is now Saskatchewan was administered by the dominion government as part of the North-West Territories (NWT). No legislation existed concerning the insane in the NWT before 1879. In that year an Act Respecting the Safekeeping of Dangerous Lunatics in the North-West Territories was passed by the House of Commons and Senate of Canada. Under this act, a person adjudged to be "insane and dangerous to be at large" could be removed to the penitentiary at Stony Mountain, Manitoba. Such persons were "therein detained at the pleasure of the Governor General in Council or until discharged by law."[1] In the same year, the lieutenant governor of the NWT passed an Ordinance Respecting Dangerous Lunatics. Under this ordinance, a person charged with being "insane and dangerous to be at large" was brought before a justice of the peace. Upon hearing evidence the justice could "commit the prisoner to gaol awaiting the pleasure of the Lieutenant Governor or until the prisoner was discharged by law."[2] Detention in gaol was to be a temporary arrangement, as plans were being developed to build a "Dominion Lunatic Asylum, or Hospital" in Regina. According to the federal minister of public works the proposed institution was to be made suitable for either purpose.[3] Such an institution, however, was never built and until the opening of the mental institution near North Battleford in 1914, no facility for the insane existed in Saskatchewan.

When Saskatchewan became a province, the provisions enacted by the Canadian government for the management and care of the insane were included in the provincial statutes.[4] At that time the provincial attorney general was assigned, among other duties, "the superintendence of asylums, prisons, houses of correction and other places of confinement within the province [as well as] the examination of papers in connection with the admission and discharge of lunatics to and from asylums."[5] In 1906 the Saskatchewan legislature passed the Insanity Act. Under this act, the determination of insanity remained a legal prerogative. In Saskatchewan "insanity" had not yet become "mental illness." The dominance of the view that insanity was a legal matter, and not a medical matter, is attested to by the fact that until 1913 the costs of caring for and maintaining the insane were recorded under the heading "Administration of Justice."[6] One significant change wrought by the 1906 act, however, was the transfer of financial responsibility for the insane from the federal to the provincial government.

In 1907 the new provincial government, under Premier Walter Scott, requested that the provincial health officer, Dr. David Low, visit mental hospitals in eastern Canada and the United States with the view to making recommendations for the construction of a facility in Saskatchewan. Dr. Low conducted the survey and duly submitted his report. The most interesting recommendation made, in light of subsequent developments, was that the planned facility be constructed on the basis of a cottage system:

> I believe the cottage system to be most suitable for the requirements of this Province, because a building suitable for the present population may be erected now and others can be added as required. Thus only buildings actually needed are provided. These are complete in themselves and will not be interfered with by subsequent additions.[7]

This recommendation was not implemented, presumably because of the counterrecommendations of a Toronto-based architectural firm. These were given added weight by the support of Dr. C.K. Clarke, a well-known Canadian psychiatrist and superintendent of the Toronto Asylum:

> We notice that Dr. Low, in his valuable report advises the adoption of the cottage system. While we agree with him that this system gives ideal conditions for the patients themselves, and provides means for breaking up the patients into smaller distinct groups, and that this system has been used successfully in Europe and elsewhere, we think that its use would be questionable in this case for both economic and climatic reasons.[8]

In spite of Dr. Low's argument that the cottage system would be less expensive, the government opted for the construction of a pavilion-style institution near the towns of Battleford and North Battleford (see Figure 1). The choice of what appears to have been a more expensive and less functional option for the first provincial mental institution is interesting, particularly in light of the 1914 Haultain Royal Commission to investigate allegations of patronage and unfair tendering practices surrounding its construction.[9]

The choice of a site for the proposed institution was not an easy matter. Representations from many towns and cities were made which extolled the virtues of locating the asylum in their vicinity. The location of the institution would, of course, have significant social, political and economic consequences for the life of the community chosen. Thus, the final

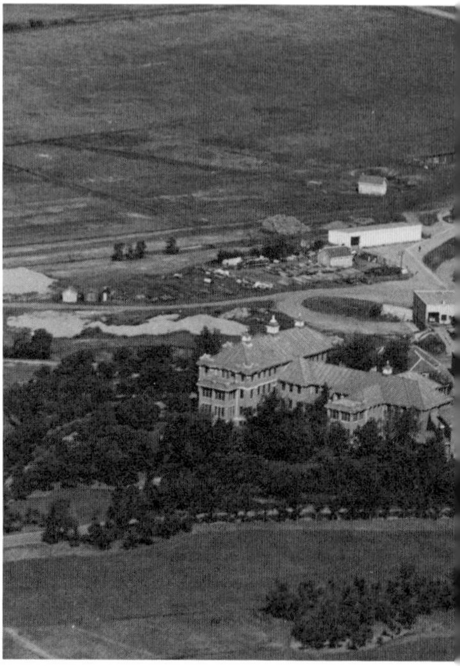

*Figure 1*
*Saskatchewan Hospital,*
*North Battleford c. 1960*
*Source: SAB Photograph Number*
*R-B 5008(2)*

decision to locate the institution "near" the towns of Battleford and North Battleford was apparently political. This aside, the briefs submitted to the government recommending the virtues of locating the institution in one district as opposed to another are interesting insofar as they provide an insight into lay conceptions of the nature of insanity:

> As life itself is at stake the Asylum should be located at the place in the Province, wherever it be situated, which would best consult the interests of its inmates. The location which tends to best assist them to restoration of mind and body should be selected. Environment and surroundings have the greatest influence over the mind, and when this environment is suitable, it alone unaided by medical science is frequently sufficient to restore both the mind and body to their normal healthy condition. What this environment should be needs hardly to be pointed out. Beauty, scenery, trees, lakes, rivers, valleys, quiet rest, air, climate, health, etc., are all factors which go together to constitute a suitable

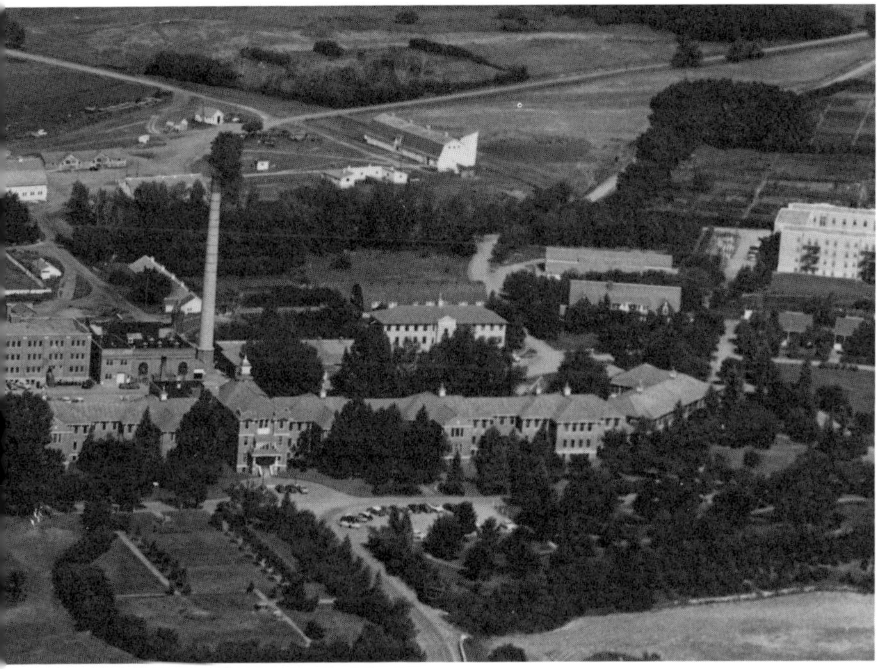

> location. Such environment will do more for the patients than medical treatment.[10]

The view that insanity was not primarily a medical condition and therefore not particularly amenable to medical treatment was prevalent. It was, however, a view which was attacked by medical superintendents of asylums as they struggled for control of the definition of insanity and treatment of the insane. Support for the medicalization of insanity, for example, is to be found in the 1907 Low Report:

> I find that the modern idea is to remove all evidence of restraint in the management of the insane; and instead of insane people being treated as criminals they are regarded as sick people whose disease is some lesion in the brain and treated accordingly.[11]

In spite of this conceptualization among those with medical training, legislative recognition of medical dominance in the definition of insanity was not forthcoming in Saskatchewan until 1950 (see Table 1).

**Table 1**
**Selected Legislation Relevant to the Treatment of Mental Disorders in Saskatchewan**

| Date | Title of Act | Comments |
|---|---|---|
| 1906 | The Insanity Act | Committal was on the order of a provincial magistrate upon finding a person to be insane and dangerous to be at large. |
| 1917 | The Insanity Act is amended | Responsibility for a committal was transferred from the attorney general to the minister of public works. |
| 1919 | The Dangerous Lunatics Act | Committal was still the responsibility of a magistrate. |
| 1922 | The Mental Diseases Act | In the eighth annual report of the North Battleford Mental Hospital the superintendent wrote: "I am pleased to note that the legislation takes into account that a disease process is being dealt with, rather than a criminal prosecution." All committals were, however, still by court order. |
| 1936 | The Mental Hygiene Act | Featured provisions for voluntary admissions and certification by physician in addition to magistrate's committal. |
| 1950 | The Mental Hygiene Act | A court order was no longer required for admission, certification by two physicians was sufficient. Insanity had become mental illness. |
| 1961 | The Mental Health Act | This act was based on the British Mental Health Act, 1959. The admissions process was further liberalized, "voluntary" admissions were abolished and replaced with "informal" admissions which were patterned, in most cases, after the admissions and discharge procedures operative in general hospitals. |

Throughout the first part of this century mental hospitals were primarily custodial institutions. Unless one was fortunate enough to be restored to sanity by "environment and surroundings," the chance of being discharged as cured was slim. In fact, it was not until after World War II that the annual reports of the two provincial mental hospitals included a category for discharges. Prior to that time, the only officially reported ways to leave the hospitals were death, deportation, elopement, transfer or parole. This seems to be an indictment of the dominant modes of treatment of the time, which consisted primarily of "water and work."

"Water" refers to the various forms of hydrotherapy and baths which were employed for their calming effect on agitated patients (see Figures 2 and 3). The Low Report had recommended the use of hydrotherapy for disturbed patients instead of various mechanical constraints or padded cells. A 1918 survey of the Battleford institution, conducted by C.M. Hincks of the National Committee for Mental Hygiene (NCMH), commented favourably on the extensive use of hydrotherapy:

> The medical staff at the Battleford Hospital shows a keen interest in the scientific study and care of their patients and the absence of excitement in the wards was to be explained largely by the fact that hydrotherapeutic treatment is employed intelligently and with good effect. No less than ten continuous baths are to be found in the hospital, and at the time of our visit, they were nearly all occupied by restless patients. Sometimes between forty and fifty hydro treatments per day are given, and the arrangements for the administration of different forms of special douches and electric light baths are admirable.[12]

The ability to work, however, was considered the *sine qua non* of sanity and the most likely route by which a person would be returned to that state. According to the Low Report, agricultural employment was the most effective form of work therapy:

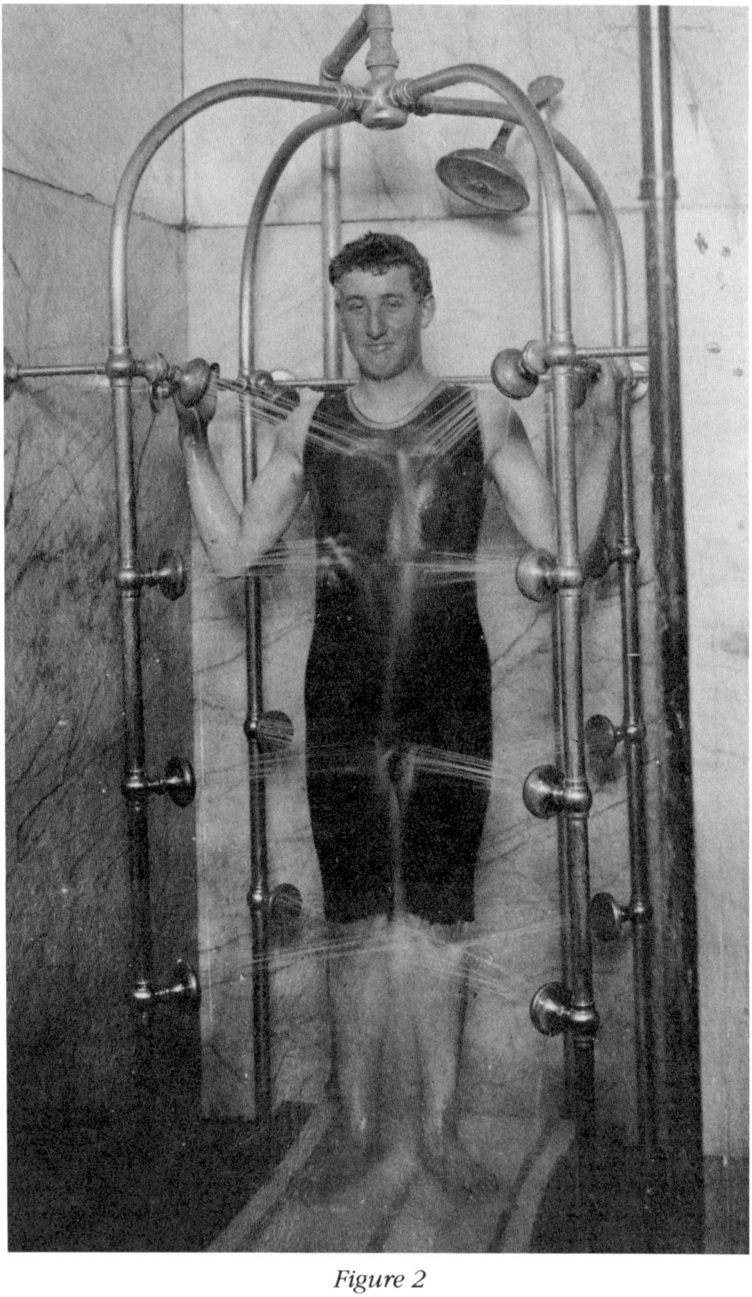

*Figure 2*
*Water Therapy — Relaxing Spray Bath, SHNB c. 1915*
*Source: SAB Photograph Number R-A 6404*

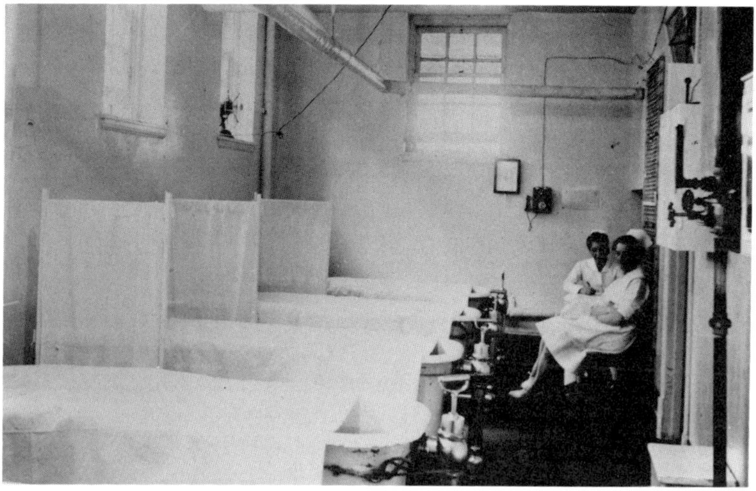

*Figure 3*
*Water Therapy — Prolonged Bath, SHNB c. 1940*
*Source: SAB Photograph Number R-4 6434(2)*

> Employment in the open air has been found one of the most efficient methods of bringing about recovery in the insane; and the various employments of agriculture constitute the most easily provided means of supplying this essential in the pleasantest and most acceptable way to the patients.[13]

The centrality of work in effecting a cure for insanity was further attested to in a small pamphlet given to inmates upon admission to Saskatchewan Hospital North Battleford (SHNB). The new inmate was told:

> Occupation keeps the troublesome thoughts away, keeps you interested in useful things and gives the necessary exercise to your mind and body. *Work* for your own sake and peace of mind — if your physician finds that you are physically able. To take an interest in some occupation is the best and surest way to convince the physician that you are well enough to be at home.[14] [emphasis in original]

Inmates were provided with plenty of opportunities to convince the physician they were well enough to be at home. Unpaid inmate labour power was, in fact, used in all

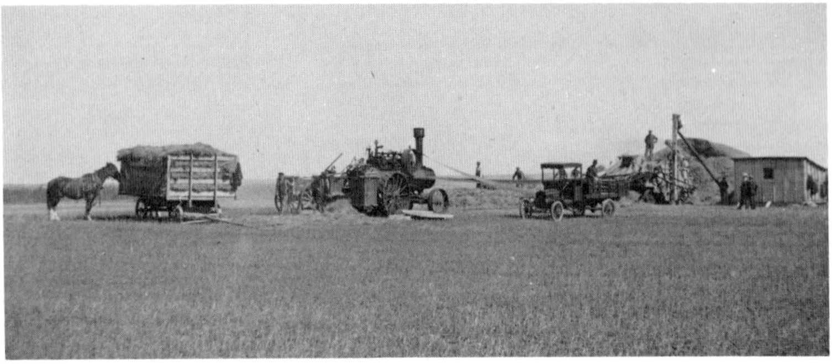

*Figure 4*
*Work Therapy — Threshing on the Farm, SHNB c. 1915*
*Source: SAB Photograph Number R-A 6409*

aspects of running the mental institutions except the custody and care of other inmates. They were employed in the kitchens and laundries, and performed everyday housekeeping chores on the wards. They were also employed to construct and maintain buildings and roads, and to help operate institution power plants. Inmates were even used as private servants by the in-hospital management and medical staff. The principal occupation, however, particularly for males, was as labourer on the institution farms which produced agricultural commodities for sale, as well as for immediate consumption by both institutional staff and inmates (see Figures 4 and 5).

The practice of using unpaid patient labour had consequences for both inmates and paid hospital workers.[15] First, it resulted in the contradictory situation wherein the more able an inmate was to work, the less likely he or she would be paroled. This not only contributed to the interconnected problems of overcrowding and rising costs, it also gave rise to intermittent charges of slavery and unjust internment by inmates, their relatives and disgruntled hospital employees. Public criticism of this sort, to the extent that it had the potential to develop into a "political crisis," was something which elected state officials were keen to avoid. As such, the way in which patient labour power was utilized became a continual source of conflict between in-hospital management

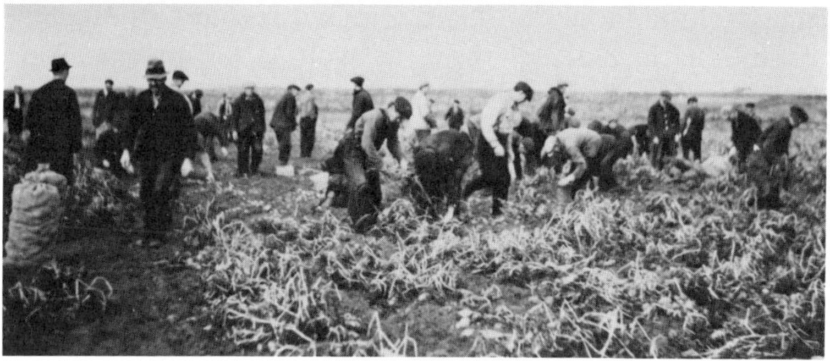

*Figure 5*
*Work Therapy — Potato Croppers, SHNB c. 1940*
*Source: SAB Photograph Number R-A 16,441(11)*

and the government department to which they were responsible. The use of patient labour for private ends was particularly criticized, although it was a practice vigorously defended by in-hospital management. The following excerpt from a letter to the deputy minister of public works from the superintendent of SHNB provides an example of this. Responding to criticisms of this practice contained in an anonymous letter sent to the Department of Public Works (DPW), he stated:

> It is . . . true that I employed patient labour in putting in my garden and painting my cottage — that is a privilege which has always been extended to any member of the staff if there is any particular work to do. It is one which has been extended to any member of this staff here since the Institution opened. It is a privilege which is extended to the Superintendent and members of the staff in any place where there is an Institution of this kind.[16]

Although these practices were from time to time a source of intramanagement conflicts, the government, always keen to reduce operating costs, was prepared to turn a blind eye to the practice as long as it did not become an issue which could cost it electoral support. The use of unpaid inmate labour for institutional work was not solely a consequence of the belief in the efficacy of work for restoring a person to sanity. Throughout the first half of this century, the mental institutions in Saskatchewan, as well as the rest of North America, operated institutional farms and industrial workshops as moneymaking enterprises in an attempt to reduce operating costs. This served to perpetuate the use of unpaid patient labour and contributed to the rising incidence of "chronicity."

About mid-century, however, increasing pressure was put on in-hospital management by the state to reduce inmate populations. The explanations for this change in policy include growing humanitarian concern for the well-being of the inmates and the march of medical science. These potential explanations have well-known defects. As an alternative, Matthews suggests it is necessary to discover how the changing nature of capitalist social and productive relations during this period facilitated these developments and made them desirable.[17]

Following World War II the trend towards the concentration and centralization of agricultural production became more pronounced. The increased capitalization of agricultural production which accompanied this process undermined the capacity of the mental hospital farms to operate profitably, predicated as they were upon labour-intensive production processes. The same reason has been put forward to explain the decline in importance of the prison, a decline which is related to its demise as a profit-making institution.[18] Although mental hospital agricultural operations were never profitable in the sense that they paid for the complete operating costs of the institutions, they did generate revenues until the mid-1940s. After that time, however, the extensive mechanization of agricultural production necessitated an increased scale of operations which would have required the acquisition of additional farm lands. Not only would the purchase of additional farm lands and requisite equipment have been extremely expensive, it would have been politically impossible. The main reason for this was that the small *petit bourgeois* agricultural producers, already faced with a cost-price squeeze, would not have tolerated state-run institutions so obviously contributing to their economic demise.

As a consequence of the convergence of these economic and political factors, hospital farm lands began to be sold during the 1950s. One important consequence of this was that inmate labour was no longer required. Therefore, institutional inmates became more an expensive liability than an economic asset. This produced a powerful incentive to discharge mental patients and depopulate the mental hospitals. This tendency was compounded after 1945 when psychiatric services came to be provided "free of charge" by the Co-operative Commonwealth Federation (CCF).

The second consequence of utilizing unpaid inmate labour to operate the mental institutions was that the power base of hospital employees was undermined. This position of weakness *vis à vis* the employer contributed to the perpetuation of long hours, low pay and generally unpleasant conditions of work, factors which in turn contributed to high attrition rates among hospital workers. As a result, worker solidarity decreased, further weakening their individual and collective power base. Another consequence of this was the perpetuation of an authoritarian system of management. Within this system, management control of the in-hospital psychiatric labour process was based upon patronage, paternalism and petty tyranny. It was partially the workplace practices and the political struggles which developed within and against these relations that resulted in the transformation of the mental hospitals from custodial to treatment institutions. The successful transformation of mental hospital work, a precondition for the development of community psychiatry, necessitated the elimination of political patronage as the organizing principle of that work.

## The Struggle Against Patronage in the Saskatchewan Civil Service

The attempt to limit, although not to eliminate, patronage in the Saskatchewan civil service pre-dated the opening of SHNB by one year. In 1913 the first steps were being taken to establish a civil service commission. Similar bodies were set up throughout Canada and the United States at that time. They had two main objectives, one political and one managerial.

Politically, they were an attempt on the part of a growing civil service, and the governments that employed them, to gain credibility with the public. Some of the newly established civil service commissions, however, apparently pursued the objective with such vigour that they were criticized for powermongering and empire building. This criticism developed out of the attempt to control all government-appointed positions, even to the level of deputy minister. In a letter dated 24 September 1923 from the civil service commissioner of Saskatchewan to the joint secretaries of the Quebec Civil Service Commission, this problem was made explicit:

> Not a little of the suspicion in which the public service is held is laid at the door of the advocates of civil service reform; — the very men who have done so much to help it — They have been so anxious to get rid of political patronage that they have lost sight of the point at which they are usurping the power of government by seeking control over positions of a policy forming or confidential character, or wrangling over border line cases so that the whole system has been subjected to criticism that has retarded its development.[19]

In further reference to this issue, the civil service commissioner of Saskatchewan stated:

> If it is admitted that the people and their representatives are fit to administer; then we must admit that these representatives shall be allowed to select unhampered those officials by and through whom promised results are to be put into effect, otherwise a political issue has been created, and not a civil service question raised.[20]

In an attempt to avoid this problem, the civil service of Saskatchewan was divided into a governmental group and an administrative group.

The governmental group included "executive positions, and positions responsible for the installation of new and important undertakings." Appointments to these positions (the superintendents of the mental hospitals fell into this category) were recognized as being beyond the scope of the civil service commission, although it did try to standardize salaries and control pay raises.

The administrative group included all other government employees. This group, described as "the large body of civil servants who carry on the administration as laid down by the government,"[21] was the object of civil service commission standardization plans; an undertaking which proved problematic for a number of reasons.

The first obstacle faced in trying to standardize job descriptions, salaries, promotions and discipline was the patronage system itself. In the pre-1913 period, each government department operated as a separate entity in matters of appointments, salaries, transfers, promotions, staffing levels and discipline. As a consequence, there was no standardization between the various departments or branches of the government. Examination of the correspondence exchanged between various provincial civil service commissions, as well as comparable commissions being established in the United States, reveals a generalized strategy for dealing with this — the application of private sector management techniques to public sector work. A good example of the above mentioned trends is found in a letter dated 24 April 1923 from the civil service commission of Saskatchewan to the joint secretaries of the Quebec Civil Service Commission:

> The knowledge by the staff that efficiency or inefficiency in the Public Service is treated exactly as it is in private service has had a most beneficial effect and [it] is largely due to this that we have an efficient and satisfied service in this Province.
>
> At the time of the appointment of the first Civil Service Commission in Saskatchewan in 1913, there was an equalization of salaries and an effort to bring salaries up to the standard paid for similar work in private life, taking into consideration, of course, conditions such as hours of labour, sick, and recreation leave, etc.[22]

It can be argued that private sector and public sector labour processes are both characterized by similar management objectives: increased productivity and reduced production costs. These objectives are pursued by similar managerial strategies.

The implementation of the Civil Service Commission Act met concerted opposition from the administrators of several departments, especially concerning the matter of hiring. Attempts were made to undermine the commission: "for a year or so there were several occasions in some departments where the provisions of the Act and regulations under the Act were openly violated."[23]

The ostensible reason for opposing the civil service commission's control of hiring was that it would make it impossible to secure suitable and politically sympathetic employees. This fear, coupled with resentment of the commission's usurpation of power, led to a general strategy of passive resistance within the various government departments. In fact, the only thing that made it possible for the civil service commission to operate at all was one provision of the act which stated that all salaries were to be paid by the commission. By effectively blocking the payment of salaries to employees not recruited, classified and appointed by the commission, the practices of bypassing and ignoring the Civil Service Act and the civil service commission were stopped.[24] This degree of legislative support makes it evident that the Saskatchewan government was anxious to centralize and standardize their civil service employment procedures.

Internal opposition was not the only obstacle to the rationalization of the civil service. There was also a lack of financial support for civil service reform, and an acute shortage of suitable labour power. At that time, the problem of adequate revenues was occasioned, in part, by recurrent conditions of depression in Saskatchewan's wheat-dependent economy and the exigencies of World War I. The prosperity of the Saskatchewan economy, and hence the revenues available through taxation, fluctuated widely with world wheat prices. In a 1917 report the civil service commissioner commented upon the shortage of suitable labour power:

"Although the Commissioner takes application from all comers, *there are at least one half of them that are entirely unsuited* for positions in the classified service under his jurisdiction. . . ."[25] [emphasis added]

This shortage of labour power, combined with a policy of fiscal restraint in regard to salary increases, resulted in a tense situation by the end of World War I. In order to get suitable staff, it was necessary to pay newly recruited employees more than experienced long-term workers occupying the same positions. This created antagonism between the government as employer and long-term employees, between the long-term and new employees, and between the various levels of management:

> The Commissioner has been constantly reminded that strict economy was necessary in the matter of salaries, and the salaries offered have not attracted the best material, and the annual increases have been suspended or sparingly distributed until now it would seem necessary to pay a larger salary for efficient help than is being paid to those who have been in the service for some time on the lower scale of salaries, and who occupy equally as important positions, which makes an awkward situation. The placing of new employees on higher salaries than that paid for similar positions in the same office or any other branch . . . is resented by the head of the Branch and other employees. . . .[26]

An unintended consequence of this was the further destabilization of the civil service. The resulting reduction of staff morale increased staff turnover and attrition rates. As a result, the Saskatchewan civil service was increasingly staffed by relatively more expensive and less experienced labour power.

These conditions, and the problems generated by them, prevailed within SHNB. In fact, the attrition rate was so high among the attendants that it was impossible for the civil service commission to centralize control of appointments and standardize credentials:

> There is so much of a turnover in the 'attendants' class of the asylum staff, it is found impractical for the

> Commissioner to handle such appointments on account of delays, etc., and this is left to the Superintendent, who secures the necessary assistance if he can, and reports to the Commissioner who certifies the appointments to the Auditor. . . .[27]

This is significant insofar as it shows that management strength and autonomy prevailed. The in-hospital management was able to retain and extend its control of the provincial psychiatric labour process even in the face of a generalized and legislatively supported trend towards centralization. This situation was of significance for the position of medically trained labour power within the psychiatric division of labour because the top administrative positions were all occupied by medically trained persons (men). This occupational identity manifests itself in many instances as an isomorphism of interests between management and medically trained labour power. It is not surprising, therefore, that the relationship between management and medically trained labour power was generally harmonious throughout the 1914-44 period. The major difficulty arose from the high rate of attrition among doctors. A number of interrelated reasons can be found for this phenomenon.

### Medical Men and Psychiatry

One reason for the high attrition rate among doctors was the inaccessibility of social and cultural amenities. This was partially a result of the hospitals being situated at a considerable distance from the major urban centres of the province. It was often felt, especially by immigrant doctors from the British Isles, Europe and eastern North America, that working in Saskatchewan entailed too great a sacrifice. Another contributing factor was the ceiling placed on incomes of government employees. A number of doctors left public sector employment to enter private practice where they could earn higher incomes. Due to the nature of Saskatchewan, leaving public sector psychiatric employment invariably entailed leaving the province or leaving the practice of psychiatry, since the sparse, predominantly rural population rendered private medical practice generally problematic and private practice psychiatry infeasible. As a result, virtually no private sector psychiatry existed in the province until the mid-1950s.

The challenge of ensuring adequate medical services for a sparse rural population characterized by widely fluctuating incomes gave rise to a number of municipal doctor plans. These plans, begun in 1915, were an early form of socialized medicine that gained support even from the provincial medical profession. A 1938 report of the Saskatchewan Medical Association's Committee on Economics referred to them as "a unique system of socialized medicine which had served a definite purpose and provided a service which could not easily have been obtained on the then prevalent basis of private practice."[28]

Non-specialist medical practitioners within a municipal doctor plan provided some psychiatric services, as did those in private practice. The major locus of psychiatric work, however, was the mental institution. It was within the institutional work context that a major source of occupational frustration emerged.

The prognosis for individuals committed to the large human warehouses was not good. Inexorable overcrowding reduced the possibility of providing active, effective treatment programmes. The medically trained employees of the institutions were in the unhappy position of providing physical care for an increasing population of ever-aging inmates (see Figure 6). Dr. C.M. Hincks, from NCMH, described conditions at SHNB in 1937:

> Conditions in the Men's Annex could not be worse. At night more than 265 patients are crowded together in dormitories with beds touching each other and the entire floor space is occupied. There is insufficient air and the ventilation is bad. In the day time conditions are no better. The day-rooms are crowded and one of the rooms is used for both dormitory and day-room. The patients are huddled together in a pitiful way and opportunities for improvement are almost negligible. All in all arrangements would be considered inadequate for animals, and the fact that the Annex is a fire trap causes great anxiety.[29]

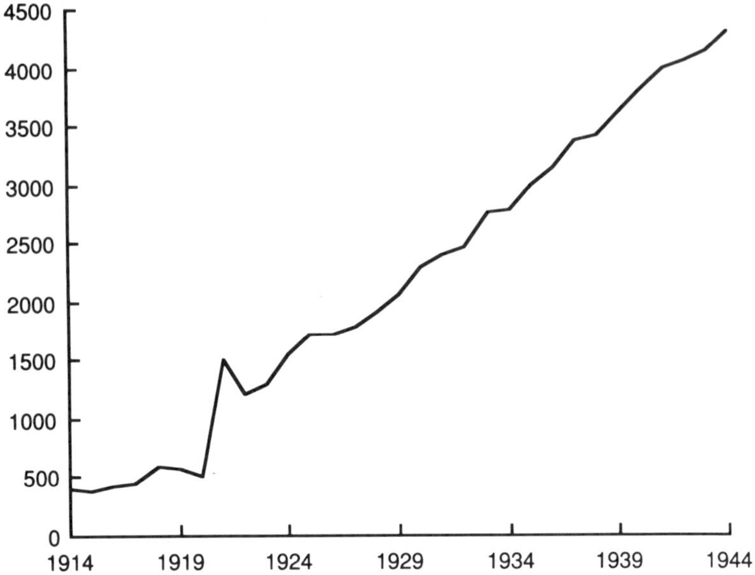


*Figure 6*

*Patients on Register by Year From 1914 to 1944*

*Source: Saskatchewan Department of Public Health Annual Reports*

Although Hincks's report referred to the conditions in 1937, overcrowding had consistently characterized the provincial mental institutions. The doctors were confronted with their professional impotence daily. Many found the situation intolerable and responded by attempting to change their working conditions. One response was to move out of the institutions into private practice. Another response was to try to move into administrative positions. This, however, was also somewhat problematic due to the limited numbers of administrative positions and the extreme stability among in-hospital management. A third response was to move from institution to institution in search of better working conditions but not necessarily in search of better wages.

The institution-hopping response was the major cause of physician attrition rates. It cannot be fully explained in terms of a search for higher wages since there was a conscious attempt to standardize wages and other conditions of employment on an interprovincial basis. From the earliest days of Canadian psychiatry there were extensive communications among the superintendents of the institutions; later, the same existed between the various provincial civil service commissions. One of the primary aims of this communication network was to strengthen the position of management *vis-à-vis* the potential labour force. This plan for interprovincial standardization was not entirely workable, however, due primarily to the differences between the various provincial economies.

Standardization of certain public sector wages was effective in minimizing the impact wage differentials would have as an incentive for mobility, at least in the four western provinces. The attempt to standardize interprovincial conditions of employment can be seen in a letter dated 8 October 1918 from the civil service commissioner of British Columbia to his counterpart in Saskatchewan:

> My object in writing to you now is with the view to securing information in regard to the salaries in force in the Western Provinces in the hope that it may be possible for us to work along similar lines, and that there may be no unfavourable comparison as between one Province and another.[30]

He stated he was "looking forward to receiving . . . a free expression of opinion in regard to a standard basis of salaries to be paid to Provincial employees in the four Western Provinces."[31]

Thus it appears a major motivating factor underlying the high rates of attrition among physicians within the institutions was discontent with working conditions. Added to this was the generally low status and prestige accorded psychiatry within the medical profession. In fact, psychiatry was not recognized as a *bona fide* medical specialty by the Royal College of Physicians and Surgeons of Canada until 1941. Within the occupational hierarchy of the mental institutions, however, the medically trained employees were in an undisputed position of dominance. This position was achieved and maintained through the support received by the occupation from all levels of management. This support was, in part, the consequence of occupational identity. That is, doctors were managers and managers were doctors. It was also, in part, the consequence of winning a major battle in the war for control of the psychiatric commitment process.

By 1922, Saskatchewan medical doctors had made some progress in the struggle to transform "insanity" into "mental illness." The winning of this battle, however, did not signal the end of the war. A key participant in these continuing struggles was the NCMH.

## The Canadian NCMH and Psychiatry in Saskatchewan

The Canadian NCMH was founded in 1918, four years after its American counterpart. Both had close personnel and funding arrangements with the large American philanthropies, particularly the Rockefeller Foundation. The Rockefeller Foundation financed many of the mental hygiene surveys performed by the NCMH, both in the United States and Canada.[32] According to the NCMH, the purpose of these surveys was to "secure popular support for Governments in the introduction of progressive legislation."[33] To help achieve this objective, the NCMH followed an organizational strategy of recruiting a limited number of influential persons as members. The NCMH in Canada was organized under the patronage of the duke and duchess of Devonshire; the duke of Devonshire was then the governor general of Canada. Also recruited were the ministers of health in each province, the leading educationalists, physicians and other "outstanding persons," including businessmen and political figures. Premier W.M. Martin of Saskatchewan received and accepted an invitation to become a member of the Canadian NCMH. According to the provisional constitution and bylaws of the Canadian NCMH, adopted 26 April 1918, it was established that total membership would not exceed 120 persons at any one time. Furthermore, it was established that at least one-third of the active membership at any given time would be physicians, and at least one-third would be non-physicians.[34]

By the second year of its existence, the NCMH was ready to begin surveying the various provincial facilities for the mentally ill. The first Canadian survey was conducted in Manitoba. Given the objective of the NCMH to influence legislation in a particular direction, the survey was very successful. In a letter dated 20 March 1919 to Premier Martin from C.M. Hincks, the associate medical director and secretary of the Canadian NCMH, it was pointed out that the survey "had been instrumental in securing legislation that will put into operation practically all of our recommendations."[35]

In July 1919, the NCMH completed a survey of British Columbia.[36] This survey resulted in the construction of a new facility for the feeble-minded. At the same time, initial arrangements were being made to conduct similar surveys in Alberta, Saskatchewan, New Brunswick, Prince Edward Island and Nova Scotia. It was thought by the NCMH that a survey of Saskatchewan would not be possible until 1921. Circumstances changed, however, and a mental hygiene survey was carried out in the summer of 1920, the first of three conducted between 1920 and 1944.

The 1920 survey was conducted by Hincks and Dr. C.K. Clarke, the Toronto psychiatrist who had opposed the cottage system asylum plan recommended in the 1907 Low Report. At Premier Martin's request Dr. MacNeill, superintendent of SHNB, assisted them. Overall, the report of the Saskatchewan survey was favourable. In fact, Hincks stated in a letter to Premier Martin:

> we were greatly impressed by the excellence of your institutions — in many instances the finest we have seen in the Dominion. Our recommendations, therefore, will be in the nature for the most part of an elaboration of your system that will raise the general level of efficiency.[37]

Although the report was favourable, it was never published. It was, however, presented as Sessional Paper No. 5 in the 1921-22 sitting of the legislature. The recommendations were significant for two reasons. First, it recommended the further medicalization and liberalization of the admission procedures to allow for voluntary admissions. It was argued that by having the admission process under the control of magistrates, the asylums were transformed into expensive custodial institutions. The medically dominated NCMH argued costs could be substantially reduced by making the admissions procedure a medical, rather than a legal, matter.

The proposed cost reduction was to be achieved through the application of public health principles to psychiatric practice:

> It is universally conceded that early treatment is the *sine qua non* in mental cases, and it is admitted that the majority of developing cases will not go to hospital for the insane for treatment even under the voluntary system of admission. It is not difficult to sympathize with this point of view because the prejudice is founded on the old tradition which made it a species of disgrace or even a crime to be insane and to require legal commitment to a public or even private institution. Frequently the patient who was sent to a public institution became one of the herd — his individuality was lost and opportunities for special treatment missed. The whole asylum system tended to magnify evils, and prejudice frequently found a basis in fact. These points are so well recognized that it is not necessary to waste time on further argument. It is now very clearly established that in prevention and early treatment in cases of insanity, the building of small psychopathic hospitals provides the ideal plan for meeting the situation.[38]

The NCMH was clearly intent on redefining insanity as mental illness. One of the tactics employed in this struggle was the argument that mental illness was no different than physical illness and was therefore best left to the care of physicians. Not only would medical treatment provide the insane with better care, it was also supposed to save money. In Saskatchewan in 1920, this was to be achieved via the construction of two sixty-bed psychopathic hospitals located in Regina and Saskatoon. The proposed hospitals, although intended to be free-standing, were to be constructed close to general hospitals. The hospital in Saskatoon was to be affiliated with the university in order to make full use of the planned research and educational facilities. The hospitals were intended to accommodate short-term, voluntary patients who would receive early medical intervention and thereby be diverted from the large, expensive custodial institutions. MacNeill had been advocating the construction of small psychopathic hospitals for a number of years, but to no avail.[39] Even NCMH endorsement of this idea failed to convince legislators.

Between the 1907 recommendation that the provincial mental hospital be constructed on a cottage plan, and the 1920 recommendation for the construction of small psychopathic hospitals, all the principal elements of the Saskatchewan Plan had been suggested. This is interesting because when the Saskatchewan Plan was first enunciated in the mid-1950s, it was heralded as the epitome of all things new and innovative in psychiatry.[40]

These recommendations were not accepted in 1920. As a result another large pavilion-style mental hospital was constructed at Weyburn (see Figure 7). This reflected the fact that medicalization of mental illness, endorsed by the NCMH, was not universally regarded as favourable. Although the proposal that psychiatric treatment be available on a voluntary basis had been under discussion during the 1919 session of the provincial legislature, it was opposed on the grounds that it would encourage "malingerers and deprive the public of protection from people who are dangerous to be at large."[41]

Thus, there was political opposition to the medicalization of psychiatric work. In spite of the opposition, the legislature passed the Mental Diseases Act in 1922. In his annual report

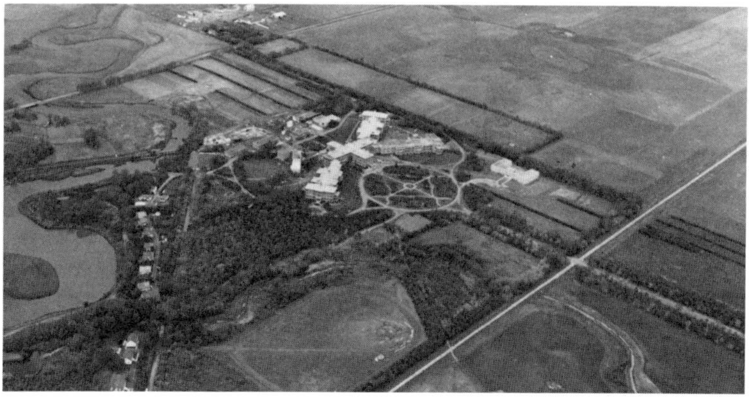

*Figure 7*
*Saskatchewan Hospital, Weyburn, June 1957*
*Source: SAB Photograph Number R-A 11385(1)*

for that year, MacNeill wrote: "I am pleased to note that the legislation takes into account that a disease process is being dealt with, rather than a criminal prosecution."[42]

The second significant implication of the 1920 NCMH recommendations is related to the points raised above: the transformation of psychiatric practice was to be achieved through the creation of new occupations, or at least widely expanded functions for already existing occupations. In particular, the NCMH at this time was keen to create and demonstrate the efficacy of psychiatric social workers in reducing the costs of psychiatric services.

The Canadian NCMH, therefore, in cooperation with the University of Toronto, established a "Course of Training for Social Workers in the Field of Mental Hygiene" in 1918. This eight-week training programme consisted of approximately thirteen hours of course work per week, supplemented by field work. In 1919 the training programme was expanded to Montreal. The NCMH also provided bursaries for the training of psychiatric social workers. In some instances, the NCMH paid the salary of these psychiatric social workers in an attempt to demonstrate their utility in the provision of psychiatric services. In 1918, for example, the NCMH paid for the training and salary of a psychiatric social worker to be attached to the St. Jean de Dieu Hospital, at that time the largest mental hospital in Canada. She was given an initial salary of $80.00 per month for three months with the proviso that

> If, at the conclusion of this time she proves valuable, and suitable for the work, she should be granted $100 a month. At the conclusion of six months or a years work, the Hospital St. Jean de Dieu will be requested to furnish her with her salary.[43]

A similar arrangement was made with an institution in Halifax.

This, however, was not the case in Saskatchewan. MacNeill, with the backing of the NCMH, suggested in a 1921 letter to Premier Martin that a social service worker be employed at SHNB to "look into the situation at the [inmates'] homes, and . . . adjust matters there so as to get patients out of this place thereby relieving the burden on the Province."[44]

He went on to make some interesting observations regarding the trend toward increasing in-patient populations and what the proposed social service worker could do to reverse that tendency:

> It is a fact that a number of families are leaving their relatives here, although they could be taken care of at home . . . . The popular conception is that everybody is falling all over themselves to take their friends home, my experience has been that this is not so, and my intention was to insist on some of these people being taken home and looked after by their people at home, provided I had the right kind of an individual who could to [*sic*] the work diplomatically and with judgement . . . a little pressure on the relatives of these patients sometimes makes them see things as they would not otherwise see them, and that pressure cannot be made by me at this distance.[45]

Premier Martin was not convinced and stated that as far as he was concerned the appointment of such a person was simply an unjustifiable expense. He also suggested to MacNeill that the matter best be left, as it was.[46] No follow-up services were provided in the province prior to 1944 and it was not until 1950 that both provincial hospitals had a social worker attached to them for the follow-up of discharged patients.

Although both Dr. MacNeill and Dr. Uhrich, the first provincial minister of public health (see Table 2), supported the NCMH's recommendations for the transformation of psychiatric work, they were unable to generate the political support necessary to realize that goal. Thus, in the pre-1944 period the mental hospital psychiatric labour process remained largely custodial, performed by unskilled attendants dominated by medically trained physicians.

## Relations and Conditions of Psychiatric Work

When the provincial mental hospitals were constructed it was generally thought that a major element in the cure for

**Table 2**
**Provincial Ministers of Public Health, Saskatchewan, 1923-1982**

| Minister | Party | Term of Office |
|---|---|---|
| John Michael Uhrich | Liberal | March 22, 1923 – September 9, 1929 |
| Frederick Dennis Munroe[1] | Conservative | September 9, 1929 – July 19, 1934 |
| J.M. Uhrich | Liberal | July 19, 1934 – July 10, 1944 |
| Thomas Clement Douglas | CCF | July 10, 1944 – November 14, 1949 |
| Thomas John Bentley | CCF | November 14, 1949 – July 27, 1956 |
| Jacob Walter Erb | CCF | July 27, 1956 – November 21, 1961 |
| William Gwynne Davies | CCF | November 21, 1961 – September 7, 1962 |
| Allan Emrys Blakeney | NDP | September 7, 1962 – May 22, 1964 |
| David Gordon Steuart | Liberal | May 22, 1964 – October 18, 1966 |
| Gordon Burton Grant | Liberal | October 18, 1966 – June 30, 1971 |
| Walter Edmund Smishek | NDP | June 30, 1971 – November 5, 1975 |
| Wesley Albert Robbins | NDP | November 5, 1975 – August 2, 1977 |
| Edwin Laurence Tchorzewski | NDP | August 2, 1977 – June 18, 1979 |
| Herman Rolfes | NDP | June 18, 1979 – May 8, 1982 |

[1]No archival records exist for this term.

mental illness was asylum from the rigours of social life. Regarding the location of the mental hospitals, the Low Report thus recommended that

> The building should be situated at a sufficient distance from town to discourage too frequent intercourse between the town and the institution, and yet not too far away for those really compelled for various reasons to visit the institution.[47]

Not only did such a location minimize too frequent intercourse, it also made it difficult to recruit adequate numbers of workers. For those recruited, it was difficult to get to and from work, especially during the winter.

This was particularly onerous for the nursing and attendant staff who worked shifts. For these workers, the day was divided into two twelve-hour shifts. The first shift was from 7:00 A.M. to 7:00 P.M. and the second shift from 7:00 P.M. to 7:00 A.M. The day shift was given forty-five minutes for the noon meal and thirty minutes for supper. The night shift was granted thirty minutes for supper at midnight. Meals were to be taken at the hospital and their value was included in calculating the employee's wage. It was not until 1936 that the Public Service Commission agreed to allow married staff living outside the institutions to supply their own meals, and to pay cash in lieu of meals.[48]

Also included in the calculation of wages were lodgings, laundry and uniforms. These perquisites, along with others such as the right to requisition food and other goods from hospital stores and the right to purchase coal at a discount rate, constituted a substantial proportion of an employee's total wage. In fact, calculations based on figures available from as late as 1936, indicate that the non-cash segment for a female ward supervisor at Saskatchewan Hospital Weyburn (SHW) accounted for between 36 and 54 percent of the total wage. This calculation is based on figures taken from the following:

> the girls going on the nursing staff here receive an initial salary of $660 per year, increasing to $725 in three months and $830 in six months. There is no subsequent increase unless the nurse becomes a Ward Supervisor. Ward Supervisors are paid $988 per annum. Included in this total salary are perquisites of $300 per annum for board and room so that the initial salary on that basis is $30 per month cash and board and room. Their laundry is done by the institution and they receive uniforms when they commence work here.[49]

Given that a large proportion of every employee's total wage was received in non-cash form, employees, especially attendants and nursing attendants ('attendants' refers to male and 'nursing attendants' to female workers), who did not live in accommodation on the institution grounds were financially penalized, since they had to pay for their housing out of the meagre cash portion of their wage. This affected a significant number of hospital employees as adequate on-site housing was not provided. This shortage of housing had reached crisis proportions by 1918 and threatened to become a major source of management-worker conflict. Within the context of post-World War I labour unrest, this was something hospital management wished to avoid.

The general mood of unrest among the western Canadian working class culminated in the 1919 Winnipeg General Strike[50] as well as a number of support strikes, including one in Saskatoon.[51] The post-World War I labour unrest did not escape the notice of MacNeill who, in addition to being an able administrator, was an astute political observer. He was aware of the unrest within the western labour movement and he was intent on forestalling radical unionism, or any other kind of independent unionism, at the hospitals. This goal was achieved for a number of years through the twin management tactics of co-optation and direct control.

## Co-optation and Control

The tactic of co-optation was implemented in a number of ways. As previously noted, the housing situation had reached crisis proportions by 1918. The provision of housing constituted a significant proportion of an employee's total wage and could easily have developed into a major source of conflict between management and workers. MacNeill, however, took the stance that the provision of adequate housing not only helped procure a stable work force, it also served to undermine rising demands for a union. Thus, it was MacNeill who instigated and pursued demands for the construction of adequate accommodation with the government:

> I am within my rights to bring your attention to the condition of affairs under which the people who work here suffer.

> Had these people a Labour Union, they would not stand, nor would the Union of which they formed a part, stand for them working 12 hours a day and housed in hovels (for I could not call them by any other name) that they are at present living in. It is impossible to expect the people who work here for a small salary (of which it takes every dollar to supply themselves with the necessities of life) to build for themselves cottages to live in, as the outlay would not be justified even if they were able to do so, which they are not.[52]

The government apparently concurred with MacNeill, for in 1919 several new cottages were constructed for hospital employees. The cottages, however, were not totally satisfactory as a letter from the chief engineer to the superintendent states:

> The work done on these cottages was of very inferior quality, both the painting and the plastering also the plumbing in some cases. The furnaces are very poorly installed . . . .[53]

Shoddy construction, combined with a continued lack of adequate on-site accommodation, served to generate management-worker conflict over a new issue of housing quality.

MacNeill demonstrated his co-optative management techniques again in 1919. MacNeill was aware of the general labour unrest and was concerned about the impact it might have on management-worker relations at SHNB. The following excerpt from a letter dated 7 June 1919 provides an excellent example of his anticipatory approach to labour relations:

> there is a strike on at Brandon for an eight hour day and an increase of pay. This is a matter which has never been discussed here, the eight hour day proposition. This has been tried in some Hospitals in the United States, and in a number of places that I know of, at least, it has not been a very satisfactory arrangement.
>
> This is a matter which the Administration should know something about and in the event of anything transpiring, they would be in a position to advise what course I should pursue at least they should know that

> such a demand is a possibility, as I would not like to wake up some day to the fact that we had a strike on our hands for an eight hour day, without any thought having been given to the matter.
>
> In the meantime, there is nothing here in the way of a demand for this, and perhaps will not be, but in the event of any such thing happening, it would be well for the Government to have some line mapped out which I should follow.[54]

In addition to demonstrating an alertness to potential sources of labour conflict, MacNeill also demonstrated an astute political mind and an awareness of his own self-interest. If a politically explosive labour situation had developed in the institution, MacNeill could not easily have been made the government's scapegoat; he had clearly placed the responsibility for laying down policy guidelines with them. Unfortunately, no record exists of the government's response to this request for guidance. An examination of the available evidence, however, indicates that no organized labour unrest occurred in SHNB at that time.

As has been seen, a new institution had been opened at Weyburn in 1921, temporarily reducing the crowding and thereby improving working conditions. Around the same time, unemployment rates were so high in Canada that labour's power base was effectively eliminated.

Of course, the reverse of this was increased power and stronger bargaining positions for management. Evidence of this can be found in the following letter to MacNeill, who had requested information concerning two men who had applied for jobs at SHNB, from the superintendent of an Ontario mental hospital:

> I have no objection to them going out to your place. I do not know why they should wish to leave here, unless the desire for a change. Men are so plentiful with us this year that it is quite immaterial to me whether they go or not.[55]

MacNeill responded by saying conditions in Saskatchewan were similar, and that he would not be taking the two men on. He went on to state that he was primarily concerned to let the medical superintendent of the Ontario Hospital in London know that the men were thinking of leaving.[56]

The potential for mental hospital employees to mount any effective campaign on their own behalf was further reduced in the mid-1920s with the establishment of the Government Service Association (GSA). The GSA was, in essence, a company union and, as such, provided virtually no basis for autonomous action.

Membership in this organization was open to all permanent members of the civil service. In terms of hospital employees, this included all persons who had at least one year of satisfactory service, as well as nurses and attendants who, after 1930, had completed the three-year diploma course. This membership criterion had the effect of fragmenting the hospital workers on the basis of length of service and, after 1930, on the basis of credentials. Furthermore, GSA membership was entirely voluntary and probably never included as much as 50 percent of all government employees, and only on rare occasions 50 percent or more of the mental hospital employees.[57]

The GSA, with its voluntary membership, made it easy for management to intimidate, and thereby control, hospital workers. It also permitted management to forestall any attempts at independent worker unionization. As the acting superintendent of SHNB wrote in 1945, the GSA "was not a trade union in the present day sense at all and never pretended to be."[58] In fact, he added, "In the years prior to 1944, it was an understood thing that the government employees could not form or join a trade union . . . ."[59]

In terms of making demands and presenting grievances, the power of the GSA proved to be more illusory than real. The normal procedure was that hospital locals would approach the superintendent of the institution in question with any demands or grievances. If a satisfactory resolution was not achieved, the matter would be referred to the central executive of the GSA. The GSA would then deal directly with the DPH. This, however, would have been unlikely to result in any substantial change in the decision made by the hospital superintendent, since it was the superintendent who provided government officials with guidelines for the most appropriate course of action regarding labour relations in the hospital. MacNeill effectively employed this technique from his earliest days as an administrator. Decisions which he felt would be unpopular, or generate opposition, he often presented to the workers as being beyond his control. He did this by writing letters to government officials telling them what he wanted established as policy. If the suggested policy was implemented, MacNeill could present himself, not as the initiator, but as an unwilling enforcer who, like all other employees, was a victim of the faceless bureaucrats in Regina.[60]

Co-optation and these other managerial techniques and tactics, important as they may have been, all took place against a backdrop of rigid, military-like control of the pre-1944 psychiatric labour process. MacNeill was the author of this strategy of control in Saskatchewan.

Even though MacNeill was not the only mental hospital superintendent in the province after 1921, it was his administrative style which dominated the province until 1945. The *Rules and Regulations for Employees of Mental Hospitals* apparently were, for example, drafted by MacNeill around 1914, passed by the government and used until the mid-1940s. The regulations were derived from those in effect at the time both in Canada and England.[61]

The centralization of administrative power in the office of the superintendent was solidly entrenched in the *Rules and Regulations.* This was, of course, intentional. It was a position MacNeill defended against even the slightest hint of encroachment. In 1914, for example, when it was recommended by the deputy provincial treasurer that the bursar at SHNB be responsible for seeing that the institution store kept the stock as ordered, MacNeill quickly responded:

> Now this virtually puts some of the administration into the hands of the Bursar. That is not his duty at all, — the administration is my duty, if I don't fulfill that properly, it is your duty to get one who will, but the administration and taking of orders can only come from me.[62]

The *Rules and Regulations* provided an explicit set of duties for all administrative positions in the hospital(s). Regarding the duties and responsibilities of the assistant superintendent, for example, it was stated:

> *Subject to the approval of the Superintendent*, he shall have entire charge of the medical service. It shall be his duty to divide the service into assignments for the various members of the medical staff, taking into account that recently admitted patients and those in the infirmaries and hospital wards require a larger degree of attention, and the number of patients assigned to the various members of the medical staff shall be in suitable proportion to the requirements of the patients. Assignments in the various departments of the medical service of the institution may be changed from time to time at the discretion of the Assistant Superintendent *with the approval of the Superintendent.*[63] [emphasis added]

As can be seen, even for the assistant superintendent, one of the chief executive officers of the institution, there was a sharp curtailment of on-the-job autonomy.

The rigid authoritarianism of the *Rules and Regulations* was more evident in the duties and responsibilities set out for attendants and nurse attendants. Control even extended to certain aspects of their *non-working lives.* Examples of the nature of this control can be seen in the following extracts from the original *Rules and Regulations*:

> Employees;
>
> Nurses and attendants must be in the dining room from 6:30 a.m.
>
> All resident employees must be in the building at 10 p.m. Lights out at 10:30 p.m.
>
> Late leave may be obtained by applying to the heads of the departments before 9 a.m. on the day on which it is required, and special permission must be obtained for all night leave. Late leave slips must be left with those in charge of sleeping quarters.
>
> Employees' rooms must be kept tidy and open for inspection at anytime.

> All gossip is strictly forbidden. Employees must not make the affairs of the institution the subject of conversation while off duty, must not give any information concerning the institution to any outsider; an infraction of this rule will be punished by instant dismissal from the service.[64]

The same authoritarian control was evidenced in management-worker relations at SHW:

> Gentlemen are not permitted to sit on the steps of Nurses' quarters with residents.
>
> The Night Staff must be in bed not later than 9 a.m. and to remain there until 3 p.m. at least.[65]

The first rule listed above refers to the fact that meals were considered to be a non-cash portion of the employee's total wage — a perquisite of the job. The day shift staff, who began work at 7:00 A.M., were to be at breakfast at 6:30 A.M., whether they lived at the institution(s) or not. Although one would not be fired for being late for breakfast, as one would for "gossiping," the names of offenders and the time they arrived for breakfast were publicly posted as a form of reprimand. More serious than mealtime tardiness was the receipt of medical care outside the institution. This act was subject to dismissal. The following is taken from a letter dated 13 June 1922 from the superintendent of SHW to an employee about to be dismissed:

> If you are sick you should have gone into our Hospital and we would have treated you here. We do not permit our attendants to be outside. If they wish outside treatment, they have the privilege of resigning and employing any person they wish. Will you kindly send me your resignation.[66]

The extent and nature of control within the context of working relations assumed a military-like dimension. Also, like the military labour process, there was a very clearly defined set of status differentials. This helped fragment employees into numerous status groups, thus constituting part of a "divide and rule" strategy. Again, extracting from a copy of the *Rules and Regulations*, it was stated that

> Nurses and attendants must not leave wards while on duty without obtaining permission from the chief attendant on the male side and assistant head nurse on the female side.
>
> Respect must be paid to all officials of the institution.
>
> Nurses and attendants will rise when officers enter wards and remain standing while they are in the wards. Senior nurse or attendant will go through the ward with officers and give any information they may ask for, concerning patients, wards, etc.
>
> All due respect must be paid to those in charge of wards by their subordinates.[67]

The control and organization of the workplace involved a strict segregation of male and female wards. The segregation also applied to male and female ward workers. This meant men worked on male wards, and women on female wards. This segregation was not maintained because male and female workers performed different kinds of work, for they did not, but because it was believed to be physically and morally dangerous for women to work on the male wards. Not only did management fear women might be physically injured by agitated male patients, they were also concerned that their finer sensibilities might well be permanently damaged by the sight of men masturbating, a pastime that was apparently widely favoured on certain wards.

More materially damaging to women workers, however, was the pay differential. Women were paid less for no other reason than they were women. This is, of course, a state of affairs which still confronts women in the workplace. One does not usually find the reasons for such inequitable treatment as clearly expressed as in the following letter which discusses the grading and classification of workers:

> My experience in working with and employing women, both in business concerns and in the Government leads me to believe that it is physically impossible for a woman to be of the same relative value and service as a man, although she may be just as efficient and perform the same work.[68]

There were further differentials along gender lines between institutions, with women employed at SHNB receiving both a lower minimum and maximum wage than women employed at SHW. The starting wage for nurse attendants at SHNB was $25.00 per month, while at SHW it was $35.00. After seven months of probationary employment the respective figures were $40.00 and $50.00 per month, this being the maximum wage for that category at the time. For male attendants the situation was different. They started $5.00 per month higher at SHW than at SHNB, at $45.00 per month compared to $40.00. Although the maximum of $60.00 per month was the same at both institutions, it was achieved four months earlier at SHNB than at SHW.[69]

These wages remained the maximum until a person moved into a supervisory position. As a result of this, the policy of ward segregation discriminated against women. Although this may not appear to discriminate against women advancing into supervisory positions, set against the structure of the inmate population it had that effect, since in the early years there were consistently fewer female than male patients in the institutions (see Table 3). This, combined with the tendency to have more female than male attendants, meant that female workers faced reduced prospects of advancement compared to male workers. The situation could have been rectified, of course, if the policy of males on male wards and females on female wards had not been so adamantly embraced by hospital management. They were, however, firmly committed to this division of labour:

> While a great deal has been stressed about Nurses — by that I mean Female Nurses — in Mental Hospitals, the time is not arrived and the time, in my judgment never will arrive when you can do without men taking care of the Male Patients in Mental Hospitals.[70]

The proposed solution to what was perceived by the administration as a problem of too few male workers in the attendant classification was an attempt to transform the job into a "career." This general management strategy for achieving labour force stability and increased control of workers has been usefully discussed by Edwards in terms of career

**Table 3**
**Inmate Population by Institution and Sex, Showing Females as Proportion of Male Inmates, Saskatchewan Mental Hospitals**

| | Saskatchewan Hospital North Battleford | | | Saskatchewan Hospital Weyburn | | | Total Inmate Population | | |
|---|---|---|---|---|---|---|---|---|---|
| | Inmates on Register | | Proportion Female to | Inmates on Register* | | Proportion Female to | | | Proportion Female to |
| Year | Male | Female | Male | Male | Female | Male | Male | Female | Male |
| 1930-31 | 669 | 355 | .5306 | 689 | 394 | .5718 | 1,358 | 749 | .5515 |
| 1931-32 | 697 | 378 | .5423 | 868 | 468 | .5392 | 1,565 | 846 | .5406 |
| 1932-33 | 768 | 412 | .5365 | 915 | 501 | .5475 | 1,683 | 913 | .5425 |
| 1933-34 | 781 | 421 | .5391 | 959 | 566 | .5902 | 1,740 | 987 | .5672 |
| 1934-35 | 822 | 430 | .5231 | 997 | 593 | .5948 | 1,819 | 1,023 | .5624 |
| 1935-36 | 875 | 467 | .5237 | 1,027 | 637 | .6203 | 1,902 | 1,104 | .5804 |
| 1936-37 | 923 | 484 | .5244 | 1,106 | 674 | .6094 | 2,029 | 1,158 | .5707 |
| 1937-38 | 957 | 493 | .5152 | 1,177 | 718 | .6100 | 2,134 | 1,211 | .5675 |
| 1938-39 | 993 | 512 | .5156 | 1,238 | 743 | .6002 | 2,231 | 1,255 | .5625 |
| 1939-40 | 1,016 | 538 | .5295 | 1,282 | 794 | .6193 | 2,298 | 1,332 | .5796 |
| 1940-41 | 1,056 | 541 | .5123 | 1,348 | 859 | .6372 | 2,404 | 1,400 | .5824 |
| 1941-42 | 1,062 | 578 | .5443 | 1,427 | 919 | .6440 | 2,489 | 1,497 | .6014 |
| 1942-43 | 1,079 | 604 | .5598 | 1,431 | 960 | .6709 | 2,510 | 1,564 | .6231 |
| 1943+ | 1,069 | 620 | .5800 | 1,463 | 999 | .6828 | 2,532 | 1,619 | .6394 |
| 1944+ | 1,083 | 604 | .5577 | 1,475 | 1,013 | .6868 | 2,558 | 1,617 | .6321 |

*Includes Mental Defectives
+Calendar Year
*Source: Saskatchewan Department of Public Health Annual Reports*

building and bureaucratic control.[71] Addressing precisely this issue, MacNeill stated in 1930:

> the only way to cope with the situation is to give the men training in the care of the patient, both when they are physically well, and physically ill, and pay them a salary to make it worth their while to continue in the business as a Profession, and at the end of their usefulness, to give them a pension on which they could live comfortably for the rest of their days.[72]

As a consequence of this management strategy, wages increased by the early 1940s for both male and female workers, although differentials were not eliminated.

Besides being paid less than their male counterparts, women workers were expected to have higher educational attainment. Prior to 1944, when the local labour market allowed it, females were expected to have a grade ten education in comparison to grade eight for males.[73] The views of administration regarding the nature and complexity of the work of nurse attendants is made quite clear in the following letter from the civil service commission to the superintendents of both mental hospitals:

> It is thought by the Commission that the salaries paid for Nurse Attendants in the Institution should be a little above that paid for domestic help, as it is realized that girls who undertake to perform these duties should possess a little higher intellect than the average of domestic helpers.[74]

With regard to educational credentials, one of the reasons for discrimination, besides sexism, was that it served as a screening mechanism to help keep married women out of the institutional labour force. The political demand for this was particularly strong during periods of high unemployment. Thus in 1930 the following memo was circulated to women employees by the superintendent of SHW:

> I am instructed by the Public Service Commission to call your attention to the fact that under Section 36 of the Public Service Act recently passed, they are obliged to dispense with the services of the married women on the staff whose husbands are engaged in remunerative employment.[75]

The government, realizing the negative effect this attack on women and their families would likely have on worker morale, was equivocal with regard to the enforcement of this new regulation. Thus, the superintendent's memo went on to state that the government was not insisting

> on immediate dismissal or even the three months mentioned in the Act, but set the time for the termination of their services as at the end of February, 1931.[76]

The attack on married women workers was received with little opposition from hospital workers. This was, in part, a testimonial to the efficacy of the management tactics of control and co-optation. The death knell of this coerced and co-opted labour peace, however, was about to be sounded. Ironically, the bell-ringer was the redoubtable Clarence Hincks of the NCMH.

## The Transformation of Mental Hospital Work: The First Steps

By the late 1920s both mental hospitals were grossly overcrowded, and the cost of maintaining these huge psychiatric warehouses was becoming prohibitive. Furthermore, based upon past experience, the future promised more of the same. Added to the fiscal burdens of paying for the apparently inevitable expansion of the inmate population were the political liabilities of being responsible for an inadequate psychiatric system. The Liberal government of the day was apparently cognizant of the potential political dangers, for in 1929 the NCMH was commissioned to undertake yet another mental hygiene survey. The Liberals were defeated at the polls later that year, and replaced by a Conservative-Progressive coalition government. The new government received and published the Report of the Mental Hygiene Survey in 1930.

The NCMH had argued in the 1920 survey that costs could be reduced through early intervention and the provision of treatment and follow-up services. The 1920 survey called for the construction of two small psychopathic hospitals wherein trained psychiatric attendants would provide active treatment, rather than simply custodial care. It was felt that this would reduce the average length of stay and hence the costs of service provision. The NCMH also recommended the hiring of trained psychiatric social workers to provide follow-up treatment for paroled inmates in the community. It was argued that this would allow the rate of readmission to be kept as low as possible. However, nothing was done at the time to implement any of these recommendations. In fact, the report of the 1920 survey was never published, although the government of the day did make political mileage out of the many laudatory comments contained therein.

The report of the 1930 survey was made public. In essence, it reiterated the findings and recommendations of the 1920 report and advocated the adoption of a preventive approach to mental disorders. This time, however, some action was taken. In particular, a small thirty-five-bed psychopathic ward was opened in the Regina General Hospital. This ward, in keeping with the recommendations of the NCMH, was for acute, short-term patients; the average length of stay was about thirty days.

Selective sterilization was also advocated as an effective and economical form of prevention. Pressure was coming from several sources, including sitting members of the provincial legislature, for the implementation of such a programme. On 4 April 1930 a motion was put before the legislature:

> Be it resolved, that in the opinion of this Assembly the function of parenthood should be denied to mental defectives. To this end strict regulations for the issuance of marriage licenses should be combined with social supervision of the mentally incompetent, together with sterilization, in the interest of eugenics.[77]

Dr. Uhrich, the former minister of public health, spoke at length against this motion and it was subsequently defeated. Although the issue arose from time to time throughout the 1930s, it never gained the necessary political support in Saskatchewan to be enacted as government policy. This is interesting insofar as it demonstrates quite clearly that the autonomy of the medical profession to determine its therapeutic techniques is limited. This becomes especially clear in those instances where medically trained doctors are employees of the state. State policy, or even ministerial preference, can determine which medical techniques are permitted.

In this case, if provincially employed psychiatrists had tried to insist on their professional autonomy to determine the most appropriate treatment technique, their employment status would have been jeopardized. Within the context of limited employment alternatives, the reality of professional autonomy is curtailed.

As another corollary to the preventive approach being advocated, training programmes for attendants and nurse attendants were instituted in the mental hospitals. The object was to produce a labour force able to provide active therapeutic treatment directed towards achieving increased rates of discharge, and thereby preventing long-term hospitalization. The training programmes were not standardized either between institutions or from year to year. Over the three-year period of the training course some groups received 125 hours of instruction while others received only 60.[78] This programme was the precursor to the creation of the occupation of psychiatric nursing. It was also the preferred solution to the problems of recruiting and retaining on-ward labour power. For example, the Alberta commissioner of mental institutions stated in a 1932 letter to the superintendent of SHW:

> a number of men in the east and particularly Dr. William Russel who was last year President of the American Psychiatric Association, and all those who have had prolonged experience are in agreement that for the solution of mental hospital nursing problems, the best nurses are those who receive their initial training in the mental hospital.[79]

Mental hospital management in Saskatchewan agreed with this evaluation. The superintendent of SHW, for example, stated in a 1932 letter that although he had recently been able to recruit several general nurses,

> My experience in the past has not been particularly satisfactory insofar as graduate nurses [RNs] are concerned, from the standpoint that it always seems to me that these girls have been more or less imbued with the attitude that it is a step down in life for them to work in mental hospitals. There is a little tendency it seems to me for them to approach this work rather apologetically, that is, that they are taking a position that is inferior to their qualifications.[80]

Although RNs could not be recruited to, or retained in, mental hospital work except during periods of high unemployment, the Saskatchewan Registered Nurses' Association

(SRNA) and other nursing associations across Canada opposed the establishment of the in-hospital training programmes for attendants. The Alberta commissioner of mental institutions mentioned this in a letter to the superintendent of SHW:

> there appears to be developing a very definite opposition on the part of registered general nurses to mental hospitals continuing training schools at all. They appear to feel that these institutions should be reserved for the undergraduate or post-graduate training of general nurses.[81]

The registered nurses were unable to thwart the development of the training schools largely because of the support given the idea by the medical superintendents of the mental hospitals. By 1930, MacNeill had become such an avid supporter of the training programmes that he reversed his position on the desirability of the eight-hour day. In a letter to the civil service commission he stated:

> speaking of the Training School, I do not believe that we can do justice to this work and continue a twelve hour day. I am of the belief that an eight hour day system will have to be adopted if we are going to have a Training School. In the first place, it is very difficult to get the time to attend lectures, and in the next place, I do not think that any person who is on duty for twelve hours a day, at the kind of work our Attendants and Nurses are doing, can take in Lectures and make the material their own so that it would be useful for them. I think that the future of our work demands that some arrangement be made so that we will be able to continue this Training School which we have started here.[82]

Although the eight-hour day was still some years away, MacNeill's change of position indicates the strength of management support for the training programmes. This was to have consequences for future developments.

It is interesting to note that, as was the case with housing, the impetus for improved working conditions came from management, not from the workers. That is to say, the transformation of the mental hospital labour process and conditions of work cannot properly be seen to be the outcome of workers' struggles. These changes are more properly understood as the outcome of management initiatives to reduce the cost and medicalize psychiatric services. MacNeill in particular was convinced that there was no room for worker input into the organization or control of work:

> I am not a believer in the doctrine that the employees are the best judges of how an Institution or an Industrial Plant should be run. I believe that there must be a management, and the Manager must be experienced and qualified to run the place — the time may come when the employees will be qualified enough to know how an Institution should be run, but certainly not the class of people I have around me. . . .[83]

It was not simply the administration's domination of the mental hospital labour force that resulted in a long reign of labour peace, although this clearly was an important factor. The authoritarian management system could not ensure labour peace if the labour power involved was not able to ensure personal and extended reproduction. As was seen previously, an elaborate system of perquisites had been developed in order to reduce the cash portion of the mental hospital workers' total wage. This system of perquisites included low rents, cheap meals and free light and water. Even including these non-cash considerations, however, wages were very low. To augment these wages, an extensive system of "income supplementation" developed from the highest levels of the hospital administration down. This system of income supplementation involved the extensive use of free patient labour and hospital supplies and facilities. Income supplementation was not unique to Saskatchewan. Indeed, it seems to have been widespread throughout North America, largely as a consequence of the patronage system which underlay the development of mental hospital psychiatry on this continent.[84]

Although it appears that initially this income supplementation system was semi-official, it was also the focus of repeated criticisms and complaints. The first indication of opposition to it came as early as September 1915. At that time there were several criticisms made of the superintendent's personal expenditures and alleged misuse of hospital resources. In a letter dated 1 October 1915 the superintendent replied to queries from the Department of Public Works (DPW):

> When I was hired here I made a bargain with the Premier, and he said I should be allowed my sustenance. I have never at any time taken anything but my sustenance out of this place. I have lived always as well as I live now, when I was a General Practitioner. I do not propose to live any worse than I am living now. If I do not suit you, get somebody else and I do not propose . . . to be harassed by a bunch out of the Auditor's Department, who could not give themselves a bran mash three times a day if they were not in the Government Service.[85]

The issue of alleged misuse of hospital resources was raised again in 1932. One of the criticisms included in an anonymous letter sent to the DPW was that the superintendent painted his cottage at the lake with paint supplied by the institution. His reply to the deputy minister is interesting:

> The first matter is that of painting my cottage at the Lake, which is true. I did paint my cottage at the Lake, and I got the paint from the supply of paint kept in stock at this Institution, which is the privilege of everybody who is an employee in this Institution, and the head of a family, according to your letter of March 6, 1931.[86]

The last sentence is instructive, for it indicates that the use of hospital resources for personal consumption was condoned all the way to the departmental level. Regarding another issue raised at the same time, the superintendent's use of a hospital employee as a personal chauffeur, he went on to state: "I am prepared to meet any investigation you may care to make, but I feel that I have the right to a Chauffeur."[87]

Although there was no investigation launched at that time, a royal commission was established in 1946 to investigate the illegitimate use and consumption of hospital resources. Evidence presented before the commission indicated that up to 90 percent of hospital employees were involved in an extensive, largely non-cash economy involving hospital resources. The following extract from a letter of confession written by a former employee indicates the extent of this subterranean economy:

> When the police arrived at my house and searched for liquor they did not find any of same because my wife had it hidden in the clothes basket (and this while they were in the house). However, I had in my possession and sitting in the open: a kitchen table from your carpenters and delivered to our home by hospital van, five gallons of shingle stain from the paint shop, two or three quarts of other enamel as well as a few gallons of flat wall finish which was used on the walls, one door bell complete from Electrician Shop, two boxes of floor wax from [ward] Supervisors, one suit of clothes from [ward] Supervisors, two sets of drapes for windows from tailor shop, one woollen blanket from men's hydro-bath, about twelve yards of window screen. Then, besides this, it is impossible for me to remember how many pounds of butter, pounds of meat, quarts of cream, and other things I had given to me while I was in your employment, such as bread, cakes, cookies, groceries of all kinds, yes, and even some goods from the workshop such as children's toys; in other words, I am ashamed to say that *we practically lived on goods given to me by others of your staff.*[88] [emphasis added]

Also included in this hospital-based barter economy were drugs and toiletries. The trading was not, however, confined to barter, nor to hospital workers. There is evidence that cash changed hands for some of the hospital goods. There is also evidence to indicate the operations extended to include a black market supplying local businesses and restaurants.

The length of the Depression and the outbreak of World War II undoubtedly contributed to the mental hospital perquisite system growing into a criminal racket. Although World War II marked a turnaround for much of the world capitalist economy, for Saskatchewan it resulted in new depths of economic depression. This was largely because it closed the European market for wheat, Saskatchewan's major export, and thereby contributed to a further decline in provincial government revenues. This in turn had a negative impact on mental hospital budgets, the largest portion of which went on wages and salaries. The perquisite system thus expanded to supplement incomes. In fact, this expansion was encouraged by management in an attempt to ensure a cooperative and peaceful labour force.

A number of factors converged during the late 1930s and early 1940s which undermined the autocratic system of mental hospital management and facilitated the transformation of psychiatric work. These included inexorable overcrowding exacerbated by shortages of labour power and increased worker strength. The new strength of hospital workers was manifested as unionization, a process given further impetus by the election of the CCF in 1944.

The CCF not only gave workers the power to effectively undermine the autocratic, patronage-based system of management, they provided the political will and the financial resources to proceed with the transformation of the psychiatric labour process. This process had begun in 1930. With the passage of the 1936 Mental Hygiene Act another major step in that direction was taken. This act, which allowed for voluntary admissions and certification by physicians, also provided for the "holding of mental health clinics and the boarding out of mental patients in approved homes."[89] Thus by 1936 significant progress had been made in establishing the legislative preconditions for the medicalization of mental hospital work and the development of community psychiatry. However, lack of political will, revenues and appropriately trained labour power delayed further progress in this regard.

All the while the conditions of overcrowding worsened. Commenting on the situation in 1937, C.M. Hincks told the provincial cabinet in a private meeting:

> the present Mental Hospital situation constitutes a crisis. If nothing is done . . . it is evident that the therapeutic work will become paralyzed. They will be reduced from

> the status of active hospitals to custodial institutions where even the comfort of the patients will be jeopardized. Recovery rates will drop and this will mean, not only a lack of adequate service to the public, but will prove costly in dollars and cents. This will ensue because there will be an accumulation of chronic uncured patients who will constitute a perpetual charge on the State.[90]

By characterizing the two provincial institutions as "active hospitals" engaged in therapeutic work, Hincks was not providing an accurate description so much as he was providing support for his staunch allies, Dr. MacNeill and Dr. J.M. Uhrich. Both Hincks and Uhrich were committed to the development of a mental hygiene programme based on public health principles. This is attested to in a 1940 letter to Hincks, wherein Uhrich stated "Mental Hygiene is, to my mind one of the most vital problems of Public Health in Canada today. . . . my Department . . . proposes as soon as possible to develop a community program essentially preventive in character."[91] Although both Uhrich and the NCMH had the transformation of mental hospital work and the development of community psychiatry as ultimate goals, the problem of overcrowding was given immediate priority. Three possible solutions were considered: (1) additions to existing hospitals; (2) boarding-out programmes; and, (3) the construction of a new hospital.

The first solution was rejected because of the "prohibitive costs [involved] in the duplication or enlargement of existing power, water and other plants."[92] Boarding-out, although strongly supported by both the minister of public health and the NCMH, was not seen as a viable solution to the immediate crisis of overcrowding. This was due to the feeling that

> Successful boarding-out demands preliminary public education and a cautious policy of placing a relatively small number of patients in private homes at a time. Public approval must be won gradually through the demonstration afforded by successful placements.[93]

This warning against rushing headlong into an extensive programme of depopulation was prophetic in light of subsequent developments in Saskatchewan. At the time, however, it was superfluous since, for political reasons, very few legislators seriously considered turning the insane loose on the community. This is attested to by the fact that the rate of parole was relatively stable throughout the whole of the 1914-44 period. The only major fluctuation occurred in 1921 with the opening of SHW. That event was marked by a major reduction in the parole rate, underlining the predominantly custodial nature of psychiatry. In the face of political opposition to releasing mental patients, the major impetus for increasing the rate of parole in the pre-1944 period came from the physical lack of space (see Figure 8).

The only viable solution to the crisis of overcrowding was thought to be the construction of a new mental hospital. It was eventually to accommodate a total population of two thousand persons. In order to deal with the immediate crisis,

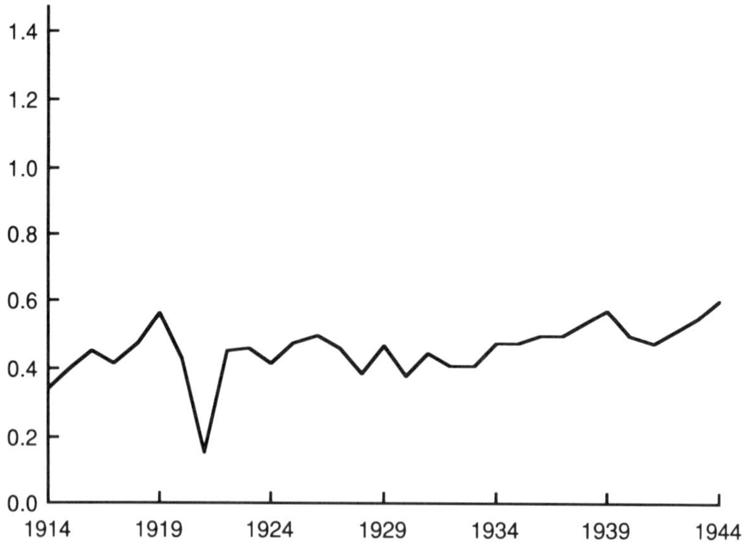


*Figure 8*

*Total Paroles as Proportion of Total Admissions by Year, 1914 to 1944*

*Source: Saskatchewan Department of Public Health Annual Reports*

however, plans to construct accommodation for fifteen hundred patients were to be implemented.

Although the construction of a new mental hospital was thought to be imperative, it was not conceived as the total solution to the problem. Rather, it was conceived by the minister of public health as "a link in a chain of needed mental health services."[94] In his 1937 presentation to the provincial cabinet, Hincks stated that "support should be given to the plans of the Minister of Health."[95] These plans included: (1) the development of clinics throughout the province; (2) public education; (3) the training and supervision of the feeble-minded; (4) the guarding of the mental health of school children; (5) the boarding out of mental patients; and (6) the strengthening of psychiatric services in mental and general hosptials. In summarizing the "Uhrich Plan," Hincks stated: "There are involved arrangements for prevention as well as treatment, and for the prosecution of scientific research in extending our knowledge."[96]

In order for Saskatchewan to contribute to, and gain from, the prosecution of scientific research, it was argued that the proposed mental hospital be located in close proximity to the university in Saskatoon. There were, however, more immediate reasons for choosing to locate the new institution in Saskatoon. As Hincks reported:

> There have been suggestions that financial assistance might be forthcoming from one of the largest American Foundations towards the training of psychiatric personnel, and this assistance might well be contingent upon the hospital's association with an accepted seat of learning.[97]

The large American foundation was likely the Rockefeller Foundation, although there was no specific mention of this. In light of chronic shortages of trained psychiatric labour power, a problem exacerbated by wartime enlistment, these suggestions carried some weight.

Military enlistment had decimated the provincial psychiatric labour force. The number of trained attendants employed at SHNB, for example, declined from a high of 104 in 1939 to 40 in 1944. In addition the total number of attendants had been reduced from 161 to 147 between 1942 and 1944. A 1944 report to Dr. MacNeill on conditions at SHNB reported that

> when our experienced supervisors are off duty, it is frequently necessary to place inexperienced Attendants in charge of wards, who are not familiar with the condition of the various types of patients nor the general management of these wards. Conditions have made it necessary to employ almost anyone available. . . .[98]

At SHW the situation was even worse.[99] From management's point of view these conditions translated into crises of efficiency and control. From the workers' point of view it meant increased power.

Hospital workers took advantage of this position of strength. Besides a slight increase in wages, they achieved two consecutive days off per week. This exacerbated the already critical labour shortage. Management responded by reducing the customary three-week holiday period to one week per year. Workers simply booked off more sick time:

> from July 1, 1943, to July 1, 1944, time off for sickness amounted to 902 days. There appears to have been more sickness amongst the staff since the holiday period has been reduced. . . .[100]

Hospital workers also used their increased bargaining strength to eliminate GSA membership restrictions. Following the outbreak of the war, all government employees, permanent and temporary, were eligible for membership. MacNeill and the in-hospital management were losing their iron grip on the mental hospital work force.

The election of the CCF government late in 1944 completed the shift in the balance of power. The CCF, drawing its principal support from a farmer-worker alliance, had particularly close ties with the Canadian Confederation of Labour (CCL). This was an industrial union organization which advocated the political education of workers and legislative lobbying.[101] With the election of the CCF much of the political intimidation which had kept labour cooperative disappeared. As a result, the CCL supporters achieved majority support in the two mental hospitals and immediately struck a deal with the CCF government.

The agreement gave the CCL union exclusive bargaining rights for mental hospital employees. It also specified that all employees hired after the effective date of the agreement must join the CCL within thirty days, although workers employed before that date could join or remain apart as they saw fit.

Many hospital employees comfortable with the old patronage system opposed the union and its attempts to alter the status quo. Union supporters, in an attempt to strengthen their position in the hospital, undertook to dislodge their rivals by exposing the existence of racketeering. The CCF government saw this as a good method to revamp the management structure of the mental hospitals and used the union's information to institute a royal commission into the administration of SHNB. The immediate result was the arrest and conviction of four employees on charges of theft and the replacement of key personnel in the mental hospital management hierarchy. Ironically, this close cooperation between government and union in the pursuit of common goals was subsequently to result in various problems of management for the CCF government.

Changes with far-reaching consequences had been set in motion. A new labour order was about to emerge, one in which workers not only had increased power within the work setting, but strong political backing as well. Community psychiatry, which had long had strong ideological support in Saskatchewan, was about to emerge as a new working reality.

# Chapter Three

# From Custody to Therapy: The Transformation of Mental Hospital Work, 1944-1963

The election to office of the CCF in 1944 was the culmination of a long series of populist struggles characteristic of the economic development of the North American west. The CCF (as a political party) was primarily an alliance of *petit bourgeois* agricultural producers (mostly wheat farmers) and a growing urban wage-labouring class. The main political enemies identified by the CCF were eastern-based industrial and financial capitalists, particularly the banks, and farm machinery, railroad and grain companies. The CCF forged a tenuous political alliance between farmers and urban wage-workers on the basis of a promise to protect them from their common capitalist enemies.[1]

The CCF, in a further attempt to solder this tenuous alliance, put forward an ideology which paralleled the security of farm tenure to the rights of workers to organize and bargain collectively.[2] This presumed isomorphism of interest was untenable: the security of farm tenure was a commitment to the preservation and defence of private property, while the rights of workers to organize and bargain collectively was seen, by the CCF, as a necessary first step in the transition to socialism. The CCF was never able to resolve this contradiction characteristic of all social democratic/ populist political parties.

The position of the party on labour rights eventually manifested itself as a problem of management in government-operated enterprises including the mental hospitals. The 1933 Regina Manifesto, which was the product of the CCF's first national convention held in Regina, contained the roots of this problem. In that document the CCF advocated the creation of a national labour code which included state regulation of wages, "equal reward and equal opportunity of advancement for equal services, irrespective of sex,"[3] unemployment insurance, and a limitation of hours of work. The manifesto asserted that

> workers must be guaranteed the undisputed right to freedom of association, and should be encouraged and assisted by the state to organize themselves in trade unions. By means of collective agreements and participation in work councils, the workers can achieve fair working rules and *share in the control of industry and profession*; and their organizations will be indispensible elements in a system of genuine industrial democracy.[4] [emphasis added]

In an effort to fulfill these commitments, the provincial CCF, upon election in 1944, immediately passed the Trade Union Act wherein the above-mentioned rights and principles were given explicit legislative expression. This legislation gave the trade unions an unprecedented degree of power, both politically and within the workplace. It was in part through the newly strengthened trade unions that the CCF planned to overthrow the capitalist system, a goal which it had also set for itself in the 1933 manifesto: "No C.C.F. Government will rest content until it has eradicated capitalism and put into operation the full program of socialized planning."[5] Having pledged itself to this rather ambitious objective, the CCF was soon confronted with a major contradiction between political theory and practice:

> This government, despite its socialist aims and objectives, is still forced to function within the framework of a capitalist economy. Not only may it be forced to compete with capitalist institutions, it may even be dependent on these institutions . . . to attain some of its immediate objectives.[6]

It was in fact dependent on those institutions to achieve *all* its immediate objectives. These included the prevention-oriented system of socialized medicine promised in the 1944 provincial election campaign.[7]

The implementation of such an ambitious plan would require considerable revenues, which were not available in Saskatchewan at that time. Speaking of economic conditions in 1944, T.C. Douglas told the author:

> Saskatchewan had the unfortunate distinction of being one of the poorest provinces in Canada. We had the highest per capita debt. We had one of the lowest per capita incomes. The province had never paid off a dollar of its debt from the day it was formed in 1905.[8]

He pointed out that as a consequence of the Depression and seven years of drought, which was particularly severe in the southern half of the province, Saskatchewan was characterized by a "great despondency and great poverty."[9]

This poverty, combined with the fact that no federal health insurance scheme existed, made inauspicious the prospects of successful implementation of a complete system of socialized medicine. These fiscal problems were exacerbated when the CCF adopted a policy of "free" psychiatric services in 1945. Saskatchewan was the first province in Canada to implement this policy. One of the consequences of so doing, however, was to further drain already limited revenues.

Initially the CCF followed two strategies in an attempt to ease the fiscal burden which resulted from the implementation of these ambitious programmes. The first was to try to secure federal cost-sharing agreements. This proved to be the most important influence on the transformation of psychiatry and the organization of psychiatric work in the province. The second was to seek financial and organizational assistance from the large American philanthropies. Thus, partly out of necessity and partly out of a pragmatic approach to politics, Premier Douglas, leader of a government avowedly dedicated to the eradication of capitalism, approached the Rockefeller Foundation, an archetypical capitalist institution, requesting support for the implementation of a planned programme of socialized medicine. The request met with the following response:

> In general, the policy of the International Health Division is to collaborate with official health agencies in the development of new services when suitable opportunities occur. In some instances, our assistance is limited to granting fellowships for the training of personnel for key positions; in other cases financial assistance is granted for limited periods. Any assistance on our part is undertaken only on the recommendations of a representative of our organization who has had an opportunity to visit the community concerned and study its needs and the opportunities presented. Naturally, we desire to employ the limited funds at our disposal so as to obtain the most significant results.[10]

These conditions were apparently acceptable to the CCF government, for over the course of the next decade the Rockefeller Foundation and other large American philanthropies became involved in several aspects of the province's mental health system. These included training segments of the psychiatric work force, the financing of psychiatric research and the development of psychiatric education programmes.

The collaboration of a government dedicated to the overthrow of the capitalist system and a foundation financed by one of the most powerful bourgeois families in the world may seem odd, but the ideological basis for this relationship was a shared belief in the possibility of planned social change. The CCF, with its Fabian roots, its socialist rhetoric and its vision of perfectibility of the human species, was dedicated to the planned elimination of capitalism and the orderly transition to socialism. The Rockefeller Foundation, although not so optimistic about the perfectibility of the species, was likewise committed to a programme of planned social change. It was a plan for the perfection of the capitalist system, however, not its elimination.

It was expected that the perfection of the capitalist system would be achieved through the application of scientific knowledge, including psychiatric knowledge, to the orderly control of human relations. Raymond Fosdick, president of the Rockefeller Foundation, provided a succinct summary of the nature and function of psychiatry as seen from the point of view of the foundation:

> Psychiatry as a science is still primitive and imperfect, but enough has been accomplished to justify the application of some of its principles to wider fields than the treatment of the mentally ill. Most of the pressing questions which confront us today, from the settlement of strikes to the formation of a world order, are fundamentally problems in human relations. The search is for institutions which will provide satisfaction for man's needs while compensating and controlling his ineradicable defects. The old method of allowing these institutions to grow out of a struggle of opposing forces is no longer possible when the power at our command is so easily capable of destroying everything we have inherited. In the future we shall have to provide social arrangements through conscious planning and mutual agreement. Such processes may reasonably look for help from those who make a profession of studying the impulses and frustrations of individual human beings. Psychiatry is a tool of evolving importance in building a new kind of stability in human society.[11]

Thus both the CCF and the Rockefeller Foundation were committed to improving the effectiveness of psychiatric theory and the efficiency of psychiatric practice as part of an effort to rationalize the processes of social reproduction. This shared commitment formed the basis for a rather incongruous working alliance.

### The Sigerist and Hincks Commissions

In 1944 the CCF commissioned two major studies of the provincial health care system intended to establish some guidelines for the proposed system of socialized medicine. The first of these, a survey of the complete health care system, including an examination of psychiatric services, was a royal commission. This survey, commonly known as the Sigerist Commission, was conducted by Dr. Henry E. Sigerist from Johns Hopkins University. He was assisted by Mr. Clarence Gibson, former superintendent of Regina General Hospital, Dr. Lloyd Brown, a Regina pediatrician and chairman of the Health Insurance Committee of the Saskatchewan Medical Association, Mrs. Ann Heffel, an RN with considerable experience in public health work, and Dr. Mindel Sheps as secretary.[12] The second survey was exclusively concerned with the province's psychiatric system. It was personally conducted by the ubiquitous Clarence Hincks of the NCMH.

Both the Sigerist and Hincks surveys duly noted and commented on the extent of overcrowding within the two provincial mental hospitals. Hincks stated:

> The greatest handicap at the present time is the unfortunate degree of overcrowding at both institutions. The North Battleford Hospital with a normal capacity of 1,174 patients is caring for 1,716; and the Weyburn Hospital with a normal capacity for 1,040 patients is sheltering 2,485. In other words, at both institutions there are 4,201 patients with adequate accommodations for 2,214. This represents overcrowding to the extent of 89%.[13]

The first recommendation made by Sigerist was for increased specialization in the provision of services. He recommended that services and facilities for the mentally ill be separated from those for mental defectives and epileptics. This was to be accompanied by the transfer of exclusive administrative responsibility to the DPH, instead of having it split between the Departments of Public Health and Public Works. He also recommended the establishment of mental hygiene clinics in Saskatoon and Regina which were to be operated in conjunction with general hospitals in those centres. In addition, the creation of travelling mental hygiene clinics was proposed, as it had been in the 1920 Hincks Report. These travelling clinics were to be staffed by a psychiatrist and a nurse, who were to tour the province providing consultative and diagnostic services for municipal doctors and school teachers. They were conceptualized as a mainstay in the prevention of mental disorder. It was thought by Sigerist that "such a measure would decrease the need for hospitalization and would permit the treatment of milder cases in their homes."[14] This was a clear statement of one of the primary goals of community psychiatry. The public health principles of early intervention and mobilization of community resources were fundamental to Sigerist's recommendations.

It was recognized that successful implementation of these recommendations depended upon the availability of sufficient labour power "fully trained in modern methods of *psychiatry and psychology.*"[15] [emphasis added] Here one sees evidence of the medical-psychological dualism discussed by Ray as characteristic of nineteenth-century psychiatric practice in England. Ray argues that the conceptualization of mental illness as a disease, curable by appropriate medical intervention, is mediated by an ambiguity regarding etiology. That is, mental illnesses are viewed as being both physically and psychologically caused. This is not only central to the development of psychiatric theory but, as Ray also argues, it relates to the way in which nineteenth-century psychiatry was constituted as a form of practice (work).[16] It is my contention that this dualism remains central to the organization of psychiatric work in the twentieth century and underpins the de-medicalization of community psychiatry.[17]

The report of the Hincks survey, published in 1945, reiterated the recommendations which he and the NCMH had been making for a quarter of a century. It also closely paralleled Sigerist's recommendations.

Hincks, like Sigerist, recommended the centralization of administration within the DPH, and the specialization of treatment. Thus, he recommended the development of a training school for mental defectives to accommodate an initial population of one thousand. He also recommended the creation of a geriatric centre to accommodate three hundred patients. Reiterating the recommendations he had made to the provincial cabinet in 1937, he called for the construction of a twelve hundred-bed mental hospital and for the "development of a 50 bed Psychiatric Division at the General Hospital in Saskatoon" which was to be used for medical teaching purposes by the University of Saskatchewan.

Hincks also recommended the construction of two mental hygiene clinics, one in Saskatoon and one in Regina. It was suggested that besides serving these two major urban centres, a travelling clinic service should be organized to serve the six other cities and two larger towns in the province. These clinics, as conceived by Hincks, were to perform several functions. These included:

> (a) Provision of diagnostic services in connection with all types of mental and nervous disabilities; (b) Provision of therapeutic services in collaboration with the physicians of the province, in regard to cases that can be treated with advantage in the general community; (c) Provision of guidance for children with emotional and behavioural problems; (d) Furnishing mental hygiene training to health, educational and welfare personnel; and (e) collaboration with mental hospitals in securing histories of new admissions and in the rehabilitation of discharged patients.[18]

These recommendations represent the attempted implementation of public health principles in the provision of psychiatric services. One can also see the basic dualism of psychiatry in the recommendation that each clinic be staffed by a psychiatrist, a psychologist and one or more psychiatric social workers. The community psychiatric division of labour in the province did not develop along these lines for a number of reasons. This proposed division of labour contained the seeds of a series of unanticipated conflicts between medical and non-medical labour power that continue to influence the development of community psychiatry.

The establishment of mental hygiene clinics was to form one of the fundamental bases of community psychiatry. Another major foundation of community psychiatry was to be the strengthening and extending of psychiatric services in general hospitals. As Hincks stated, "The ultimate aim in Saskatchewan should be the inclusion of psychiatric services in all the general hospitals in the province."[19] It was thought that the implementation of this recommendation would encourage people to voluntarily seek early treatment, and involve general practioners (GPs) in the treatment of mental illness:

> Through such a plan, there will be secured the interest of the medical profession as a whole in psychiatric problems; and there will be promoted a greater readiness on the part of patients with incipient mental illness to seek prompt treatment when it will be of greatest avail.[20]

It was reasoned that by medicalizing psychiatric treatment and shifting the primary locus of treatment from the traditional mental hospitals to general hospitals and mental hygiene clinics (i.e., to the community), much of the stigma associated with psychiatric disorder and treatment could be eliminated. What was not apparent to the proponents of community psychiatry at the time was that the transformation of the forces of psychiatric production, entailed in the shift from the mental hospitals to the general hospitals, would produce a corresponding shift in the social relations of production. This was to have a profound impact on the nature of psychiatric work, particularly as practiced in the large mental hospitals. The success of this proposed shift in the nature and location of psychiatric service delivery depended, in large part, upon convincing GPs that mental disorders were no different than physical disorders, and could be effectively treated in the community. It was not until the introduction of the psychotropic drugs in the mid-1950s, however, that this was to take effect.

Sigerist and Hincks also concurred on the issue of selective sterilization of the mentally ill and mental defectives as a form of prevention. This issue was somewhat problematic from the political perspective because of the widely publicized programme of eugenics undertaken by the Nazis. Sigerist was aware of this and attempted to dissociate his recommendation from the practices of the German fascists:

> The sterilization of mental defectives should be given careful consideration. Much experience has been gained in this field during the last 50 years in America and Europe. One should not be deterred by the fact that Nazi Germany has practiced sterilization in a brutal and wholesale manner, but should study the results obtained in such countries as the Scandinavian countries, Switzerland, and some of the American states where sterilization has been practiced humanely and cautiously with good results.[21]

Hincks also recommended selective sterilization as an economical form of prevention following the 1944 defeat of the Liberal government and the removal of Dr. Uhrich, the former provincial minister of public health, who had been a vigorous opponent of sterilization. Hincks, not wishing to alienate a powerful political ally, had refrained from vigorously advocating sterilization in Saskatchewan while Uhrich was in office. In 1945, however, he stated that since "50% or more of mental defectives come from poor stock, a contribution can be made to prevention through the sterilization of selected cases who without the precaution of this operative procedure transmit their mental defect to offspring. . . . There is a special indication for sterilization in connection with physically attractive moron girls prior to their discharge from the residential training school."[22] The recommendation seems to betray a sexist bias on the part of the NCMH, insofar as enforced sterilization is specifically recommended for women and not men.

This form of treatment was never given broad legislative sanction in Saskatchewan. This provides one example of how political rather than simply "professional" considerations determine the form and content of psychiatric work.

Sigerist and Hincks both outlined comprehensive plans for the transformation of psychiatric work and the transition to community psychiatry in Saskatchewan. The historical realization of these recommendations was only achieved, however, through a series of interconnected struggles. In the course of these struggles the plan for community psychiatry underwent a series of transmutations.[23] One of the consequences of this process was the mobilization of new interest groups, which in turn influenced the concrete transformations which took place.

The balance of this chapter is an examination of the various struggles and events which surrounded the transformation of the in-hospital labour process, and the development of a new on-ward division of labour between 1944 and 1963.

## Changing the In-Hospital Management — A Beginning

In an attempt to realize the recommendations put forward by Sigerist and Hincks, the DPH gave top priority to the reorganization of the mental hospitals. This was part of a general CCF programme which was aimed at the elimination of political patronage within the civil service.[24]

Political patronage had characterized the provincial civil service since its inception. Attempts had been made to minimize the extent of this practice by the establishment of the Public Service Commission (PSC) in 1913. However, the mental hospital management had successfully circumvented PSC controls, and consequently patronage was the norm. The prolonged Depression in Saskatchewan had resulted in the extension of the patronage system to virtually all levels of the mental hospital's division of labour, since economic conditions were so bad that the previous government had traded scarce jobs for political support. Speaking of this process as it applied to the mental hospitals in 1944, T.C. Douglas stated that unemployment had become so bad that any job

> was a political plum to be handed out to some of their supporters. Nearly all the people who were appointed had been appointed by some politician who had recommended them. Some fellow would go to them and say, "My boy is 19-20, can't get anything to do, nothing on the farm. Could you get him into the hospital?" If he happened to be chairman of a local committee, or had

> some influence, municipal reeve, or municipal councillor and carried some weight in the community, the politician was very anxious to get one of his sons on staff. The fact that the son wasn't interested in psychiatry, and couldn't care less about looking after the patients had nothing to do with it.[25]

The general feeling within the CCF leadership was that this kind of political patronage produced a work force largely uninterested and uncommitted to their work. This in turn was thought to result in an inefficient and uneconomical mental hospital system. In order to counteract these tendencies, it was thought the replacement of political appointees in key decision-making positions was necessary.[26] To this end, government employees suspected of actively obstructing government policies within the mental hospitals were blacklisted.[27]

The easiest solution, of course, would have been simply to replace one set of political appointees with another, and although this was done to a limited extent, it was a practice which was largely curtailed by Douglas. In a 1945 letter, referring to people named on the mental hospital blacklist, he stated his position quite clearly:

> As you know, I am adamantly opposed to taking action against these or other persons because of their political opinions. I believe they are entitled to hold whatever political opinions they choose, but I do not think that any person is entitled to use a government position to sabotage and undermine the government's position, whose policy they are supposed to be carrying out.[28]

The in-hospital management's opposition to government attempts to increase the rate of discharge did not derive from stubbornness or malevolence towards the inmates. The mental hospitals depended on unpaid patient labour for their existence and it was rightly feared that if they were made more like general hospitals (i.e., if mental hospital work were increasingly medicalized), those inmates capable of working would be discharged first. One of the consequences of this would be to amplify the tendency for the mental hospitals to become increasingly decrepit warehouses for the chronic and aged insane. Thus, paradoxically, physicians employed in the mental hospitals, although generally supportive of the claim that mental illness was no different than physical illness at the ideological level, opposed the convergence in treatment at the practical level because of the fear that it would result in a further loss of status for mental hospital doctors compared to their colleagues in other branches of medical work.

Non-medical mental hospital workers also opposed the transition from custody to treatment because of the fear of job loss, although they too espoused support for the idea that physical and mental illnesses were identical. The government, however, was committed to the transformation, and had to find a politically acceptable solution to the dilemma of how to replace obstructionist in-hospital management and uninterested and untrained ward workers without appearing to undertake a political purge.

For some, the solution to this problem appeared to lie with the newly created union. The previous management structure, built as it was on personal patronage and tyranny, had generated internal rifts and tensions at all levels of the in-hospital division of labour. Discussing the nature of work relations in the pre-1944 period, a psychiatric nurse stated: "Junior staff were afraid to speak to the head nurse on the ward usually, and the atmosphere was very tense. I think you were more afraid of the staff than you were of the patients."[29] As a consequence, there were many who were willing to do whatever they could to bring down the old autocratic system of management. The union provided the means to do this.

In 1944 the provincial mental hospitals were organized as Locals 2 and 3 of the United Civil Servants of Canada (UCSC), an industrial union affiliated with the pro-CCF Canadian Congress of Labour (CCL). The CCL was dedicated to securing traditional "trade-union" gains for its members through lobbying and negotiation, an objective apparently achieved when the CCF government, in an unprecedented move in Canada,[30] signed collective agreements with its own civil service in 1945.

As a consequence of this historic agreement, the government recognized the union as "the sole collective agency for hospital employees."[31] The government also agreed to negotiate with the union, or its designated agents, "in any and all matters affecting the relationship between the government as employer and its employees."[32] This gave the union a significant degree of power, for in effect *all* aspects of work within the mental hospitals were subject to negotiation.

At that time there was no "management rights" clause in the collective agreement. This situation was agreeable to both the administration of the DPH and the union executive, who joined forces to purge the in-hospital management. It looked as if the government was making good on its 1933 promise to establish a system of genuine industrial democracy, starting with its own civil service.

In July 1945, three members of the UCSC Local Number 3 from SHNB made a voluntary statement to a legal advisor in the premier's office. It was claimed that the acting superintendent of SHNB, who had been appointed after MacNeill's retirement, was engaged in a "concerted attempt to impede the work of the Union, and to obstruct the policy of the Government."[33] The union representatives went on to state that the acting superintendent

> has not been co-operating either with the trade union, its members, or with the Government in any way. Appointments have not been made according to seniority, and we are of the opinion that a concerted effort is being made to appoint persons unsympathetic with the present Government's policy, and that persons well known for their political activity in opposition to the CCF have been appointed.[34]

The acting superintendent and others on the hospital's management staff were further accused of "continually delaying and obstructing the implementation of all clauses of the collective agreement."[35]

This statement provided the government with the justification needed to replace the in-hospital management. At the same 12 July meeting a plan was proposed to undermine the existing in-hospital management structure. The plan was to have the union expose the existence of an extensive system of criminal racketeering which was operating at SHNB. This union-instigated investigation resulted in the establishment of the Royal Commission into the Administration and Financial Affairs of the North Battleford Mental Hospital, and culminated with criminal charges being laid against four hospital employees.

This was, of course, precisely what the government needed to enable it to revamp the in-hospital management without appearing to be simply replacing one set of appointees with another of a different political stripe. This was important to the government for two reasons: first, the CCF, for political reasons, wanted to be recognized as ending the patronage system in the civil service, and second, because patronage had extended into every level of the hospital system it was important, especially in light of chronic shortages of labour power and the high attrition rate among workers, not to aggravate the already critical situation by raising the fear of wholesale dismissals and/or criminal prosecutions. The following quotation can be seen as an attempt to allay the fears of mental hospital workers in that regard:

> We are not interested in prosecuting or persecuting these people simply to obtain convictions. I believe that for the most part, they are simply the victims of a vicious system which years of neglect and inefficiency produced.[36]

It was made clear, however, that the continuation of these practices would not be tolerated:

> It is high time that we have a thorough house cleaning at the mental hospital and that those responsible for thefts, and those whose neglect made theft a simple business, be made to account to the people of the province for their misconduct.[37]

The government concluded that the result of the investigation "will be a saving in operating costs which will amaze the public." Furthermore, it was to lead to "the establishment of a new and healthy labour-management relationship, which will substitute mutual trust and co-operation for the suspicion and coercion which has not been uncommon."[38]

These assertions proved to be more wishful than prophetic. However, having started to reorganize the in-hospital management structure and to replace key personnel, a process made easier by Dr. MacNeill's retirement in 1945, the DPH, under the control of Premier Douglas, undertook to further implement the recommendations of the Sigerist and Hincks reports. To this end, Dr. D.G. McKerracher was appointed as the commissioner of mental services in 1946.

Dr. McKerracher seemed to be well suited for the task at hand. His vision of how best to organize the production of psychiatric services was compatible with the prevention-oriented public health model long advocated by the NCMH, and endorsed by the new CCF government. In addition, he had had extensive experience with the organization and delivery of psychiatric services in the armed forces during World War II. His military experiences were to provide the inspiration for many of the organizational innovations subsequently implemented in Saskatchewan. Indeed, military experiences, and the exigencies of World War II, constitute what might be considered one of the proximate causes of the major changes in the nature and organization of psychiatric work in general. Under pressure to ensure an adequate supply of military labour power able to function reliably under conditions of intense and prolonged stress, the military authorities turned to psychiatry. The nature and organization of psychiatric work as it existed, however, was inadequate for the task at hand. Therefore, according to Dr. William Menninger, the famous psychiatrist,

> The use of auxiliary personnel had to be augmented to include not only clinical psychologists and psychiatric social workers but also an increased number of psychiatric nurses and recreational, educational and occupational therapists.[39]

Based upon the efficacy of this new psychiatric division of labour, Menninger stated that those in the civilian practice of psychiatry would find their work greatly altered following the war. The postwar transformation of psychiatric work in Saskatchewan, under the guidance of Dr. McKerracher, proved him correct.

Upon arriving in the province, McKerracher immediately set out three interrelated goals:

1. Co-ordination of the mental health services provided by the two Saskatchewan Hospitals, the Saskatchewan Training School and the Psychopathic Unit.
2. Assistance in the improvement and development of programs in therapy and care in the four facilities mentioned above.
3. The development of a community program of mental health directed at the prevention and alleviation of mental disorder.[40]

The various attempts to fulfill the first two functions, and the struggles thereby generated, resulted in the reorganization and transformation of the in-hospital psychiatric labour process.

## Coordination of Mental Health Services

To adequately fulfill the first function, it was necessary to centralize decision-making and control. The two provincial mental hospitals, under the direction of Dr. MacNeill, had been able to secure and maintain a significant degree of autonomy and self-direction. The CCF, committed to planned social change and increased efficiency in the civil service, set out to change this.

To end this autonomy, the mental hospitals were put under the exclusive control of the DPH and the office of the commissioner of mental services. In-hospital management, however, was accustomed to independence in running the hospitals, and did not willingly relinquish power. In an effort to retain managerial autonomy, attempts were made to bypass the new commissioner of mental services, a practice which was opposed by the DPH. In a 1949 memo to the superintendents of the provincial institutions, the deputy minister of public health stated where administrative power lay:

> there never, at any time, was any doubt in the minds of the Minister or myself that Dr. McKerracher, since his appointment as Commissioner of Mental Services, was in complete charge of the Division of Mental Services and

> that he was over each and every Superintendent of an institution. . . . I want it understood by all that Dr. McKerracher is in complete charge of the mental hospitals and responsible through me to the Minister.[41]

Although this memo was sent to the superintendents of both SHNB and SHW, it was intended primarily for the superintendent of SHW. Following the administrative house-cleaning of the 1946 royal commission, the situation at SHNB *seemed* to be well in hand, although not as unproblematic as one would expect; the situation at SHW was of more immediate concern to the DPH. At that time SHW was "run by two very conservative people";[42] the superintendent and the business manager. Both men felt threatened by the proposed changes entailed in the transition from a custodial to a therapeutic psychiatric labour process. Consequently, they opposed many of the changes put forward by the commissioner of mental services.

This opposition impeded the attempted reduction of inmate populations and the DPH wanted it stopped. However, the government did not want to be seen to be conducting political purges within the civil service and wished to avoid simply firing these employees. The situation was further complicated by the fact that T.C. Douglas was the sitting member from Weyburn, and it was known that any internal power struggle at the mental hospital would eventually manifest itself in the political arena. This was of special concern because the superintendent reportedly had "some political clout."[43] This came from two sources, the hospital employees who justifiably feared that the proposed changes threatened their jobs, and the local business community which benefitted by servicing both institutional needs and the needs of hospital employees.

With significant forces opposed to the planned transformation of mental hospital work, it took considerable political will to proceed. As has been seen, the commissioner of mental services had both the administrative and political support needed to push ahead, and a concerted effort to change the nature and organization of psychiatric work was begun.

As part of that process, the commissioner of mental services stationed himself in Weyburn for the winter of 1946 in an attempt to overcome the recalcitrance of the in-hospital management.[44] Opposition to the proposed changes remained strong, and in a further attempt to gain control the DPH reorganized the Division of Mental Services into the Psychiatric Services Branch (PSB) in 1950. This resulted in a concentration of power in the hands of the director of PSB. Even with this change, the struggle for control of the mental hospitals was long and bitter, and not completed until the early 1960s.

One of the major intramanagement struggles in this attempt to coordinate mental health services occurred over the control of hiring, firing and promotions. Under the previous regime the in-hospital management at both institutions had achieved complete control of these matters. As a consequence, there was a lack of standardization regarding conditions of employment between the two mental hospitals. Premier Douglas and the director of PSB were determined to rationalize the civil service by centralizing all hiring in the office of the PSC. High attrition rates among ward workers, combined with obstructionist in-hospital managers, made this difficult. Premier Douglas was adamant, insisting all public sector hiring was to be carried out by the PSC according to a clearly specified procedure. It was felt that this was the only way to eliminate patronage in the civil service and thereby improve the efficiency and economy of its operation.

The opposition was so strong that a compromise finally had to be reached. This compromise allowed the in-hospital management to hire certain categories of ward personnel as casual employees. Casual appointments covered a twenty-six-day period during which the process of selection by the PSC could be completed. It was argued that "this would permit the hospital authorities to hire likely looking prospects on the spot and at the same time allow the usual screening process to be used."[45]

The autonomy of the in-hospital management prior to 1945 had resulted in differentials in pay ranges, job classifications and perquisites. Indeed, since the existence of the perquisite system and the privilege of requisitioning goods for personal consumption was thought to be a factor which contributed to inefficiency in the operation of the mental hospitals, it was to be eliminated:

> it is the government's intention to make uniform the privileges of staff at the two mental hospitals in the province and for this reason, it is its intention to discontinue the practice of permitting members of the permanent staff to requisition goods for their personal use. . . .[46]

In the context of critical on-ward staff shortages and high attrition rates, this necessitated an increase in the cash portion of hospital workers' income. As well as being an attempt to standardize the conditions of employment between the two mental hospitals, the increase in pay, combined with the reduction of the working day from twelve to eight hours, was part of the plan to develop and improve the mental hospitals' therapeutic programmes.

## The Improvement and Development of Programmes in Therapy and Care

The government believed the only long-term solution to the problem of overcrowding in the provincial mental hospitals was to increase the rate of discharge. It was also thought this strategy could only be effective if the mental hospitals ceased to be mere warehouses for the insane, and engaged in the provision of active therapeutic treatment. In order to do this, however, it was necessary to have a sufficient supply of appropriately trained labour power. The commissioner of mental services employed a number of tactics to achieve this goal: extensive national and international recruitment campaigns; the establishment of local training programmes; and the creation of a bursary system to assist DPH employees wishing to upgrade their credentials.

### *Psychiatrists*

The provincial mental hospitals had always experienced difficulty in recruiting and retaining an adequate supply of medically trained labour power due to Saskatchewan's geographical remoteness and the physical isolation of the mental hospitals. Regarding this, the deputy minister of public health opined that "given a choice no psychiatrist would come to Weyburn, North Battleford or any other smaller centre in this province because of the weather, the social and cultural amenities or the living conditions."[47] This seemed self-evident to many. In 1944, for example, of the twelve doctors in the provincial mental hospitals only four or five were trained psychiatrists.[48] This was only half the American Psychiatric Association's recommended contingent of medical staff, and clearly insufficient to provide adequate custodial care, let alone active psychiatric treatment. This point was made by the commissioner of mental services in a letter to the deputy minister of public health at the time:

> I also wish to call your attention to the lack of Medical staff here [SHNB], as well as at Weyburn. According to the American Psychiatric Association, the standard we are endeavouring to work with is only fifty percent of the Medical staff required in a hospital of this population. At the present time, we are hopelessly behind in our mental examinations, not because the Medical staff are not working hard but because they cannot reach the work that should be done in a hospital of this kind.[49]

In an attempt to remedy this situation, the commissioner of mental services attempted by recruitment drives and training programmes to increase the number of psychiatrists employed by the DPH.

In 1949 the two provincial mental hospitals, the Munroe Wing of the Regina General Hospital and the mental health clinics were incorporated as "training centres for persons receiving certification as specialists in psychiatry."[50] The post-graduate resident training programme, which was recognized by the Royal College of Physicians and Surgeons, was four years in length. Each year the programme graduated from five to seven PSB doctors, and appeared to be a great success. Commenting on this programme in 1955, a CMHA brief to the provincial cabinet stated: "The success of

Saskatchewan candidates in the Royal College examinations has been outstanding and psychiatrists are now coming from other provinces in order to complete their training in Saskatchewan."[51] Although this was encouraging to the DPH, the rate of increase was less than desired when set against the continued high attrition rate.

In an attempt to supplement the supply of locally trained psychiatrists, an overseas recruitment campaign was undertaken. This too failed to achieve the hoped-for results. The Saskatchewan Psychiatric Association (SPA), in a 1956 brief to the minister of public health, commented on this situation:

> Over the past ten years there has been a rapid and large turnover of Medical Personnel in Psychiatric Services. Much of this can be laid at the door of the policy of employing unlicensed Medical Practitioners coming to the Province from overseas, who following their one year's rotating internship require a "job" to tide them over that difficult period between the end of their internship and their Dominion Council Examination. These men come to the Hospitals and clinics having no interest in Psychiatry and are only of value in taking some of the routine general medical work off the shoulders of the few Doctors who have the psychiatric knowledge necessary to help their patients. Following success in their examinations these men hurry off to the more lucrative field of private practice.[52]

From the SPA's point of view, the solution to the problem of retention was higher salaries — a position PSB management consistently supported. This is not surprising since, at that time, all upper-level management positions in PSB were still held by psychiatrists. The arguments put forward in support of higher pay, and the explanations for high attrition rates (intemperate climate, underdeveloped social and cultural amenities) can only be accepted as legitimate in relation to particular conditions, one of the most important of which is the existence of a labour market wherein demand exceeds supply. Such was the case for psychiatrists.

"Professionalization" has been usefully conceptualized as the process whereby an occupation seeks to "constitute *and control* a market for their expertise."[53] [emphasis in original] Similarly, Parry and Parry argue professionalism is most usefully defined as a control strategy wherein an occupation attempts to secure self-government and restrict entry to the occupation through educational recruitment, training and licensing procedures.[54]

This approach to the sociology of the professions is much more useful than the widely discredited attribute approach, and there would be no particular problem with it if researchers within this tradition did not overextend its analytical applicability by assuming that control of a labour market automatically entails autonomy within a labour process. The control of the market for particular occupational skills does not automatically result in autonomy within, and control of, work organization. It is, rather, the specific nature of the labour process within which professional work is practiced which will determine if a profession has autonomy or not.[55] This point is often recognized, as when Larson points out that within the Anglo-Saxon tradition "profession is presented . . . as the antithesis of bureaucracy and the bureaucratic mode of work organization."[56] However, having recognized this, the analytical implications are most often ignored. As a consequence, labour market practices and labour process practices are conflated, conceptually confusing much sociological work on the professions.

Arguing for the *analytical* distinction between labour market and labour process analysis is not to deny that the two are inextricably intertwined. It is simply to suggest that the various occupational practices undertaken to secure monopoly in a labour market[57] are not necessarily the same as those undertaken to achieve autonomy, job security and improved working conditions. However, it must be noted that an occupation with a strong market position, and a range of employment alternatives, will use that situation in an attempt to achieve the above-mentioned workplace objectives.[58]

This is significant for the purposes at hand insofar as it provides the basis for another potential explanation of the cause of the rapid and large turnover of medical personnel. Although the immediate problem may have been the policy of employing unlicensed medical practitioners coming from overseas, the fundamental problem could be argued to be one of occupation generated and maintained scarcity. The practioners recruited from overseas were unlicensed because the College of Physicians and Surgeons would not recognize their previous training and credentials. Although this was legitimated in the name of protecting the quality of services, the effect was to perpetuate the scarcity of fully qualified psychiatric labour power, a scarcity psychiatrists used to enhance and protect their position within the psychiatric division of labour.[59] In particular, PSB psychiatrists used their position of strength to attain three interconnected objectives: increased remuneration, improved working conditions, and what was described as a morale-building "emotional climate."[60]

Increased remuneration was always an object of struggle, although given the uncompetitive nature of the province with regard to its climatic, social and cultural amenities, it was accepted by the government that psychiatrists' salaries had to be relatively high in order to compensate. Consequently, although psychiatrists constantly sought more money, salaries were not the major source of conflict. The deputy minister of public health, himself a medically trained doctor, stated in a memo to the minister of public health: "So far as our people are concerned there is no major complaint about salaries; our salaries are competitive and compare favourably with other jurisdictions."[61]

Working conditions, or what might more accurately be referred to as non-salary benefits, were similarly not of crucial significance in employer-employee relations. Some of the central elements of this category which did occasion limited struggle were employer-provided housing, pension benefits, holidays, educational leave and early retirement.

In the previous chapter it was shown that the quality as well as the quantity of housing provided had been a source of conflict; this remained the case. In an effort to deal with criticism emanating from hospital workers and others,[62] the government initiated both construction and repair programmes in the 1950s.

The repair programme was financed out of revenues derived from increased rents.[63] Not surprisingly, the increased rents themselves became a source of employer-employee tension. Discussing the level of satisfaction of PSB psychiatrists with their working conditions, the president of the SPA advised the premier: "This recent sudden increase in rentals alters this for the worse."[64] The issue of accommodation remained a source of conflict and dissatisfaction until the early 1970s, when the government finally stopped providing employee housing altogether.

The primary source of antagonism between PSB psychiatrists and the government developed around what has been termed the "emotional climate." This may best be understood as a euphemism for the definition and control of, as well as autonomy within, the psychiatric labour process.

When the CCF government undertook to increase the rate of discharge from the mental hospitals, and thereby reduce inmate populations to rated capacities, it was also decided to give the commissioner of mental services a free hand in his attempts to achieve this. This freedom was extended, in large part, to all PSB psychiatrists who supported DPH objectives. These psychiatrists were encouraged to innovate in the treatment of the mentally ill and this innovation became articulated as a complete system of psychiatric care for the province known as the Saskatchewan Plan. Psychiatrists viewed their autonomy as indicative of "a progressive, dynamic attractive program . . . in the forefront on this continent."[65]

The autonomy of PSB psychiatrists to determine the nature and organization of psychiatric work, however, depended upon government policy. When the government's refusal to endorse the Saskatchewan Plan established the limits to "professional sovereignty," psychiatrists responded by leaving PSB, and/or publicly attacking the government and its psychiatric policies. The first response was, within limits, tolerable to the government. The second tactic, however, was interpreted as insubordination or obstructionism and, in either case, something that would not be tolerated from government employees. The government thus took steps to assert its control of the psychiatric labour process.

In one case, for example, the government refused to promote a psychiatrist recommended by the director of PSB, and delayed the appointment and reclassification of another who had successfully achieved certification. This raised charges of political interference from the psychiatrists, who argued that they alone were able to determine who was best suited to perform psychiatric work. The deputy minister of public health commented on this in a memo to the minister:

> To understand this complaint one must keep in mind two aspects of institutional life. The first is that any large institution and particularly a mental hospital, is characterized by the fact that there are few secrets, a great amount of speculation and 'scuttlebut' and an interest of everyone in everyone else's business. The second characteristic of the mental institution is a very vivid recollection of the old-time mental hospital where appointments were based on patronage rather than merit, with the result that it often became a refuge for incompetent and fundamentally disinterested employees; any suggestion of an increasing amount of political influence in appointments is greatly feared and results in damaged morale.[66]

The struggle between psychiatrists and the government for control of the psychiatric labour process became so intense that the SPA accused the government of engaging in McCarthy-like political repression,[67] and intimated mass resignations would be the consequence.[68]

The premier did not back down in this struggle for control, and his reply to the SPA showed clearly where power lay: "Where two or three persons have been declared eligible for a position, then *the final decision as to the appointment must rest with the Minister of the Department*."[69] [emphasis added]

These struggles, and that over the implementation of the Saskatchewan Plan, which was also partially a struggle between government as employer and psychiatrists as employees for control of the psychiatric labour process, were to shape the development of community psychiatry in

Saskatchewan. Before examining these developments in any more detail, however, attention will be returned to developments within the in-hospital labour process.

*Psychiatric Nurses and the Union*

In 1944 "there was a large staff turnover and the educational requirements were not high."[70] The nursing staff was on a twelve-hour day, six-day week and "the starting salary was $75.00 per month."[71] These were low wages and long hours, even at the time, which made it difficult to recruit and retain ward workers. This in turn created severe shortages of on-ward labour power, and made the work of those employed even more difficult. The extent of these shortages, and the burden they created for the existing staffs, was incredible. The commissioner of mental services wrote to the deputy minister of public health:

> That night you and I were down at the Hospital, you will recall that one ward had only one woman to handle 150 patients and another slip of a girl had 111, which is not only dreadfully hard work but a dangerous situation to be in.[72]

It was thought that the only way to overcome this situation would be to increase the level of remuneration and reduce the hours of work. Management reasoned that by so doing, a stable work force of trained ward workers could be produced, and enticed to stay in the government's employ. The superintendent of SHW stated:

> I consider this proposed [wage] schedule as a fine bit of mental hygiene work. It would mean that a young married man can commence work here and be reasonably free from worry. It should also ensure that everyone going into the service will remain and it should do away with the constant changing of staff.[73]

The shortening of the working day made it necessary to staff three shifts as compared to two under the previous structure. Even though this increased the costs of producing psychiatric services, it was accepted by the DPH and PSB

### Table 4
### Schedule of Mental Hospital Wage Range by Job Classification and Sex

| | Pre-1942 | | 1942-43 | | 1943-44 | | 1945 | |
|---|---|---|---|---|---|---|---|---|
| | Monthly | Annually | Monthly | Annually | Monthly | Annually | Monthly | Annually |
| | $ | $ | $ | $ | $ | $ | $ | $ |
| Nurse Attendants – Female */Attendants | 60-80 | 720-960 | 60-100 | 720-1200 | 77.50-105 | 930-1260 | 100-155 | 1200-1860 |
| Attendants – Male | 80-90 | 840-1080 | 75-105 | 900-1260 | 77.50-105 | 930-1260 | 100-155 | 1200-1860 |
| Supervisors – Female | 85-95 | 1020-1140 | 105-125 | 1260-1500 | 110-130 | 1320-1560 | 175- | 2100- |
| Supervisors – Male | 105-115 | 1260-1380 | 110-130 | 1320-1560 | 110-130 | 1320-1560 | 175- | 2100- |
| Head Nurse – Female */Chief Attendant | 117.50-125 | 1410-1500 | 130-150 | 1560-1800 | 165- | 1980- | 180-225 | 2160-2700 |
| 1st Asst. Head Nurse – */1st Asst. Chief Attendant | 110- | 1320- | 115-135 | 1380-1620 | 150- | 1800- | 164-205 | 1968-2460 |
| 2nd Asst. Head Nurse – */2nd Asst. Chief Attendant | 95- | 1140- | 110-130 | 1320-1560 | 135- | 1620- | 183-190 | 2196-2280 |
| Chief Attendant – Male | 125-140 | 1500-1680 | 135-150 | 1620-1800 | 165- | 1980- | 180-225 | 2160-2700 |
| 1st Chief Attendant | 114-125 | 1372-1500 | 115-135 | 1380-1620 | 150- | 1800- | 164-205 | 1968-2460 |

*In 1945 nomenclature changed to reflect implementation of equal pay for equal work government policy.

*Source:* Derived from SAB, R-97, l.a. Uhrich Papers: Staff General and SAB, R-33.4, 98.(13-4-1-4); Douglas Papers: Mental Hospitals and United Civil Servants of Canada.

management that this extra financial burden was necessary in order to transform the nature of in-hospital psychiatric work.

This is the same reasoning as that put forward by MacNeill in the mid-1930s. In fact, a policy of increased wages had been implemented prior to the election of the CCF, as can be seen from Table 4. It was probably this policy of increased wages, combined with reduced hours, that served to postpone construction of the proposed twelve hundred-bed mental hospital in Saskatoon. Had this hospital been constructed, although labour power shortages would have been exacerbated, the overcrowding would have been significantly reduced, and the historical development and the organizational transformation of psychiatry in the province would have been dramatically altered.

The new hospital never was constructed, and the newly acquired strength of the psychiatric work force *vis-à-vis* the government as employer manifested itself in the form of a crisis of management within the psychiatric services system. Initially, the union demanded even more money and shorter hours of work; demands which the government resisted, not in principle, but for pragmatic reasons, as can be seen from the following excerpt from a letter from the premier's office to the regional representative of the CCL:

> I am further instructed [by the premier] to advise you that by reason of the fact that the 44 hour week was not provided in the Collective Agreement now effective, the Government is of the opinion that no action can be validly taken to adjust the working hours according to that schedule at this time. The Government has subscribed to the principle of the 8 hour day, which, coupled with the 6 day working week results in a 48 hour week. You are well aware of the difficulties which the Department of Health is now experiencing in securing personnel for these mental hospitals who are capable of absorbing the necessary information, conducting sufficient study and writing such examinations as will qualify them for attendants and nurse attendants. This is the only type of employee which the Government hopes to retain in the classifications of attendants and nurse attendants. To date it has been impossible to secure suitable personnel to fill all positions properly. When the time comes, I have no doubt that the Government will subscribe to the 44 hour week.[74]

Even after the union secured the forty-four-hour week, the issue of hours remained a point of contention in management-worker relations. In 1953, for example, the union took the DPH before a conciliation board in an attempt to institute a forty-hour week with two consective days off for ward workers. The conciliation board ruled against the union at that time. The government's opposition to the forty-hour week was primarily due to the prohibitive costs involved, combined with "the great difficulty of obtaining sufficient staff for even existing establishments."[75] The government also rejected "the union's contention that a shorter work week would contribute materially to solving the problem of obtaining staff."[76] This item was not taken off the union's agenda until 1958, the year the forty-hour week was finally introduced for all on-ward workers.

The issues of increased pay and shorter hours of work were not simply a source of management-worker conflict. It was around these two issues that the isomorphism of *petit bourgeois* farmers' interests and the interests of (public sector) wage workers, posited by the CCF, broke down. The internal contradiction of the CCF political alliance manifested itself in the form of opposition to the shortened hours and increased pay associated with the transformation of in-hospital psychiatric work. The principal opposition came from the predominantly rural constituencies.

The following letter, from a CCF party member who later became an advisor to the premier's office, expresses the strength of opposition to further wage increases for mental hospital workers, both within and outside the CCF:

> I have interviewed several hospital employees, of both Liberal and CCF persuasion, and they have agreed with me that the demands presently to be made are unreasonable. A few of the lower paid employees . . . should no doubt receive a bit of a raise, but as for the rest they are now getting more for less than they could get anywhere else in Canada . . . . The upper strata are well paid right now — don't let them bamboozle you.[77]

The union assumed opponents simply did not fully understand the situation and, therefore, proposed to educate them regarding the dangerous and arduous nature of mental hospital work. In a letter to the minister of public health it was stated that the union membership felt:

> if the farm population did not now feel that these employees in their hazardous occupation did not earn the right to better wages and working conditions it was because of the fact that they were not familiar with the true conditions surrounding the question, and therefore the Unions should embark on an educational campaign

> regarding this matter and so aid in smoothing away the opposition which the Government representatives claimed they were meeting in this regard.[78]

This was the last thing the DPH and the PSC wanted. They were already confronted with a critical shortage of labour power, and certainly did not wish to have the union frightening off prospective employees:

> We must recognize the fact it [the proposed advertising/educational campaign] is apt to have a very unfavourable reaction upon the employees in the Hospitals in that it might discourage applicants from accepting positions in those institutions thereby causing understaffing.[79]

Although in this instance the union was persuaded not to take its struggle for improved working conditions and increased pay into the public forum, the government was not always able to convince it to keep its struggles within the hospitals. This was largely a consequence of the fact that the executive of the union local at SHNB was highly politicized. This politicization manifested itself in the form of a commitment to the general socialist objectives espoused by the CCF, rather than to the lobby tactics of the CCL-dominated locals in Weyburn. This had two consequences for management-union relations: first, the North Battleford local adopted a generally collaborative stance *vis à vis* the government, although not necessarily with the in-hospital management, and second, as a consequence of adherence to CCF political goals, failure of the union to achieve its more specific workplace objectives was perceived to be a consequence of obstructionist tactics on the part of political enemies of the government and its union supporters.

An example of this can be seen in a letter from the union to the premier's office explaining a one-month delay in the implementation of a retroactive pay agreement:

> there are certain strategically placed minor officials in the Government offices who belong whole heartedly to the old school of reaction politics, and these people will not leave any stone unturned in their efforts to very slyly and discreetly estrange the Government with many of

> the voting electorate in and during the course of their duties as civil servants. I feel sure that the obstructionist policies is [*sic*] only a part of the preconceived plan on the part of the enemies of the Government to discredit a Union, which openly supports the CCF Party, in the eyes of the Union's own membership. They are working very subversively with their eyes on a certain election date some three or four years distant.[80]

This perception led the North Battleford local constantly to petition the government to intervene in hospital affairs. The expectation that the government and the union would collaborate to defeat common enemies had been established in 1946 when the government used the union to undermine the in-hospital management structure. After achieving that goal, however, the government was not anxious to help the union undermine the new management structures being developed, and consistently rejected requests from the union and others to intervene in management-union disputes, thereby tacitly supporting management and management's right to control the psychiatric labour process.

The Psychiatric Nurse Training Program, organized by PSB management as part of its process of creating the occupation of psychiatric nursing, was also the object of intense conflict. In particular, curriculum content and methods of evaluation were contentious issues. These conflicts were usually manifested as dissatisfaction with particular teachers. In one instance the union attempted to get PSB management to fire a teacher with whom it was dissatisfied. Management refused, and the union attempted to bring political pressure to bear by staging mass demonstrations. These were reported to the premier:

> It appears that a large meeting of Union members, over one hundred strong, had gathered on Friday evening at North Battleford, when the contentious issue of [the teacher] was again raised. It was the unanimous decision of those assembled that the Union executive should resign as a body as a protest to the Government over the retention of [the teacher] and that [the local MLA] be asked to resign as government representative in further protest. . . .[81]

The DPH viewed this as an illegitimate infringement on management rights. In the above-quoted report, the acting deputy minister of public health went on to state:

> I . . . told [the local MLA] that I thought the Union were [*sic*] going far outside their powers in attempting to dictate to the Government who should or should not be an employee of the Government, especially those who were outside the scope of the agreement. . . .[82]

It had thus become clear to the CCF government, if not the CCF party, that democracy in the workplace was not feasible. Due to the base of CCF political support, however, it simply could not abandon its commitment to union goals, or rescind its support of the union movement, even had it been so inclined. Rather, the government attempted to depoliticize the union and restrict its sphere of interest to economistic concerns. Therefore the response of the government to various demands for intervention, from the union, the party constituency executive, or the MLA, was always the same: the collective agreement had established procedures for dealing with grievances, and they should be used. The following comments from the minister of public health to the local MLA are typical:

> I can fully appreciate your feelings of frustration when you are subjected to so many complaints . . . by dissatisfied persons employed at the Hospital, but again I want to remind you that dissatisfied employees have a Union to represent them and the Union has all the necessary procedures set out in the agreement for dealing with these matters of dissatisfaction.[83]

The depoliticization of the North Battleford local was not easy. Besides generating much management-worker conflict, the highly politicized nature of the North Battleford local produced much intraunion antagonism, the extent of which can be seen in the following letter sent to the premier's office from the union executive at North Battleford:

> I would like to say that we are very dissatisfied, and very disturbed, over the anti-social and anti-government attitude of the two Locals of this Union in those two institutions [i.e., Saskatchewan Hospital Weyburn and

> Saskatchewan Training School Weyburn]. We have found them to be positively antagonistic towards the employer in a sullen and unreasoning manner which so far we have been unable to break down. . . . We have spoken to [the regional director of the CCL] about this situation . . . for the purpose of clearing up and improving the employer-employee relations there. We have found however to our dismay, that he was inclined to favor [the] Local which is causing the trouble, and that he wasn't much impressed with our presentations. He has even hinted that we were inclined to be too easy going and soft. We are now at that stage where we wonder if he is not encouraging [that] local in its ugly and wayward attitude.[84]

The intraunion conflicts became so intense the North Battleford local considered disaffiliating from the other two locals and the CCL. The premier's office advised against taking such action. It was suggested to the North Battleford union executive that disaffiliation would diminish their influence, which derived from being in one bargaining unit.[85]

The government, by phrasing its request that disaffiliation not occur in order that the union and government would unite to defeat common enemies within the union movement, was able to convince the union executive at North Battleford to remain affiliated. This made the institutionalization of management-union conflict more likely because the non-politicized Weyburn locals, with almost twice the membership, were able to exert a considerable depoliticizing effect on the North Battleford local. Thus institutionalized, the various conflicts would be effectively stabilized and less likely to escalate into political crises, or effective challenges to management, which were the major concerns of the government.

The objective of this common management strategy, which Storey refers to as "the compartmentalization of issues and the institutionalization of conflict,"[86] is to isolate and separate "legitimate" from "illegitimate" issues. As Michael Mann notes, "the institutionalization of industrial conflict is nothing more or less than the narrowing down of conflict to aggressive economism and defensive control."[87] In addition, it has been found that "inappropriate" worker demands will be resisted by "both management and the organized trade union bodies."[88]

Such was certainly the case in this instance. As early as 1946 the CCF government had decided, with respect to government-operated enterprises, that industrial democracy was unworkable since:

> If labour is allowed to make recommendations about management, it continually attempts to take on more power. When the stage is reached where management must say 'no', the labour-management machinery is bound to break down. A socialized industry, unlike a capitalist industry, cannot solve the problem by simply discontinuing the labour-management set-up.[89]

The government, therefore, was vitally interested in ensuring that the unions did not become too powerful.

The union local at North Battleford never realized that its failure to achieve an equal voice in the management of the mental hospitals was a consequence of the limitations of CCF "socialism." It consistently attributed its frustration in this regard to obstructionist practices of CCF detractors within the administration, or within the union movement itself. Kahan quotes the organizer, and charter president, of the first Trade Union of Hospital Employees:

> I had no intention of us joining the general trade unions [i.e., the TLC or the CCL], but before we had time to put our trade union on a sound basis, the Canadian Congress of Labour had organized the staff at Weyburn, *and to gain bargaining rights through the Saskatchewan Labour laws we were forced to affiliate with the CCL.* I was never too happy about this and the many disputes throughout the years with the labour organizations convinced me that my doubts were well founded.[90] [emphasis added]

It seems likely the government, by forcing affiliation with the CCL, was attempting to establish limits to union participation in management decisions. The CCL, although affiliated with the avowedly socialist CCF, pursued economistic objectives rather than attempting to achieve a system of worker self-management. This suited the CCF government in its role as employer, inasmuch as it allowed the legislative provision of concessions to the unions without abrogating traditional management prerogatives. This contradiction of CCF political theory and practice manifested itself partially in the form of management-union and intraunion conflict over the nature and scope of union power. This conflict, and the struggles thereby generated, forced the government to move more slowly than it would have liked in the transformation of in-hospital psychiatric work.

Although these intraunion struggles influenced the rate of change, management-worker struggles were most significant in influencing the transformation of the in-hospital psychiatric labour process. When the DPH decided that the only way to achieve higher rates of discharge from the mental hospitals was to provide active therapeutic treatment, it was also decided that this could only be achieved by creating a new occupation trained in therapeutic techniques. This was not a new decision; the first steps in this direction had been taken by MacNeill in 1930.

These developments were not universally embraced. There were two major sources of opposition: first, the SRNA opposed the creation of this new occupation, and second, the pretraining programme ward workers (attendants and nurse attendants) opposed these developments because it was felt, justifiably, that the transition from custody to "cure" would threaten their jobs.

Although the SRNA had long been opposed to the creation of psychiatric nursing as a distinct occupation, only in exceptional circumstances had they been willing to work in the mental hospitals. In 1947, for example, there were only six RNs in the provincial psychiatric system. They tended to be ward supervisors, however, and thereby exercised significant control over the nature of ward work.

The DPH thus expected the SRNA to oppose the creation of a new on-ward occupation. In an effort to preempt this, the commissioner of mental services asked the SRNA for two hundred nurses to work in the mental hospitals.[91] This was impossible, since two hundred RNs were not available. One provincial psychiatrist stated in an interview with the author that: "My guess is [Dr. McKerracher] knew it was impossible"[92] but, having requested labour power which the SRNA could not provide, the basis of opposition from that quarter had been undermined.

The initial problem of finding sufficient recruits for the new training programme remained, and in 1947 the Health Education Division of the DPH mounted an extensive recruitment campaign. To make the training programme more attractive, student psychiatric nurses were employed on a sliding pay scale with income increasing with length of training. The DPH was thus able to recruit a relatively large number of psychiatric nursing students, both male and female.

The recruitment drive also convinced the general population that mental illnesses were no different than physical illnesses. This generated public support for the idea that mental illnesses should be treated in the community, rather than in large, remote mental hospitals. This goal was undoubtedly facilitated by the passage of the 1950 Mental Hygiene Act. Under this act, the power to admit persons to the mental hospitals "was confined to physicians, making mental illness a medical rather than a legal problem."[93] After many decades of struggle, insanity had finally become mental illness. It was again under the complete control of physicians, much as it had been in Britain following the passage of the 1845 Insanity Act. Medical control of admissions, however, did not mean mental hospital work was completely medicalized. The hospitals remained custodial institutions due to the inability of psychiatric treatment to control symptomatic behaviour adequately. The complete medicalization of mental hospital work awaited the revolution of the forces of psychiatric production which resulted from the introduction of a new treatment technology in the form of the psychotropic drugs.

Although the 1950 legislation recognized medical control of mental illness, popular support was still insufficient to allow for the treatment of the mentally ill in the community, although significant advances had been made in that regard through the activities of the recruitment and education drives begun in 1947. Evidence of this is to be found in the comments of the commissioner of mental services, who stated:

> Not only was the recruiting drive a success. The educational results of the program are quite evident. Saskatchewan is on the way to a new day for mental health in many ways and the mounting interest and understanding of the people may be expected to bring us as much support for this work as tuberculosis eradication has had in the past two decades.[94]

This optimism may have been partly wishful thinking and partly judicious propagandizing, but it also genuinely expressed how those involved in the creation of the brave new world of psychiatry felt at the time. In a 1947 letter to the premier's office, the union executive at SHNB was enthusiastic about the creation of the occupation of psychiatric nursing: "We are . . . of the opinion that Psychiatric Nursing is now on the threshold of being universally recognized as the great new science of the age."[95]

It appeared the DPH and the psychiatric nurses were working in complete harmony towards the transformation of the in-hospital psychiatric labour process. The union executive and high-level government administrators even agreed that the job security of the newly created psychiatric nurses should be legislatively protected. In a letter to the premier's office this concern is clearly expressed:

> The Union Executive which is sponsoring this move [i.e., establishment of a Psychiatric Nurses' Association] desire to keep such an association free from any attempt at control by the Medical Association. We feel that such control though it is indirect in its nature, is the big drawback of the Registered Nurses Association . . . and that unless the Psychiatric Nurses themselves organize their own association and maintain strict control of it, they may well realize when it is too late, that the Canadian Medical Association has already taken the step and set up such an organization for them.[96]

The premier's office and the DPH both supported the union executive on this issue (it should be noted that until 1949 Premier Douglas was also minister of public health). The necessary legislation was drafted by an advisor from the premier's office, who also told the union executive how to have the proposed legislation introduced and passed by the legislature. Although the psychiatric nurses and the union were concerned that the proposed association be free of medical influence, it was McKerracher who initially cleared the way for the creation of the occupation of psychiatric nursing by making the impossible request for two hundred RNs to work in the mental hospitals. It would be naïve to suppose the DPH, or the premier's office, would not consult McKerracher when drafting and implementing legislation to create a new occupation for which he would be responsible. There is some indication, in fact, that the commissioner of mental services initiated the move to pass the 1948 Psychiatric Nurses' Act. Dr. Coburn stated that it was McKerracher who "got the legislature to establish in Saskatchewan a profession of registered psychiatric nurses on a very similar basis as registered nurses."[97]

Whether or not this was initiated by McKerracher remains unclear, but he certainly was consulted. The premier's office sent him copies of the draft legislation in February 1948, requesting that he examine the proposed bill and inform the premier's office of any suggestions for improving its provisions.[98]

The worst fears of the union executive had apparently been realized; the medical profession, primarily through the actions of McKerracher and a legal advisor from the premier's office, had created the occupation of psychiatric nursing, first by establishing a training programme, then by incorporating psychiatric nursing into a Psychiatric Nurses' Association, and finally by drafting the legislation that specified the duties and powers of the new occupation.[99]

The psychiatric nurse was clearly subordinate to medically trained DPH psychiatrists. However, without the intervention of McKerracher and other government administrators committed to the transformation of the psychiatric labour process, it is unlikely that psychiatric nursing would have existed at all. Over the years the continued security of psychiatric nursing was to be dependent upon the support of PSB management and other government-employed psychiatrists.

The creation of psychiatric nursing and the Saskatchewan Psychiatric Nurses' Association (SPNA), although marked by a degree of management-union cooperation, did not occur without conflict. The conflict between union and management centred on two interrelated issues: the in-hospital workers' fight for job security, and the struggle to protect seniority rights.

*Job Security— The "Grandfather" Clause*

The CCF announcement of the plan to transform mental hospitals from custodial institutions to active treatment centres resulted in many of the old ward workers feeling, justifiably, that their positions were in jeopardy. In 1946, for example, the premier's office, in collaboration with the PSC, established a list of hospital employees priorized "in the order in which they should be replaced."[100] The PSC was then charged with the task of creating a new job classification scheme which would

> Weed out, progressively, married women (particularly those whose husbands are on staff), persons with lower than grade 11 education, persons of forty and over, persons who have taken no qualification classes and persons who (having had time so to do) have passed no examinations.[101]

Union membership was largely comprised of those very categories of hospital workers. Therefore the union opposed, with some success, the attempts to replace "untrained" ward workers with newly trained psychiatric nurses, generally by insisting that seniority be the primary consideration in all nondisciplinary dismissals and promotions, and more specifically by insisting on the inclusion of clause seven in the 1948 Psychiatric Nurses' Act. Clause seven, which became known as the "Grandfather" clause, stated in part that

> All persons of good moral character resident in Saskatchewan who on the first day of January, 1948, were graduate psychiatric nurses at a Saskatchewan Hospital or Saskatchewan Training School established under the Mental Hygiene Act shall be admitted to the register of psychiatric nurses.[102]

The major consequence of including this clause was "that anybody who was working at North Battleford, the Training School in Weyburn (before they moved it to Moose Jaw), and the 'Big Bin' at Weyburn automatically got RPN [Registered Psychiatric Nurse] status."[103]

The DPH vigorously opposed the inclusion of this clause for it would obviously hinder the plans to transform the nature of on-ward work. The union was firm, however, and eventually prevailed. The DPH thought it would be better to accede to the union on this point in order to get the legislation passed quickly, rather than delay too long and give the SRNA enough time to come up with the two hundred nurses originally requested by McKerracher.

The government also thought it would be easier to control the new SPNA than confront the large, well-organized SRNA. The union was therefore able to have the "Grandfather" clause entrenched in the Psychiatric Nurses' Act. Although the government was not happy with this arrangement, it was thought the goal of transforming the in-hospital psychiatric labour process could be achieved by management control of promotions and transfers, especially in respect to supervisory positions. This proved to be more difficult than anticipated.

### *Seniority Rights and Promotions*

The problem from the point of view of some of the in-hospital management was the union *per se*. The strategy for dealing with this "problem" was to try to avoid the union altogether by ignoring the terms of the collective agreement. Obviously this could not be effective, and only heightened union-management conflicts. In a memo to the acting deputy minister of public health in 1949, Premier Douglas commented on the escalation of management-worker conflict:

> [The civil service commissioner] has discussed with me several instances in which [the medical superintendent, SHNB] is violating the Union Agreement which is not making for the most harmonious relations. It seems unfortunate, particularly in view of the fact that in these particular cases there was no need for disregarding the agreement.[104]

This form of antiunionism in government-operated institutions could not be tolerated by the CCF, which was purportedly the party of the working class.

Although certain in-hospital management personnel saw the union as the problem, others thought the problem lay elsewhere. Thus it was often maintained that the old Liberal appointees within the mental hospitals were using the union to protect themselves and thwart government policy. Referring to the situation at SHW, a CCF advisor stated:

> The situation here is serious. In fact, I would pronounce it rotten. We should have cleaned house ere we brought into being these unions. This is not hindsight. I maintained this much before the unions were sanctioned by the government. We had no friends among the old employees at the mental institutions, that is, among the old Liberal appointees.[105]

In a very real sense the union was a powerful tool used by mental hospital workers, in both the political arena and the workplace, to pursue workers' goals and objectives. It has already been seen that the union was successful in securing increased wages, shorter hours, better working conditions and a range of other "economic" objectives. It was also used to pursue vigorously the goal of job security, and won a major victory in this regard with the inclusion of clause seven in the Psychiatric Nurses' Act. It also attempted to secure control of hiring, firing and promotions. This, however, was an issue on which all levels of management united, and management solidarity eventually forced control of these issues off the union's agenda. The following memo illustrates the frustration felt by in-hospital management over not being able to control unilaterally the promotion process:

> There is an important common factor in all promotions covered by the Union Agreement — which means the great majority of the promotions in the mental institutions. It is that seniority determines the promotion, and management has no choice unless the senior employee is extremely incompetent. Except in these very unusual cases, experience over the years has shown that the Union will grieve in every case in which the senior person is not appointed, and management has almost no chance of winning this kind of grievance before an Arbitration board.[106]

This struggle for control was complicated by the existence of an "internal labour market." As a result, PSB employees had the right of first refusal on any positions in PSB-operated facilities. Doeringer and Piore suggest the existence of an internal labour market is viewed as a "problem" by management due to the inefficiencies it produces.[107] They fail to explore adequately the possibility that management may actively encourage the creation of internal labour markets to achieve certain of its objectives. On the other hand, Edwards does develop this theme.[108] He argues that management creates internal labour markets in an attempt to secure greater worker commitment to organizational goals. This is achieved through the creation of firm-specific careers which heighten employee dependence on employers. Edwards, however, fails to address the role, and interest, of workers in the creation of internal labour markets. For Edwards, internal labour markets are principally the result of management attempts to increase control and exploitation of employees. In the case of PSB, the establishment of an internal labour market was generally supported by both management and the union. Management was interested in creating a stable labour force in order to facilitate the transformation of mental hospital work. The union was interested in protecting job security. Conflict developed over the operation of the internal labour market, not its existence.

The internal labour market was desirable to PSB management because it lowered attrition rates, and thereby increased the stability of the on-ward psychiatric work force. The conditions surrounding the transformation of the mental hospital labour process and the creation of a suitable, stable work force, however, also resulted in a degree of management dependence because an external labour market for psychiatric nurses was non-existent.

Psychiatric nursing was specific to the mental hospitals, and only existed due to the on-the-job training programme developed and financed by the DPH. Therefore the DPH did not want to expend resources producing psychiatric nurses if they were not going to remain with PSB. Also, due to the lack of technology, psychiatric nursing work was labour-intensive. As Doeringer and Piore point out, the convergence of the above-mentioned factors — significant investment in an enterprise-specific form of labour power that entails on-the-job training for a labour-intensive work process — is often correlated with the existence of internal labour markets. Such conditions produce a degree of employer dependence on a stable and cooperative work force, and conversely, increased worker strength. In the case of Saskatchewan, especially for government employees between 1944 and 1964, this position of strength was amplified by the pro-labour legislation enacted by the CCF.

The union used this power to pursue its objectives. One consequence was support for an internal labour market. Whereas the union tried to ensure all promotions and transfers were made on the basis of seniority, the government argued that "merit and ability" were important criteria to be considered. Referring to this source of conflict, the premier stated to the minister of public health that "it has always been my understanding that seniority takes precedence provided all other things are equal and that the matter of determining merit and ability lies solely with the Government."[109]

The in-hospital management employed a number of tactics in an attempt to ensure that "all other things" were not equal. Two of the most important were refusal to promote "senior" employees to out-of-scope positions, and the use of "junior" employees in temporary substitutions. This second tactic provided the newly trained psychiatric nurses with experience denied to senior employees, thus "enabling the juniors to go around the seniors when a vacancy occurred."[110] Although management saw this as a way to speed the transformation of the mental hospital labour process, the union perceived it as a threat to job security and seniority rights.

In 1958 it was reported that twenty-five grievances per year were lodged against SHNB management alone, and that this had been going on for several years.[111] The antagonistic management-union relations which resulted also created a volatile political situation. Understandably, the sitting CCF MLA for the Battlefords was uneasy. He had no doubt, however, where the blame should be placed. In a letter to the premier he made this clear:

> I do not blame [the minister of public health] for the situation that exists. My complaint is his refusal to take any action since it has been brought to his attention. I believe that [the director of PSB] is well aware of the unhappy situation — I would go further and say he is a party to it and for reasons best known to himself, is quite content to see the morale of the institution going downhill. My humble opinion is that we must have people in responsible positions working in the best interests of the patients, the staff and the department and not carrying on personal vendettas which are bound to result in a deterioration of the whole structure.[112]

The premier and the minister of public health agreed with this evaluation of the cause of labour-management conflict at SHNB. In fact, they had previously attempted to replace the director of PSB for similar reasons. A number of factors converged to protect his position, the most important of which was the impossibility of finding a fully qualified psychiatrist with demonstrated administrative talents as a replacement. Others in management positions who were thought to be contributing to antagonistic relations were not so well protected.

### The Replacement of In-hospital Management — The End

In 1946 the government and the union local at SHNB joined forces to oust the previous hospital management. The government then needed personnel to fill the vacant positions. Unfortunately for the government, the candidate of first choice for the position of business manager did not accept the job. Consequently, one of the royal commission members was offered, and accepted, the job. This appeared to all, including the newly appointed business manager, to be a patronage appointment. Partly as a result of this, he seems to have misunderstood the nature of administrative power relations, and consequently exhibited some recalcitrance concerning the implementation of government policy. As early as 1949 the premier commented on this to the minister of public health:

> I think it is probably time that someone had a very frank talk with [the business manager, SHNB], pointing out that he must either become part of the government team or look for employment where his desire for untrammelled individualism can find wider scope.[113]

The business manager apparently was able to conform satisfactorily at that time, although the relations between different levels of in-hospital management remained problematic throughout the 1950s. A report to the minister of public health, written about 1958, stated:

> The Psychiatric Services Branch, in its efforts to improve services and produce long term economies, has been handicapped throughout the whole period by Business Managers who have lacked the necessary qualities to keep up with progress.[114]

It was suggested that the business managers at both hospitals failed to contribute to the achievement of the general objectives of PSB

> Primarily because they have been unable to grasp the purposes and goals, the raison d'etre, of the hospitals, and being unable to comprehend why different therapeutic approaches to patients are efficacious, they have

> become cynical and dis-associated themselves from the main function of the hospitals.[115]

As has been seen, the main function of the hospitals in the postwar period was the cure and/or discharge of mental patients. The position of business manager, however, had developed within the context of the mental hospitals being long-term custodial institutions run as much as possible as commercial enterprises and characterized by the extensive use of unpaid patient labour. The principal function of the business managers had been to reduce the costs of operating the institutions, and therefore an interest had developed in *not* discharging patients capable of working. The postwar discharge policy undermined the business managers' traditional method of cost reduction — the use of unpaid patient labour — and was passively resisted. To those committed to the new regime, the unenthusiastic response of the business managers appeared as obstructionism and therefore a problem requiring solution.

Several possible solutions were considered, including dismissal. The government did not feel, however, that they had sufficient grounds to justify firing the business managers. Reporting the discussions of a May 1959 meeting, the deputy minister of public health told the minister:

> It was the feeling of the meeting that it would be difficult to present a set of reasons for dismissal which would in the first instance reflect discredit on the employee. It is my opinion that the present incumbent has not committed any overt act which would justify dismissal in itself. His main fault is not that he failed to implement any regulations or orders but rather that he has been much too inflexible in the way in which he has implemented them. The chief complaints about him that have come to my attention are that he has "gone by the book" to the ultimate degree.[116]

It was finally decided that the best solution would be to create a new position in the hospitals which would be superior to that of business manager. The incumbents would be retained, but as deputies of the new appointees. This would allow the government to examine the business managers' new positions "from year to year and if the scope of their work diminished they could be downgraded to Administrative Officers III or II."[117] This would effectively remove them from power, without generating the conflict which would have surrounded outright dismissal.

It is quite clear no unity existed between the various levels of management. Differences existed not only on managerial tactics, but also on strategy. Much literature on the labour process posits management as a unified monolith endowed with prescience regarding the most economic and efficient way to organize a given labour process. This is especially true of the Marxist literature, which tends to subsume the complex and variegated strata and practices that constitute management within the concepts of capital or the capitalist class. Although E.O. Wright and others have begun to address this inadequacy through the concept of contradictory class positions and the implications of this for class politics and revolutionary practice, there is still a hiatus in the Marxist study of management.[118]

Part of the difficulty is the fact that it is often assumed that management commitment to economy and efficiency is synonymous with knowledge and consensus concerning how to achieve those objectives. It is my contention that no such prescience or consensus exists, and that management strategies are themselves the product of ongoing struggles, the end result of which may or may not be the most efficient and economic form of work organization.

Within the employment-relation, management is structurally committed to establishing and maintaining control of the work process in order to increase worker productivity and decrease the costs of production. These managerial imperatives are operative both in the private profit-making sector, and in the public, noncommodity-making sector. These managerial imperatives are not, however, pursued in a vacuum. The pursuit of profit in the private sector, and the pursuit of economy and efficiency in the public sector, occur within an historically specific social, political and cultural context. I have attempted to show that these noneconomic considerations have exerted, and continue to exert, a significant influence on the specific strategies and tactics employed. Thus, partisan political considerations have been shown to influence not only the nature of management-worker relations, and the way in which various conflicts were resolved, but also how and by whom psychiatric services would be produced.

The most significant development with regard to this point was the creation of the occupation of psychiatric nursing. This was achieved, in part, by the creation of a five-hundred-hour, three-year training programme in 1946-47. The training programme, according to the commissioner of mental services, was "about five times as intensive"[119] as the pre-1947 programme.

The creation of what amounted to a new psychiatric division of labour, working within a new psychiatric labour process, proved to be an expensive undertaking (see Figure 9). This increase in the cost of producing psychiatric services, combined with the intensified training programme for psychiatric nurses, inclines one to conclude that the creation of psychiatric nursing was not an instance of the application of the Babbage Principle to psychiatric work. That is, it does not seem to correspond to the substitution of less expensive and less skilled labour for more expensive and more skilled labour (see Appendix for a discussion of the theoretical framework).

The stated objective of the programme, however, was "to create a highly trained professional staff of ward personnel, to whom could be delegated the therapeutic procedures which were formerly considered solely within the realm of the psychiatrist."[120] This statement of management intentions is interesting inasmuch as it seems to provide unambiguous evidence to support the deskilling hypothesis. Given the examination of the pre-World War II mental hospital labour process presented in the preceding chapter, however, this conclusion does not seem to be warranted. All the evidence indicates that prewar psychiatric work in the provincial mental hospitals was primarily, although not exclusively, custodial in nature. Therapy largely consisted of "work and water."

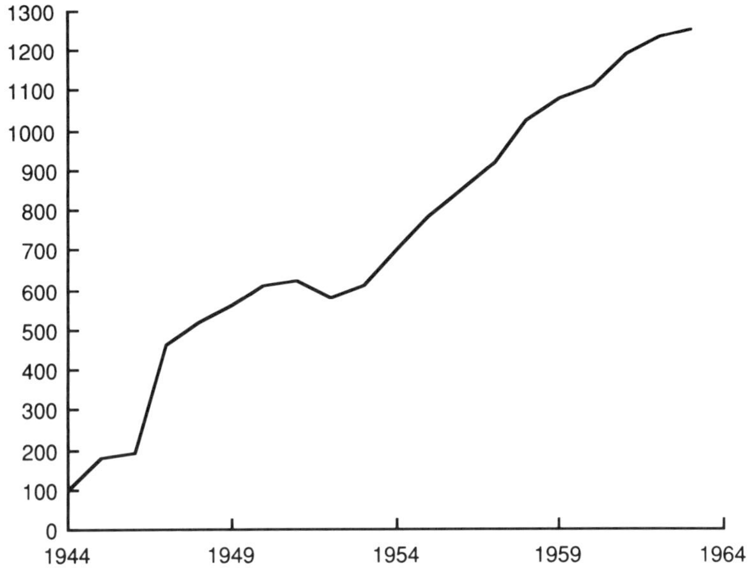


*Figure 9*
*Changes in PSB Budget controlled for Inflation*
*From 1944 to 1963*
*(Base 1944 Equals 100)*

*Source: Saskatchewan Department of Public Health Annual Reports; and Saskatchewan Public Accounts Annual Report. Indexing to inflation from Statistics Canada, Consumer Price Index.*

The work aspect of the therapy consisted, in most cases, of hard physical labour required for the operation and maintenance of the institutions themselves. Even as late as 1955 a cabinet brief from the Weyburn branch of the SPNA stated that a

> major problem which exists at Weyburn is the process whereby the hospital depends, for many of its vital functions, on unpaid patient labour. The laundry, power-house, farm, sewing-room, kitchen, bakery, upholstery shop, and many other vital departments in the hospital depend on that sort of help. While short-term and planned employment in some of these departments may be of therapeutic value, by no stretch of the imagination can we fool ourselves by saying that standing at the mangle in the laundry folding sheets day

> in and day out for weeks and months and years, is a task of therapeutic value.[121]

The brief articulated the central contradictions and pathogenic aspects of this kind of work therapy:

> 1) These tasks are frequently degrading and harmful to our patients, and result in despair and unhappiness that leads to chronic residence in hospital.
> 2) Patients become so vital to the hospital organization that a very strong vested interest develops against their discharge.
> 3) Such practice is contrary to the code of ethics of the Psychiatric Nursing profession. That patients under our care be exploited to ease the burden of the Hospital staff is a very immoral and wicked practice. Certainly in no other type of hospital must the nurses depend upon the patients to ensure a clean supply of linen for beds, nor that the fires be kept going to provide warmth.[122]

These observations are interesting given the growth of a body of literature which addresses the relationship between employment and mental illness.[123] It is also interesting in terms of Goffman's analysis of the effects of asylum life on inmates. Unremunerated work, as a factor contributing to chronic institutionalization, was one aspect of life within a total institution which he did not examine in depth.[124]

At any rate, it is plain that work therapy in the mental hospitals was certainly not solely in the realm of the psychiatrist. In fact, most work therapy was under the direction and control of virtually untrained gangmen, "*some of whom, after 1947, were psychiatric nurses.*"[125] [emphasis added]

Water therapy largely entailed putting people in baths and wet packs in an attempt to calm them when they became agitated. This form of therapy was phased out in the mid-1950s with the introduction of the psychotropic drugs. Describing this form of treatment, a long-time psychiatric nurse in the province stated:

> They used to strap a patient in a canvas bag in a large bathtub and they had water running in at one end at very high velocity going over the patient's body and out

> the other end. First you put on hot and then you put on the cold. So it was terrible. It was a very medieval form of shock therapy, called pro-baths.[126]

Regarding other forms of treatment, I was told that in the mid-1950s

> All the seclusion rooms were still in use. In 8A there were about fourteen cells down there . . . the administration didn't like it when you called them cells, but I don't know what the hell you would call them. They were fed like dogs, they were taken out and washed down with a hose and their feces and stuff was washed down a hole in the middle of the floor. Talk about treating people like animals — it was incredible.[127]

There were a few medical treatments employed, such as camphor metrozal and insulin shock therapies beginning in the late 1930s, as well as electroshock treatments and lobotomies somewhat later. However, psychiatric nurses were not employed in these therapies. It must, therefore, be concluded that the employment of psychiatric nurses did not represent the deskilling of mental hospital work. The occupation of psychiatric nursing was created to perform new therapeutic tasks within a new psychiatric labour process. Although it was generally agreed that psychiatric nurses were employed to increase the rate of discharge, there was a degree of ambiguity regarding how this was to be achieved since no one was quite sure what psychiatric nurses actually did. After 1958, this ambiguity led to insecurity among psychiatric nurses as it was becoming evident that the provision of psychiatric services was moving out of the traditional mental hospitals and into psychiatric wards of general hospitals and mental health clinics.

The insecurity of the RPNs in the face of these changes was epitomized in the debates within the SPNA. In 1961, at the SPNA annual convention, the problem of defining the occupation was addressed. The papers and presentations took on a somewhat defensive tone. For example, one paper began: "More and more people, including Doctors, Psychiatrists, Psychologists, Teachers, yes even Psychiatric Nurses, are asking the embarrassing question: What is a psychiatric nurse?"[128]

In an attempt to answer this, it was suggested that attention be given to what psychiatric nurses were doing. It was proposed that psychiatric nurses' work should be the object of time-and-motion studies. The psychiatric nurses rejected this suggestion:

> The fallacy of this method [of defining psychiatric nursing] is rather obvious. In the first place, what a nurse is doing is not necessarily an indication of what a nurse ought to be doing. Furthermore, this method, by emphasizing the technical overt aspects, does not take into consideration the real [*sic*] important aspect of Psychiatric Nursing: what happens within and between the patient and the nurse WHILE THESE TECHNICAL ROLES ARE BEING CARRIED OUT and carefully timed and charted.[129] [emphasis in original]

It was suggested that the primary function and skill of the psychiatric nurse was "establishing therapeutic relations and satisfying interactions."[130] It was also suggested "the means available to the nurse" for performing that function

> are almost unlimited. Perhaps it is alright for an aide or orderly to do the bedbathing, to give the enema, spoon-feed the patient, or comb his hair in a general hospital. In Psychiatric Nursing it is precisely this bedbath, this enema, this feeding and dressing that becomes the means to establish relationships and provide opportunities. Through these means the nurse can establish therapeutic relationships which may become the important stimulus that will remotivate the patient.[131]

It is interesting to note the juxtaposition of psychological and medical terminology in this occupational self-definition: psychiatric nursing was seen as the establishment of therapeutic relationships through which *patients* were *remotivated.* The uncertainty as to whether psychiatric nursing work was principally medical or psychological in nature reflects the continuing ambiguity about the etiology of mental disorders. This medical-psychological dualism has underpinned much of the historical development of both psychiatric theory and the organization of psychiatric work.

It is also interesting to note that the psychiatric nurses were not only anxious about the transition to community psychiatry, they were also anxious about the prospects of being replaced by psychiatric aides and orderlies. That is, they were concerned about being deskilled within their own domain.

In an attempt to forestall any development in that direction, the SPNA put forward an ideology which emphasized the "indeterminacy," rather than the "technicality," of their occupational practice. It was argued that the nature of psychiatric nursing could not be quantified because the essential element was a characteristic of *the practitioner* and not the *practices*. This is a commonly used ideological technique employed by occupations in an attempt to protect occupational existence and legitimate claims to professional status.[132] Within the context of PSB-managed mental hospitals this fear of deskilling was ungrounded, however, at least at that time. Since the mid-1940s PSB management had consistently advocated the complete staffing of mental hospitals by RPNs. In fact, it was management policy that nurses' aides were to "constitute no more than 10 percent of the 'nursing' force."[133] Thus, in 1960, psychiatric nurses constituted about 90 percent of the mental hospital on-ward workers. This was a reversal of the situation that had existed in 1950 (see Table 5).

It appears that within the mental hospitals the dominant trend throughout the 1940s and 1950s was to replace less-skilled with more-skilled workers. Referring to the Psychiatric Nursing Training Program one DPH report stated:

> It was the first of its kind to be developed in North America and remains the most intensive. It has made it possible to do away almost completely with the attendant and aide groups who, relatively untrained and with poor educational backgrounds, make up much of the staff of mental hospitals which do not train their own psychiatric nurses.[134]

**Table 5**
**Proportion of Psychiatric Nurses, Psychiatric Aides and Registered Nurses at SHW and SHNB in 1950**

| Occuptional Category | SHW Number | SHW Proportion | SHNB Number | SHNB Proportion | Total Number | Total Proportion |
|---|---|---|---|---|---|---|
| Psychiatric Nurses | 36 | 10.87 | 60 | 18.2 | 96 | 16.98 |
| Psychiatric Aides | 294 | 88.00 | 268 | 81.5 | 566 | 82.33 |
| Registered Nurses | 4 | 1.2 | 0 | 0 | 4 | .007 |
| Total Nursing Staff* | 334 | 99.9 | 329 | 99.7 | | |

*Includes the position of Superintendant of Nursing which accounted for one position at each hospital.

*Source:* Derived from Table I "Personnel Quota for the Mental Hospitals of Saskatchewan." *Report on the Provincial Mental Hospitals of Saskatchewan.* Central Inspection Board, American Psychiatric Association, September 1950.

This provides further confirmation that the creation of the occupation of psychiatric nursing, and its employment within the in-hospital psychiatric division of labour, does not constitute an instance of the deskilling of the mental hospital labour process. Obviously, the psychiatric labour process had not been mechanized or automated, and so psychiatric nurses cannot be understood as "machine tenders," as described by Braverman. In addition, the creation of the occupation of psychiatric nursing does not seem to be the result of the application of the Babbage Principle to in-hospital psychiatric work. If anything, it was the opposite of the Babbage Principle — the replacement of less-skilled and inexpensive labour power with more-skilled and expensive labour.

The creation of the occupation of psychiatric nursing, although not best understood as a manifestation of the deskilling of psychiatric work, was certainly important for the development of community psychiatry in Saskatchewan. This is not to say, however, that psychiatric nurses were employed directly in the provision of community-based services. PSB management and psychiatric nurses both perceived the occupation as part of the in-hospital work force, at least initially. Psychiatric nursing contributed to the development of community psychiatry by contributing to an increased rate of discharge of mental patients into the community (see Figure 10) which in turn contributed to the reduction of the in-hospital population levels (see Figure 11).

The sharp drop in the number of patients on register in 1946 represents the transfer of one thousand mentally retarded persons out of SHW in accordance with the recommendations of Sigerist and Hincks. Although the reduction of inpatient numbers had been government policy since 1946, the hospital populations remained relatively constant until 1954, and thereafter steadily declined. Two factors converged at that time to bring about this change. One was the effect of replacing untrained ward attendants with psychiatric nurses whose principal task was to increase the rate of discharge. The radical change in the social relations of psychiatric production, of which the creation of the occupation of psychiatric nursing was a concrete manifestation, was given form and content by a number of interconnected practices and struggles which were examined in this chapter. The second factor which influenced the transformation of the in-hospital psychiatric labour process, and thereby contributed to the reduction in patient numbers, can best be understood as a revolution in the forces of psychiatric production. This was in the form of the introduction of the psychotropic drugs into the in-hospital psychiatric labour process. The introduction of this new technology provided the material base from which the medicalization of mental hospital work was finally completed. It must be added that this is not to be interpreted as support for a form of technological determinism.

The introduction of psychotropic drugs was not a fundamental cause of the depopulation of the mental hospitals, for clearly the political and economic decision to pursue that objective must be considered the fundamental cause, the drug technology can properly be considered as a proximate cause, because of the capacity of the various drugs to produce symptom-free behaviour and maleable patients. It is the ability of these drugs to produce manageable patients

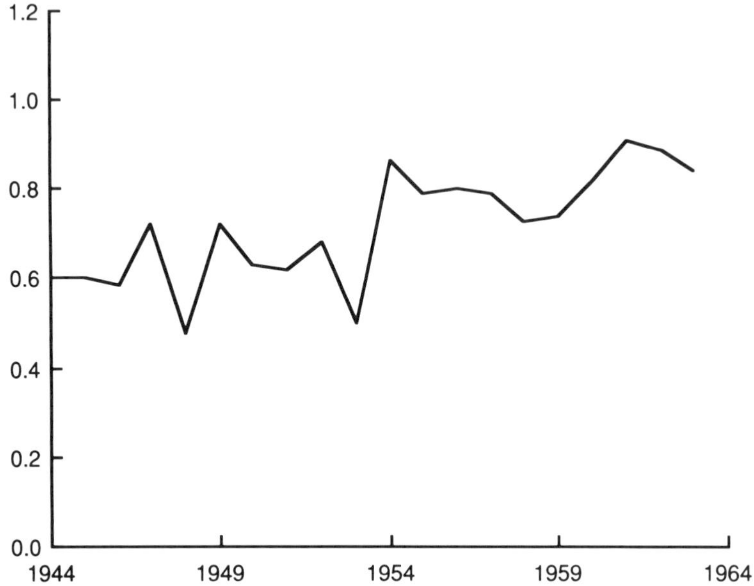


*Figure 10*
*Total Paroles plus Discharges as Proportion of Total Admissions by Year From 1944 to 1963*
*Source: Saskatchewan Department of Public Health Annual Reports*

that encouraged the shift in the locus of treatment (production) from the mental hospitals to a range of community-based alternatives, including the general hospitals. This is important, since much of the sociological literature, after having correctly concluded that the introduction of the psychotropic drugs cannot be considered as the cause of depopulation, then incorrectly presumes that it had no effect at all, or perhaps only symbolic effects. Scull, for example, states that the psychotropic drugs merely allowed physicians and psychiatrists employed in the mental hospitals "to engage in a more passable imitation of conventional medical practice" in the form of the "prescription and administration of the classic symbolic accoutrement of the modern medicine man — drugs."[135]

This somewhat facile dismissal of what must properly be considered a revolution in the forces of psychiatric production, and its concomitant transformation of both the social

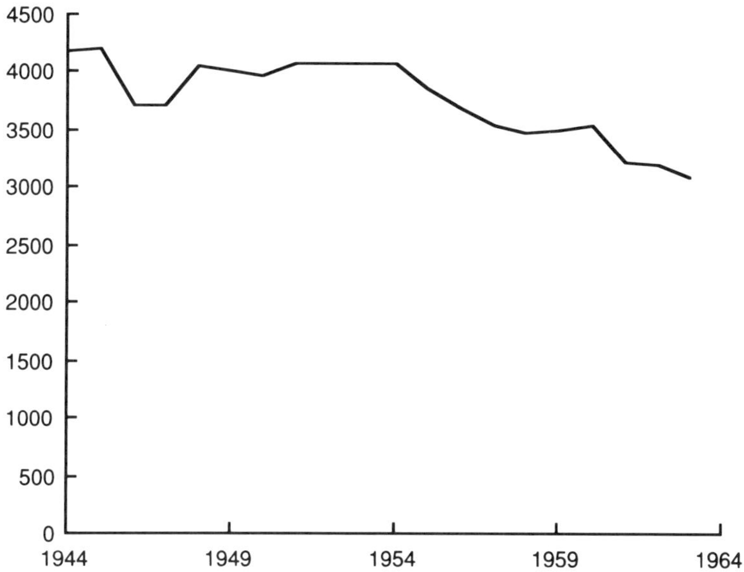


*Figure 11*
*Patients on Register by Year From 1944 to 1963*
*Source: Saskatchewan Department of Public Health Annual Reports*

relations and other forces of production, appears to be at least partially the consequence of the assumption that the medicalization of mental hospital work had been achieved by the turn of the century. Conrad and Schneider express this conception quite clearly: "In terms of the history of the medical conception of madness, the 19th century was a significant period. In the United States, as in England, madness moved once and for all into medical turf."[136] As has been seen, this was simply not true, either in Canada, the United States or England.[137] The NCMH was, in fact, originally established in the United States in 1914 to lobby for legislative changes which would ensure, among other things, that the mental hospitals would be transformed from legalized custodial institutions to medicalized treatment hospitals. Throughout most of the first half of this century the definition of insanity and the power to order incarceration in a mental hospital was either a legal prerogative, or a power shared between the legal and medical professions.

It is true that medically trained physicians dominated the mental hospital division of labour, but this was largely due to the fact that, without exception, medically trained personnel occupied the principal managerial positions within the hospitals, and not because of the medical nature of the work performed. The conflation of medical monopoly of managerial positions with the medicalization of mental hospital work is all the more surprising given that Scull and others recognize that during the eighteenth and nineteenth centuries, when medical domination of asylum management was also common, asylum work was not medical in nature. As Conrad and Schneider state with regard to that earlier time period,

> Although the mad were institutionalized, certified by physicians, and more and more were considered to be sick, there is little evidence to suggest that anything resembling *medical* treatment was carried out.[138] [emphasis in original]

The assumption that the medical domination of the mental hospital division of labour is synonymous with the performance of medical work within those facilities is not only analytically suspect, it is also empirically inaccurate. As has been seen, mental hospital work was basically performed by unskilled attendants and nurse attendants and directed toward the supervision and control of patients' behaviour.

It is only with the introduction of the psychotropic drugs that "water and work" therapies gave way to chemotherapy as the principal form of treatment. As Scull notes, "a dramatic inverse relationship quickly became established between the use of psychotropic drugs and the use of more conventional forms of constraint."[139]

As a consequence of the medical monopoly of drug prescription,[140] chemotherapy can be seen to correspond to the medicalization of mental hospital work. It is therefore the medical monopoly of this pharmaceutical technology that transformed the medical domination of the mental hospital division of labour into the medicalization of the mental hospital labour process. This process did not occur either in North America or the United Kingdom until the mid-1950s.

This revolution in pharmaceutical technology had significant consequences for other nonsocial aspects of the forces of psychiatric production. As well as being the basis for the medicalization of mental hospital work, it rendered the asylum itself, considered as an element of the nonsocial forces of production, technologically obsolete. As Scull, Rothman and others have shown, the asylum was originally developed as a technology for controlling those whose behaviour was disruptive of the functioning of other institutions, such as workhouses, gaols or hospitals. This segregation of the insane has been linked to the development of the capitalist mode of production (CMP), and the need to produce a disciplined labour force. Thus, Conrad and Schneider state:

> As the importance of a competent labour force increased, it became increasingly necessary to separate the able-bodied poor from the nonable-bodied. After all how could discipline and good work habits be instilled if lunatics were around disrupting the order of the institutions?[141]

Thus the asylum/mental hospital must be considered as more than simply a set of buildings, or a locus of treatment. It is, in fact, a significant aspect of the forces of psychiatric production, and must be considered as part of the technology of psychiatric production in the same way that the factory must be considered as part of the forces of industrial production.[142] Conceptualized thus, the asylum/mental hospital can be seen to be one of the principal technologies used in the process of producing manageable mental patients. The original proponents and supporters of the asylum system claimed confinement in a properly situated asylum would itself effect a cure for insanity.[143] The only caveat to this claim was that treatment had to take place as soon as possible after the illness was first noticed. The claim that treatment must be prompt in order to effect a cure was used by the medical superintendents of mental hospitals, and their ideological and political allies, to justify their struggle against legal/judicial involvement in the commitment process.

The psychotropic drugs made it possible to manage patients, even when they remained highly psychotic, in other settings. As Clark points out, "it is well know that patients can remain grossly psychotic and yet become passively co-operative, less overactive and destructive, or more docile."[144] He states that these are factors which may be "more important to the custodian than the patient."[145]

There seem to be two senses in which this is true. First, docile, passive patients are much easier to manage and therefore the use of drugs helps to increase the efficiency of the mental hospital labour process. In a sense, the psychotropic drugs can be considered as a labour-saving technology. To the extent that this is true one would expect the ataractic drugs would also form the base for the *potential* deskilling of psychiatric work. This, however, has not generally happened because of the continued medical monopoly of drug prescription. This monopoly formed the social basis for the medicalization of mental hospital work. This is the second sense in which chemotherapies were more important to the custodian than the patient. The medical control of drug prescription necessitated the active involvement of the physician in the psychiatric treatment process. Thus the medical dominance of the mental hospital division of labour was enhanced. Paradoxically, the efficacy of the physician-controlled chemotherapies in producing manageable patients greatly increased the rate of discharge from the mental hospitals, rendering them technologically obsolete. This also speeded the development of various community-based alternatives, a process which has resulted in a decline in the significance of the mental hospital, and the mental hospital labour process, in the overall production of psychiatric services. This has had profound consequences on the mental hospital division of labour, the most notable aspect of which is a marked decrease in the power of the mental hospital psychiatrist. The struggles surrounding this, and other aspects of the development of community psychiatry between 1944 and 1963, are examined in the following chapter.

# Chapter Four

# Psychiatry in the Community and the Saskatchewan Plan, 1944-1963

Sigerist and Hincks had both suggested that the development of community psychiatry in Saskatchewan required the establishment of a boarding-out system, the creation of mental hygiene clinics and the extension of psychiatric wards in general hospitals. On Hincks's advice, the DPH instigated a series of "education" programmes in an attempt to lay the groundwork for the creation of a comprehensive boarding-out plan. The intent was to prepare people for an increase in paroles and discharges, and to generate support for the plan. Public opinion was negative, however, and the education programmes appeared to have little effect in changing attitudes or lessening opposition. As a result, the plans for a comprehensive system of community placements proceeded slowly.

The proposed mental hygiene clinics were intended as the backbone of community psychiatry, for it was through them that the principles of prevention were to be implemented and hospital populations decreased. However, the clinics were opposed by private practice physicians who feared the competition, and psychiatric nurses who felt the clinics threatened their job security.

The creation of the mental hygiene clinics, combined with the extension of general hospital psychiatry, constituted part of the process of medicalizing psychiatric work. Although this had been a professed goal of PSB management-psychiatrists, they vehemently opposed the extension of general hospital psychiatry as the principal locus for psychiatric in-patient treatment. They preferred a plan for a regionalized system of small community mental hospitals, known as the Saskatchewan Plan. The most significant developments for community psychiatry in Saskatchewan emerged from the struggles surrounding the Saskatchewan Plan. The federal government's decision to exclude community mental hospitals from cost sharing under the 1957 Hospital Insurance and Diagnostic Services Act resulted in the transmutation of the Saskatchewan Plan and the rapid expansion of general hospital psychiatry, events which marked the complete medicalization of in-patient psychiatric work.

Hincks and the NCMH had been making recommendations for the medicalization of psychiatry since 1920 but lack of political will and public support had obstructed the realization of these changes. After 1944, lack of political will became less of an obstacle, for Premier Douglas and his government were committed to the transformation of psychiatric work. In 1951, for example, it was reported that every member of the provincial cabinet was a member of the Canadian Mental Health Association (CMHA), the successor to the NCMH.[1]

However, competition for limited revenues was intense, and legislators were acutely aware that there were few votes to be gained from expending large sums on the mentally ill. The CCF government, therefore, undertook an expensive propaganda campaign to generate public acceptance of the changes being made to the mental hospital labour process, and to convince voters that the development of programmes of community psychiatry was necessary.

The most well known of these educational crusades was conducted in 1951 by Elaine and John Cumming, and subsequently published under the title *Closed Ranks: An Experiment in Mental Health Education.*[2] This project, which was jointly funded by PSB and the Commonwealth Fund, an American philanthropic organization, was intended "to ascertain whether the community educational program would diminish people's feelings of distance and estrangement from former mental patients and would increase their feelings of social responsibility for the problem of mental illness."[3] This was considered a necessary step in laying the groundwork for a successful boarding-out programme. The reported findings, however, were not encouraging.

It was found that the mental health education programme had virtually no effect on the very low degree of community tolerance for the mentally ill. Furthermore, the educational programme itself produced a degree of hostility and anxiety in the community. One consequence of these findings was a significant delay in the planning and implementation of a comprehensive boarding-out programme. Instead, the DPH decided to scatter discharged and paroled patients throughout the province. This was an attempt to reduce their visibility and thereby reduce public opposition.[4]

Besides the Cummings' report, there was other evidence that fears of public outcry and political backlash were justified. By the mid-1950s, the mental hospitals had more or less accepted the theory of non-restraint, wherein the hospital was part of a therapeutic community.[5] As part of this approach, wards were unlocked and patients were granted unsupervised parole and day passes. The objective was to give them an opportunity to experience a broader range of social contacts which, by this time, was thought to be a necessary first step toward their integration into community life. The consequence of the policy, however, was the generation of fear and hostility, especially in and around the cities of Weyburn and North Battleford.

The situation reached crisis proportions in Weyburn in the mid-1950s. Just as the policy of unsupervised paroles was being implemented on a large scale, which was itself the cause of significant opposition, a man charged with the murder of a young girl in the province was found not guilty by reason of insanity. This did nothing to make the public more accepting of the new approach to psychiatric treatment, and contributed to a drastic cutback in parole and discharge rates (see Figure 12).

This public opposition to patients in the community was difficult to overcome because of the genuine fear and anxiety felt by many, and because of the partisan political struggles that developed around the operation of the mental hospitals. This second obstacle to the development of community psychiatry was to be the most difficult to surmount. The two issues were closely intertwined, with political opponents of the CCF using the fear and anxiety of the general public to their own advantage by creating what Cohen has described as "folk devils" and "moral panics."[6]

The director of PSB thought the first source of opposition to the development of community programmes, fear of the insane, was a product of the custodial nature of the mental hospitals. In a memo to the minister of public health he stated:

> the proximity of the custodial institution, where crazy people have been stored, has resulted in fear and abhorrence which has persisted in the cities of Weyburn and North Battleford, particularly the former. It is understandable that this attitude based on 30-40 years of experience with the mentally ill together with the astounding and perhaps exaggerated stories of their horrible and bizarre conduct should be difficult to change. We have always felt that the areas immediately adjacent to the large mental hospitals are among the most reactionary in the province and it has been difficult to get co-operation from them until recently in establishing an enlightened modern program for the mentally ill.[7]

It was felt that this fear and abhorrence, although a significant obstacle to the development of community psychiatry, could be resolved by the establishment of more effective public relations and education programmes.

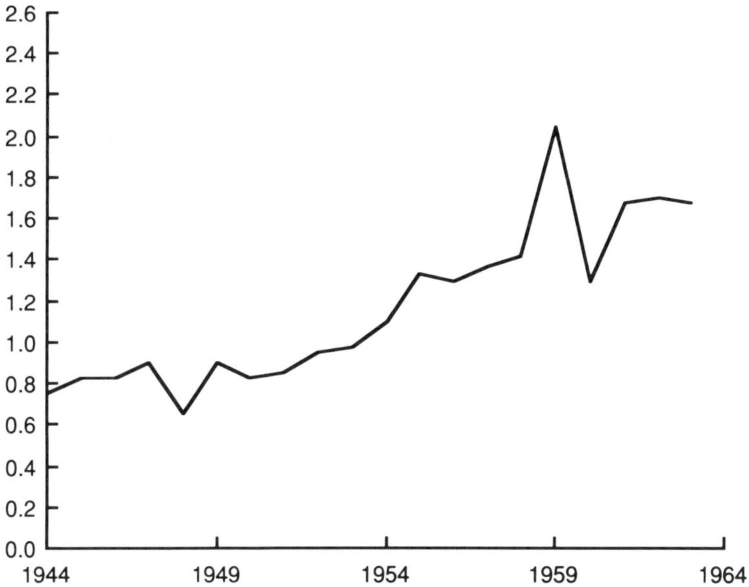


*Figure 12*
*Total Paroles plus Discharges as Proportion of First Admissions by Year From 1944 to 1963*
*Source: Saskatchewan Department of Public Health Annual Reports*

The second source of opposition was more intractable. The mental hospitals dominated the local economies and consequently local and regional politics. Addressing this issue in a letter to Premier Douglas in 1959, Humphrey Osmond, the superintendent of SHW, stated:

> Considering [the town of Weyburn's] size it might easily have become a "company" town based on the hospital. In fact it has become a businessman's town run by men who, whatever their incomes, qualify as small businessmen in the worst sense of the word.[8]

Be that as it may, there is no doubt that there were powerful forces at work in Weyburn which adamantly opposed changes to the psychiatric status quo.

However, even more powerful forces were committed to the transformation of psychiatric work and the development of community psychiatry, including the NCMH. The NCMH was an elitist organzation dedicated to securing the passage of legislation which would allow for the application of public health principles to the treatment of mental disorders, and the medicalization of psychiatric work. It was becoming increasingly clear, however, that the existence of legislation was no guarantee of its application. Thus, guided by the principle that "mass citizen participation produces the most effective force for social change,"[9] the NCMH became the Canadian Mental Health Association (CMHA). With financial support from the federal government, the first division of the CMHA was established in Saskatchewan in 1950. Many employees of PSB were members of the new CMHA, including Dr. D.G. McKerracher, who was "convinced that the politicians would only act to put up the money that was required for psychiatric services if there was some pressure from the voters, from the electorate."[10] Thus a close working relationship developed between McKerracher and the CMHA. In an attempt to educate the public regarding the need for change McKerracher, through the organizational structure of the CMHA, would organize "busloads of women to come down from Regina to [Saskatchewan Hospital] Weyburn, and one from Saskatoon to [Saskatchewan Hospital] North Battleford as visitors because this was the way to really show people how horrible the conditions were people were living in."[11] It was thought that popular support for the transformation of mental hospital work and the development of community psychiatry could be generated in this way.

This was an extremely successful tactic. In fact, from the government's point of view, perhaps it was too successful, since responsibility for inadequacies in the psychiatric system was placed at the door of the government, and consequently received a considerable amount of bad press. The government thought it could influence the nature and extent of these criticisms by encouraging DPH employees to become CMHA members. Thus, in a letter to the Manitoba minister of health and public welfare, the Saskatchewan minister stated, in spite of the bad publicity arising from the activities of the CMHA, "we will continue to encourage our psychiatrists and medical health officers to interest themselves in the activities of this organization, in an advisory capacity [because] in that way we feel that a sense of direction and proportion can be achieved."[12] Nonetheless, significant conflicts developed between the government and the CMHA, the source of which was clearly expressed in a published statement of CMHA values and principles: "Our identification is with the 'consumer' rather than with the 'provider' whenever a possible conflict of interest may be present."[13] In an attempt to represent the consumer's interests the CMHA continually publicized the inadequacies of the existing system in the form of pamphlets, public addresses and news releases wherein certain facts regarding the conditions and treatment of the mentally ill were presented. Although there was no suggestion that the information was not true, there was some concern over how it was being presented to the public. As the minister of public health pointed out to the deputy minister, "the Premier is not particularly pleased with the way the 'facts' are set out."[14]

From the premier's point of view, the main problem was political. He felt the government was not being accorded sufficient recognition for the changes which had been made, nor adequate credit for money already spent (see Figure 9).

There was nothing unusual in special lobby groups criticizing government policy. The fact that key figures in PSB management were also actively involved as executive officers of the CMHA, however, made these conflicts more significant. In their capacity as spokesmen for the CMHA, government employees were often directly involved in advocating changes which involved criticizing government policies which they were employed to implement. Referring to a newspaper account of a speech made by the director of PSB in 1957, Premier Douglas stated to the minister of public health:

> There is no Government activity which has had such a rapid increase in expenditure as the Psychiatric Branch. However, instead of telling the public how much has been done to improve conditions in mental institutions and in the treatment and care of mental patients, the

> whole aim of the Psychiatric Branch seems to be to tell the public how little we have done in this regard. Consequently all the publicity from the Mental Health Association has been critical rather than helpful. I lay the blame for this squarely on some of our own employees. . . .[15]

Apparently the sense of direction and proportion hoped for by the government was not being achieved, and this remained a source of intramanagement conflict for many years.

Although opposition to the establishment of mental hygiene clinics was not as widespread or prolonged as opposition to boarding-out programmes and patient parole, it nonetheless existed, mainly from physicians in private practice, and was economic in nature.

Although there had been legislative authority for the establishment of mental hygiene clinics since 1936, none were created until the first full-time clinic was opened in Regina in 1946. This was followed by the rapid establishment of other full-time and part-time clinics throughout the province (see Figure 13).

The mental hygiene clinics were viewed as the backbone of the preventive approach to psychiatry.[16] Their purpose was to prevent hospitalization, and thereby reduce overcrowding in the provincial hospitals. To achieve this, full-time clinics were assigned three functions: the provision of a consultative and diagnostic service to physicians and social agencies; the provision of an educational service for groups operating within the field of mental health; and the provision of an out-patient treatment service. The part-time clinics did not provide treatment services.[17]

Regarding the treatment and education functions, it appears clear that the development of the mental hygiene clinic labour process was not an instance of the deskilling of psychiatric work. These were new functions, performed in new facilities by a new occupational division of labour. In this respect, the development of the clinics represented the creation of a new labour process, characterized by new social relations and forces of psychiatric production. With regard to

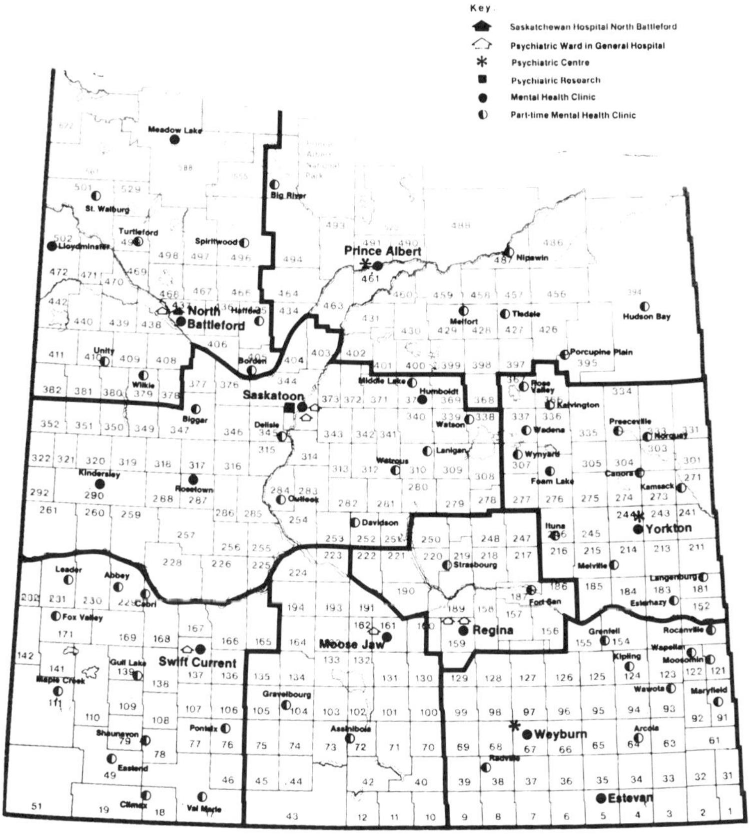


*Figure 13*
*Location of Psychiatric Facilities in Saskatchewan, 1980-1981*
*Source: Saskatchewan Department of Public Health Annual Report, 1980-81*

the provision of consultative and diagnostic services to private practice GPs, the situation is not so clear.

As conceived by McKerracher, the consultative services were designed to permit the private practice GP to provide psychiatric services on an out-patient basis or, if hospitalization was required, in the general hospital. They were intended to facilitate the expansion of GP and general hospital psychiatry and thereby reduce the rate of admission to the PSB-financed mental hospitals. In this respect, it does not appear the diagnostic and consultative services represented the deskilling of psychiatric work. By the early 1960s, however, things were changing. Given a rapidly growing demand for community psychiatric services, McKerracher realized that clinic psychiatrists would be unable to provide both treatment and consultative services. He also recognized it would be impossible to produce or otherwise recruit enough specialist psychiatrists to permit them to perform both functions. He suggested, therefore, that the most cost-effective solution to this dilemma would involve

> rearranging the duties which psychiatric specialists . . . perform. The psychiatrist would have to spend less time carrying out what is really general practice psychiatry, and thus have more time available for backing up general physicians.[18]

To the extent that the work of mental hygiene clinic psychiatrists shifted from treatment to consultation, it would appear that it represented a deskilling of community psychiatric work. The consultation function expanded in the late 1960s when the federal government established a medical care insurance plan which provided added incentive for the provincial government to develop GP and general hospital psychiatry. It thus appears that, with regard to treatment and education, the mental hygiene clinics did not represent the deskilling of psychiatric work. To the extent that the consultative and diagnostic functions supplanted treatment and encouraged the expansion of GP and general hospital psychiatry, it appears they did mark the deskilling of an aspect of community psychiatric work.

Since one function of the clinics was to facilitate the expansion of GP and general hospital psychiatry, it is ironic that the principal opponents to their development were private practice physicians, who feared the free treatment provided in the full-time clinics would result in a loss of paying patients. This fear is clearly expressed in a letter to the minister of public health from a Saskatoon psychiatrist:

> I consider free shock treatment given on an office basis, or outside the hospital by men on a salary, as civil servants interfering and competing with the private medical practitioner . . . .[19]

Because of these fears, private practice physicians lobbied for, and secured, a ban on self-referrals. All individuals receiving treatment at a mental health clinic had to be referred by a physician or some social agency. The DPH reported that 75 percent of patients seen at the clinics in 1952-53 were referred by private practice physicians.[20]

Even with physicians controlling the flow of patients, demand for clinic services outstripped capacity. As a result, the DPH reported in 1952 that it was forced to establish narrower criteria for the provision of "full-scale psychotherapy . . . . The emphasis in selection was on children and adolescents and on types of cases which could best be treated on an out-patient basis."[21]

The decision to restrict the provision of psychiatric services to children and adolescents was justified in terms of prevention and economy: "The needs of such groups are great and the rewards highest in terms of the most economical use of the facilities available and the return to society."[22]

This emphasis on prevention in children, however, was undermined by increased rates of discharge from the two mental hospitals, combined with a continuing shortage of all categories of trained psychiatric labour power. Thus, between 1949 and 1969, there was only one facility in the province for the psychiatric treatment of children and youths, the MacNeill Clinic in Saskatoon.

It is interesting to note that the increased discharge rates preceded the introduction of the psychotropic drugs in 1954. During the 1940-44 period for example, there were 2,087 discharges from the provincial mental hospitals. From 1945-49 this increased by over 40 percent, to 2,908. In 1951, the director of PSB told the minister of public health: "While we know that these figures are correct we hesitate to interpret what they mean and would not be inclined to use this information publicly."[23]

Lack of space is the most probable explanation. Such an interpretation would also be compatible with Brenner's finding that physical capacity is an important factor in determining the rate of hospitalization.[24] If lack of space was the reason the rate of discharge increased, it would certainly have been politically unwise to make such information public, especially since virtually no follow-up services existed in the province. It was not until 1950, for example, that both mental hospitals employed a social worker. After 1950, the political pressure to do something about the deplorable conditions of overcrowding increased dramatically due to the educational efforts of the CMHA and other interested individuals and groups. This pressure was not unique to Saskatchewan. In the immediate post-World War II period, pressure was generated around the world to clean up the psychiatric snake pits, a process which undoubtedly contributed to 1960 being designated Mental Health Year.

Private practice physicians were not alone in viewing the development and expansion of community psychiatry with trepidation. Throughout the 1950s, psychiatric nurses became concerned about their occupational security, a concern which was exacerbated following the introduction of the psychotropic drugs. Referring to the effect that the use of largactil had on psychiatric nurses at SHW, one long-time RPN stated:

> It caused a hell of a degree of anxiety to some of the staff because it was introduced . . . as a miracle drug that was going to cure mental illness . . . and I can remember senior staff saying "Well, isn't that a son of a gun. They are going to cure all these guys and we will all be out of jobs."[25]

These fears were amplified by the success of the mental hygiene clinics in reducing both the rate of hospitalization and inmate populations at the provincial mental hospitals. An internal DPH paper, for example, stated:

> Our own statistics show a sharp drop in the proportion of Saskatchewan Hospital Weyburn admissions coming from the Moose Jaw area after the opening of the full-time mental health clinic in Moose Jaw in 1952. Thus it

> seems clear that the extension of mental health clinics is one of the factors contributing to a decrease in our mental hospital population.[26]

High anxiety produced low morale and poor management-worker relations. In an attempt to improve the situation, PSB management decided to educate the psychiatric nurses regarding the role and function of the mental health clinics. The clinical director of the Swift Current Mental Health Clinic, in an unpublished paper entitled "The Role and Function of a Community Health Clinic in Relation to the Mental Hospital," stated:

> Community or social psychiatry is one of the new trends in this medical specialty. We are witnessing at present the development of community psychiatric services all over North America and Europe . . . I am convinced that psychiatric nurses working almost exclusively in inpatient institutions must be questioning the role and functions of a Community Mental Health Clinic.[27]

He noted that the mental health clinic had two principal functions, "the screening and prevention of hospitalization of mental patients [and] the rehabilitation of the discharged or convalescent patient following hospital psychiatric treatment,"[28] and concluded that

> This program is still at a very early stage and proceeds very empirically. There are, however, some encouraging indications, that the Mental Hospital readmission rate from the [Swift Current] Region is decreasing while the discharge rate is increasing. This strengthens my conviction that psychiatric treatment has to be given at the community level.[29]

It is unlikely that increased discharge rates and decreased readmission rates were perceived as encouraging indications by the psychiatric nurses since they were already insecure about their position within the psychiatric division of labour. In addition, it was predicted by provincial psychiatrists in 1958 that the transformation of psychiatric work associated with the transition to community psychiatry would lead to "the complete disappearance of mental institutions, as they are known today."[30] For many this was good news, heralding the end of the much vilified psychiatric warehouses. To the psychiatric nurses, however, it represented a threat to occupational security. It was thus a degree of desperation that finally led the SPNA publicly to endorse the Saskatchewan Plan in 1959.

## The Saskatchewan Plan versus General Hospital Psychiatry

In general, the Saskatchewan Plan was an attempt to transform the forces of psychiatric production by replacing large rural asylums with small community mental hospitals. It was developed in the early 1950s as part of the attempt to medicalize psychiatry.

The 1950 Mental Hygiene Act established medical control of admission and discharge procedures, but mental hospital work was not yet completely medicalized, being still largely custodial. In an attempt to change this, psychiatrists turned their attention to the psychiatrist-patient relationship and the efficacy of psychiatric treatments. Dr. Frank Coburn discusses this point:

> When I first got into psychiatry [before World War II] the concept was that a patient had to be perfectly well before he was sent home. No other branch of medicine demands that of themselves [*sic*]. You never get a hypertensive person perfectly well. You send them home when you can manage them at home, and when they get no more benefit from the hospital.[31]

This shift in perspective implied that mental hospitals full to overflowing did not necessarily signify the impotence of psychiatry or psychiatrists. Rather, the overcrowding was thought to be the consequence of too stringent criteria for discharge, a legacy of the legal conception of insanity, poor management, and the reliance on unpaid patient labour. Dr. Humphrey Osmond, superintendent of SHW, made this point when he argued that the deplorable conditions in the mental hospitals were

> the cumulative effect of poor organization and lack of central direction since the hospital was opened in 1921.

> The lack of an adequate policy which combined with an entirely inadequate machinery for getting patients out of the hospital, has resulted in gross overcrowding for many years. . . . *And above all* by aging of a chronic population upon whose unpaid labour (scarcely distinguishable from slavery) the whole functioning of the hospitals depends . . . .[32] [emphasis in original]

The "discovery" of the iatrogenic nature of mental hospitals[33] was added to the pychiatrists' ideological arsenal. The idea that the mental hospitals themselves were a major cause of chronicity provided the impetus to look for alternatives. This resulted in the abandonment of plans for a third large mental hospital in Saskatoon and the development of the Saskatchewan Plan for community mental hospitals.

Although the plan to provide psychiatric treatment for the mentally ill in small community psychiatric hospitals was internationally heralded as a great stride forward, its seeds had been germinating for some time. Hincks and the NCMH had recommended the construction of small psychopathic hospitals for the province as early as 1920, and the 1907 Low Report had suggested the adoption of cottage-style construction. The specifics of the Saskatchewan Plan, however, apparently emerged from discussions among Saskatchewan psychiatrists in the early 1950s. As Dr. Humphrey Osmond told Kahan, "the original discussions about a community-type hospital occurred, so far as I know, between Professor Griff McKerracher, Abram Hoffer [director, psychiatric research, PSB] and myself in late 1953 or early 1954."[34]

Proponents of the Saskatchewan Plan maintained that the iatrogenic nature of traditional mental hospitals was a function of their size, design and location. The remedy thus seemed to be at hand: if large, pavillion-style hospitals in a rural setting contributed to the perpetuation and worsening of mental illness, then small, cottage-style hospitals in a community setting would undoubtedly contribute to a cure.

In a 1958 article advocating the merits of the small community mental hospitals, the director of PSB commented that the hospital must do the sick no harm, and added "we must go further than this in our conception of the mental hospital for it must not only do no harm but must actively assist in the patient's care or rehabilitation."[35] This was a common theme, as McMillan observed:

> The hospital should not make the patient worse, for instance, hospitalization in large groups leads frequently to deterioration instead of improvement; The hospital should contain facilities for adequate specific treatments; The hospital should be situated where it is readily accessible to the patient and the patient's relatives; The hospital should have facilities for segregation of various types of patients; The hospital should provide facilities to produce a milieu which will assist in the patient's recovery—embodying such items as decent human living conditions, privacy, occupational and recreational programs, good food preparation and service, social amenities, et cetera; The hospital should have sufficient staff to provide personal attention to each patient; The hospital should be small enough that the patient can feel he is a person and not an inanimate object. . . . Hospitals should be constructed in small units, each designed so that patients may be divided into smaller groups of 10 or less to allow for segregation of various types and also to allow for social relationships approximating those of the family rather than the military barracks. The type of therapeutic program which has been found most effective for a majority of mental hospital patients requires that the patients be dealt with and accommodated in groups not exceeding ten.[36]

Thus, the hospital was clearly considered to be an essential element in the treatment of mental illness. The advocates of the community mental hospital system were convinced that the design and location of the proposed facilities had significant therapeutic impact. In theoretical terms, the small community mental hospitals were considered a principal element of the means of production, and an integral component of the psychiatric labour process.

The same argument had been made by the nineteenth-century proponents of the asylum-as-cure. There are some striking similarities between nineteenth-century advocates of the asylums and twentieth-century proponents of community mental hospitals regarding what was required of a therapeutic institution. Scull, for example, points out that the model institution in the mid-nineteenth century was also to be small, providing accommodation for no more than 250 patients. It was to provide for the segregation of patients according to the severity of their disorder, and the wards were to contain no more than ten people in order to encourage the establishment of family-like relations.[37]

Other elements, however, were quite different. Nineteenth- (and early twentieth-) century proponents of the asylum system argued that the institution

> should be sited where the patients could enjoy the benefits of fresh, bracing country air, and where there was an extensive and pleasing view of the surrounding countryside to divert the mind from its morbid fantasies.[38]

It was thought a rural setting, the opportunity to engage in productive work and asylum from the pressures of social life would cure most cases of insanity. Thus, rural location and isolation were important aspects of treatment. It was for this reason that the 1907 Low Report suggested the North Battleford mental hospital

> should be situated at a sufficient distance from town to discourage too frequent intercourse between the town and the institution, and yet not too far away for those who are really compelled for various reasons to visit the institutions.[39]

By the 1950s, this isolation was viewed as pathogenic. Therefore the Saskatchewan Plan recommended that small mental hospitals be constructed as an integral part of the community, in order to encourage frequent social contacts between patients and community members. It was thought this would lead to the creation of supportive social relationships which would, in turn, minimize the need for hospitalization. By the mid-1950s, the "community" had become an almost mystical entity, exposure to which was thought to cure mental illness — an interesting inversion of the ideas prevalent in the middle of the last century. In both cases,

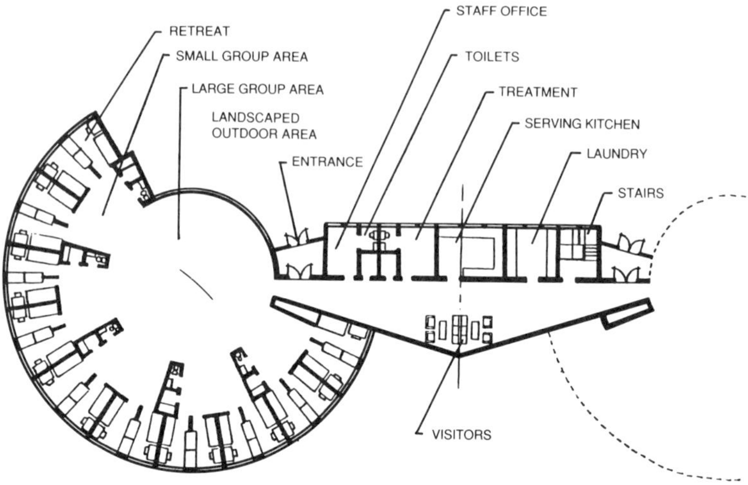


*Figure 14*
*Saskatchewan Plan Community Mental Hospital: Socio-Petal Unit*

Source: *Fanny H. Kahan, Brains and Bricks: The History of the Yorkton Psychiatric Centre (Regina, Saskatchewan: White Cross Publications, 1965), 63*

however, these are better understood as ideological claims rather than demonstrable facts.

The architecture, as well as the physical setting, was considered an essential element in the cure of mental illness in both the mid-nineteenth and mid-twentieth centuries. There was considerable conflict over the unconventional design of the community mental hospitals advocated in the Saskatchewan Plan, and major design changes resulted.

The plans for the community mental hospital were made by the firm of Izumi, Arnott and Sugiyama, architects and consulting engineers of Regina, Saskatchewan. The first plan, referred to as the socio-petal design, did away with corridors in an attempt to minimize sources of perceptual distortion, a problem frequently encountered with psychotics (see Figure 14). However, these arrangements violated established space standards of the federal government and those recommended by the American Psychiatric Association, and had to be modified.

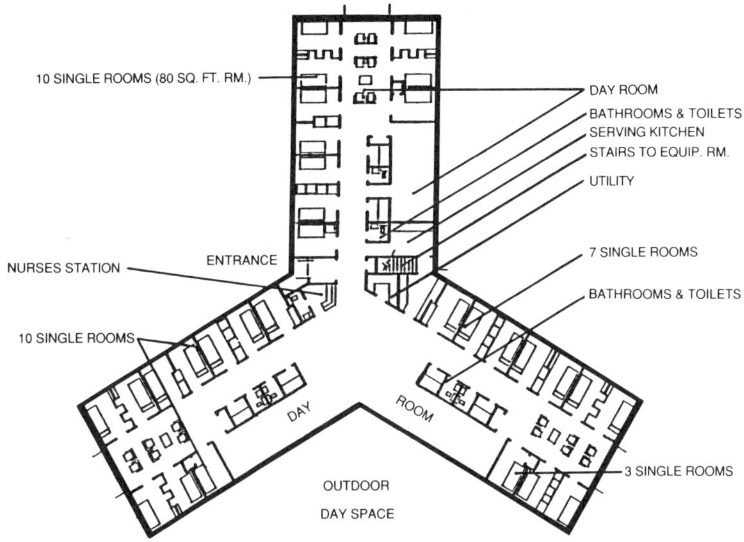


*Figure 15*
*Saskatchewan Plan Community Mental Hospital: Y-Design Unit*
*Source: SAB, R-34, 172G2. Erb Papers: Saskatchewan Plans*

In an attempt to retain what were considered the therapeutic innovations of the socio-petal design, and at the same time more closely approximate requirements of the building code, the plans were modified and emerged as the Y-design (see Figure 15).[40] These single-storey units, which accommodated thirty patients in groups of ten, were to be arranged around a central administration and service block (see Figure 16). The object was to reproduce the sense of a small village. Even this design was considered revolutionary, and met with stiff opposition from the provincial government. Mr. Izumi told Kahan that the director of PSB

> encountered an enormous number of difficulties in getting the Saskatchewan Plan brought to final realization; . . . administrative and political difficulties. I suspect that many of these sprang from the fact that people in the Health Department and the Government were unwilling to embark on what they thought was such a revolutionary program, and hoped that others would

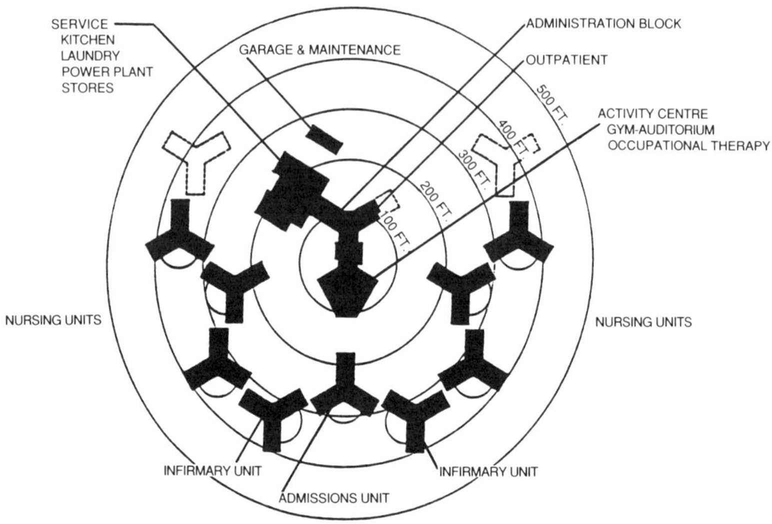


*Figure 16*
*Saskatchewan Plan Community Mental Hospital:*
*Schematic Site Plan Showing Space*
*Relationships of Functions*
*Source: SAB, R-34, 172G2. Erb Papers: Saskatchewan Plans*

> come forward and get their feet wet. It was not simply, of course, that the program was revolutionary, but the buildings were revolutionary too. So that the combination made people particularly jittery.[41]

In fact, in 1956 the DPH told the director of PSB that government support for the Saskatchewan Plan was contingent on two things: "(a) evidence that it was professionally sound, (b) evidence that the people of the province were interested in improving psychiatric facilities and would be willing to stand the cost of these."[42] Proponents set out to satisfy both these conditions, but while public and professional support were easy to demonstrate, cost proved to be a major obstacle.

There was ample evidence that the plan for community mental hospitals was considered professionally sound, conforming as it did to the Third Report of the World Health Organization (WHO) Expert Committee on Mental Health:

> It is desirable that the hospital should be composed of a group of small buildings, rather than a single block. The therapeutic community should take the village as its model. Each unit should be planned for a small group of patients, preferably about 25-30, and it should be assumed that the majority of patients will sleep, eat, and work in comparatively small groups of up to 10 patients. If economic conditions permit sleeping accommodation should include a fairly high proportion of separate rooms, and much of the remainder should be in small dormitories for 6-8 patients.[43]

This was precisely what PSB management and other psychiatrists were suggesting.

Dr. Lawson, who became the director of PSB after Griff McKerracher resigned to become the professor and head of the newly created Department of Psychiatry at the University of Saskatchewan, used the 1953 WHO report as evidence that the principles of the Saskatchewan Plan were professionally sound.[44] As further evidence of this, he stated that they had also been accepted by the senior commissioner of the Board of Control in Great Britain, a 1952 Danish commission into that country's psychiatric care requirement, the American Psychiatric Association, and the CMHA.[45]

CMHA support of the Saskatchewan Plan took many forms, including an attempt to convince the federal government to share the costs of psychiatric services in community mental hospitals, which would help convince the Saskatchewan cabinet to support the plan. A CMHA brief to the federal government emphasized the rehabilitative potential of the community mental hospital:

> the smaller mental hospital built near a general hospital, and old folks home, and co-operating with them would give an effective unit enabling the maintenance of a highly trained medical staff with specialists in all branches of medicine on its staff. It would also permit the staffs of these mental institutions to become part of the community rather than live as an isolated group. The community would be nearby and there would be a constant flow of the community into the hospital and a

> flow of patients back into the community where they would be re-established.[46]

The refusal of the provincial government to endorse the Saskatchewan Plan was more a result of the substantial costs involved than insufficient professional and popular support, or unconventional architectural design. First submitted to the provincial government in 1955, the Saskatchewan Plan called for the construction of six regional mental hospitals ranging in size from 268 to 418 beds. In addition, SHNB and SHW, besides having inmate populations reduced to rated capacities, were to be structurally modified to facilitate their use as regional mental hospitals. The province was thus to have eight regional mental hospitals with a total capacity of 2,924 beds (about five beds per thousand population). It was estimated that in fiscal year 1956, total operating costs for these regional hospitals would be $11,408,931. This was $5,702,949 more than the 1956-57 budgetary estimates for all the psychiatric facilities which then existed in the province. In addition, the proposed capital costs, including equipment, were estimated by PSB management to be between $13,158,000 and $18,835,344. Exclusive of the federal construction grant of $1,500 per bed, it was estimated that the Saskatchewan Plan would cost the provincial government between $18,860,949 and $24,538,293.[47]

Federal construction grants would have amounted to $4,386,000. This money would only be forthcoming, however, if existing building codes, fire regulations and hospital construction standards were satisfied. The Y-design units did not qualify for this money. As a result, the architectural design underwent further modification (see Figure 17).

The drastic transformation of the architectural design was not due to changing perceptions of effective psychiatric treatment. Rather, it was due to eligibility requirements for federal construction grants. Economic and political considerations continued to affect the development of the forces of psychiatric production, which in turn resulted in a transformation of the social relations of production.

Although the provincial government was anxious to secure federal government construction grants, it was even more

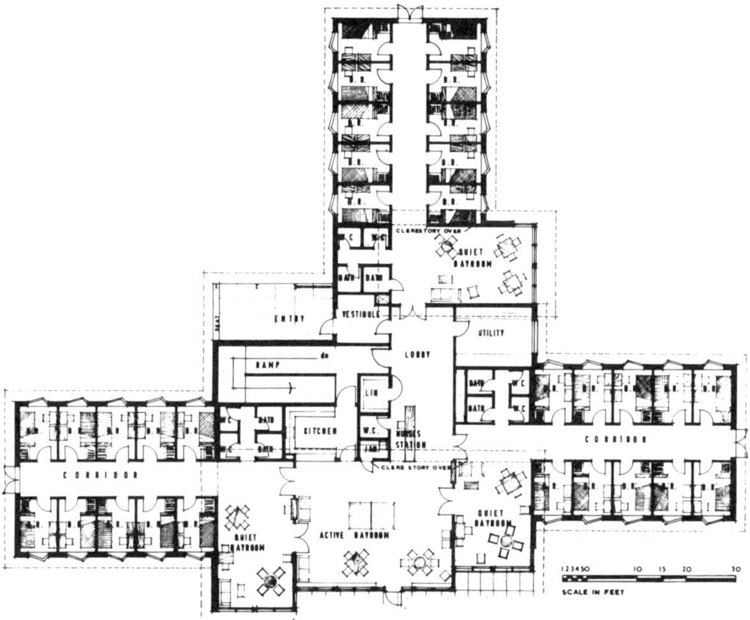


*Figure 17*
*Saskatchewan Plan Community Mental Hospital: Unit as Built*

*Source: Fanny H. Kahan, Brains and Bricks: The History of the Yorkton Psychiatric Centre (Regina, Saskatchewan: White Cross Publications, 1965), 63*

interested in establishing the principle, and maximizing the extent, of federal government cost sharing in the provision of psychiatric services. It was therefore disinclined to adopt the proposals for community mental hospitals before determining if these would be eligible for federal monies under the terms of the proposed Hospital Insurance and Diagnostic Services Act. The CCF government were thus prepared to engage in a lengthy process of negotiation and compromise. Others were not so patient or flexible.

The most avid supporter of the Saskatchewan Plan was Dr. F.S. Lawson, director of PSB from 1955 to 1965. In his efforts to bring it to fruition, he often highlighted the inadequacies of the large mental hospitals. Like McKerracher, he thought public support for the small community mental hospitals could be generated by exposing the horrors of the existing mental hospitals. There was a thin line between generating popular support for change and engaging in public criticism of government policy; from the government's point of view, proponents of the Saskatchewan Plan were often guilty of the latter. This was considered to be particularly problematic when the critics were government employees, as can be seen from Premier Douglas's response to a speech made by Lawson to the Regina branch of the CMHA in early 1957:

> I am disturbed by the attached newspaper report regarding the speech of [the director of PSB] to a meeting of the Regina Branch of the Canadian Mental Health Association. I am even more disturbed by the statements of representatives of this Branch when they appeared on television and took the Government to task because we had not proceeded to build six new 500-bed hospitals in various parts of the province.[48]

The premier pointed out that, as far as he was concerned, the major problem was PSB management, who were

> apparently trying to blackmail the government into complying with their proposals by trying to create a public demand which they think will force us into accepting their proposals. I am quite prepared to go as far as our finances will permit in extending psychiatric services but I do not propose to allow government employees to create appetites which cannot be satisfied and to encourage groups of laymen to criticize our program in order to satisfy their obsession for empire building.
>
> If you cannot restrain [the director of PSB] then I will undertake to do so. If there are any more public statements made by [the director] or any other members of the Psychiatric Services Branch I shall be compelled to make a public statement repudiating their proposals and stating the Government's true position with regard to them.[49]

Thus, the tensions between the various levels of management were high. Furthermore, because the attempts of PSB management to mobilize popular support took place primarily through the organizational structure of the CMHA, relations between the government and the CMHA were also increasingly strained.

Adding to this strain was the fact that Premier Douglas had reservations regarding the multi-hospital approach, favouring instead the centralization of psychiatric facilities. In a letter to a CCF supporter in Weyburn he stated:

> You can be sure that if there is to be any extension of mental hospital facilities, I will be on the job to see that Weyburn is not overlooked as the logical place for additional buildings rather than scattering them all over the province as was the suggestion of the Mental Health Association.[50]

Douglas favoured a "centres of excellence" approach, which he believed was more effective and economical. The stage was thus set for a protracted struggle between the government and those in the province committed to the construction of small regional mental hospitals. Commenting on these struggles Douglas stated in an interview with the author:

> Now we had, as you know, many places where they didn't want to go into larger hospital units; they wanted two or three little hospitals . . . or they wanted three or four different mental hospitals. Getting them to realize that the only way you are going to get first-class service is to have large centres where the best staff are available, and the best equipment is available and bring people a greater distance rather than getting half-baked service, and half-trained staff in every little community — that takes a lot of struggling to persuade people, and that's why . . . health education was an essential part of this whole thing.[51]

The government, although never fully committed to the Saskatchewan Plan, refrained from taking a public stance, thus adding to the confusion. Dr. McKerracher, in a letter to Premier Douglas, made this point:

> Today I had a telephone conversation with [the president] of the Canadian Mental Health Association. She said she had been told at a meeting with the Cabinet

> that the Government, on the advice of its psychiatric consultants, had abandoned the plan of constructing regional psychiatric units. She was further told that this plan was being replaced by one of constructing small psychiatric units attached to general hospitals. She asked why, if the plan had been abandoned, had none of the Provincial psychiatrists, including me, informed the C.M.H.A. with whom we have frequent meetings. Quite understandably she was confused.[52]

The premier did not want this confusion to result in further attacks on the government for failing to provide adequate care for the mentally ill. Therefore, in an attempt to make it clear to the CMHA that the government had not in fact rejected the Saskatchewan Plan, he wrote to the president of the Saskatchewan division, CMHA:

> My object in writing you . . . is to assure you that the plan for small psychiatric regions has not been rejected but the whole problem of caring for the mentally ill is under review. I can also assure you that we are anxious, insofar as finances will permit, to implement the principle of removing the differentiation in the treatment of mental patients as compared to other patients who require general nursing care.[53]

Although it is clearly stated that the plan for small psychiatric regions had not been rejected, it is not stated that the plan for small regional psychiatric hospitals had been accepted. In fact, the premier pointed out that several options for achieving psychiatric reform were being actively considered:

> One of the factors that will influence the type of plan adopted will be the decision of the Government of Canada regarding the extent to which the proposed national hospital plan will cover patients receiving psychiatric treatment. If regional psychiatric hospitals are to be excluded from the national hospital insurance plan then we may have to consider the advisability of having these units attached to general hospitals providing, of course that the national hospital plan will contribute to the cost of patients' care.

> I think you will appreciate the fact that we will want to adopt any plan which may be implemented in such a way as to enable the province to secure the maximum financial contribution possible from the national hospital insurance program. Until we have received some indication of the Federal Government's position on this question it will not be possible to decide which type of program would be advantageous to the province.[54]

The CMHA and several provincial governments, including Saskatchewan, had petitioned the federal government to include psychiatric services and mental hospitals in the proposed health insurance plan. There was some indication in July 1958 that the small regional mental hospitals built in close proximity to, and administered by, a local general hospital board would be defined as psychiatric units by the federal government. This gave the founders and proponents of the Saskatchewan Plan new hope, as can be seen in a letter from Dr. McKerracher to Premier Douglas:

> I have been assured by [a Saskatoon MP], that the Saskatchewan Plan of units from 100 to 300 beds would be eligible for inclusion. [The Saskatoon MP] after discussing this with [the federal minister of health and welfare] says that, if the Saskatchewan Government now submits a summary of its plan, a favorable ruling would result.[55]

A summary was sent to Ottawa by the minister of public health the following day:

> As you know, considerable thought has been given in this province to providing a different kind of care to the mentally ill. What has been popularly known as the "Saskatchewan Plan" consists essentially of the establishment of relatively small in-patient units for the treatment of the mentally ill, close to their home communities. . . . In some instances, some requirements would force the psychiatric unit of the general hospital to be located off the actual grounds occupied by the other units of that hospital.[56]

This was to constitute a major obstacle to securing federal support.

The federal minister responded on 22 August 1958 and unequivocally stated the position of the federal government regarding cost sharing for the treatment of the mentally ill:

> This scheme [the proposed insurance plan] takes into account the recent development of psychiatric wards in general hospitals for the active treatment of acute phases of mental illness, and includes the costs of this kind of care within the expenses to be shared by federal and provincial governments. . . .
>
> In referring to psychiatric wards in general hospitals I had in mind, of course, the generally accepted concept of this relatively new development, namely that they are units within a general hospital, specially designed for the short-term care of mental illness.
>
> You will agree, I think that the establishment of relatively small mental hospitals in close relationship to general hospitals and the home communities of patients concerned, described in your letter . . . while undoubtedly having many apparent advantages in an overall program of mental care, is different from the generally accepted concept of psychiatric wards in general hospitals to which I had reference. This difference would seem to be particularly apparent when circumstances require the location of the units at a distance from a general hospital, or where their size approaches that described in your letter. You will realize, of course, that *careful consideration must be given to these matters because of the specific exclusion of hospitals and institutions for the mentally ill from the operation of the Hospital Insurance and Diagnostic Services Act.*[57] [emphasis added]

The specific exclusion of mental hospitals marked the demise of the Saskatchewan Plan for community mental hospitals. It also marked a nadir in the relations between the government, PSB management and the CMHA. For the provincial government, there was no more indecision: the general hospital would be the primary locus for in-patient psychiatric treatment, because that was the only form of in-patient treatment eligible for federal funds.

Treatment in psychiatric wards of general hospitals had been recommended by Hincks and the NCMH in 1930 and again in 1945, as a part of a complete mental health programme, and the first psychopathic ward in Saskatchewan had been established in the Regina General Hospital in 1930 (known as the Munroe Wing after 1949). The function of the psychopathic ward was precisely as defined by the federal government, providing short-term intensive treatment to persons in acute phases of mental disorders. The intent was to provide treatment at an early stage in order to avoid the necessity of admission to either of the two large mental hospitals. In this regard, the Munroe Wing was a great success: of the 308 cases dealt with in 1945, for example, only thirty-seven were transferred to mental hospitals, whereas 213 were "returned home improved."[58] The Munroe Wing, which in 1944 had twenty-seven beds, was used primarily for the short-term stay of psychotics. By 1950 it had been increased to accommodate forty-one people. Also guided by an orientation to prevention, the scope of treatment had widened to include "intensive therapy for neurotics as well as the mild mental illnesses."[59]

Thus general hospital psychiatry was neither new in theory nor in practice. In fact, proponents of the Saskatchewan Plan had supported its development. It had never before been conceived as the primary locus of psychiatric work, however, and this generated much heated opposition. This point was clearly made by McKerracher in a letter to Premier Douglas:

> So the point of this letter is to state that there has been at no time any change in my thinking, nor as far as I know in that of other psychiatrists in this Province, as to the advisability of regional units of about 300 beds. In the eleven years that I have been associated with the service, there has been only one basic change in plan and that was from the 1200 bed hospital in Saskatoon to the 300 bed units.[60]

The commitment of both the federal and provincial governments to general hospital psychiatry, although clearly corresponding to a further medicalization of psychiatry, was actively opposed by PSB-employed psychiatrists. Dr. Lawson argued in 1958, at the first Canadian Mental Hospital Institute, that it was a regressive move: "psychiatric wings in general hospitals have set back by 10 years treatment of mental illness."[61] McKerracher, and the university psychiatrists, also saw it as a negative development:

> Never in the past six years (since the first thought of the regional plan) have I favored building more psychiatric units in general hospitals. Small units in general hospitals, while helping the short stay patient, tend to degrade further the large Provincial hospitals. Thus, I have never for a moment entertained the idea of the 50-bed unit other than as a stepping stone towards facilities in the general hospital capable of caring for *all* the mental patients in that region.[62] [emphasis in original]

Dr. McKerracher and others at the University of Saskatchewan undertook a series of studies to determine if it was feasible to provide care and treatment for all categories of mental illness in psychiatric wards in general hospitals.[63] It might be wondered, given Dr. McKerracher's commitment to the proposals of the Saskatchewan Plan, if the original motivation behind these studies was to prove that general hospital psychiatry was unfeasible. The reported findings, however, were clear: with appropriately trained ward staff, consultation by psychiatrists, and psychotropic drugs to control behaviour, *all* categories of mental illness could effectively be treated by GPs in a general hospital ward.

These were historic findings. McKerracher and the university psychiatrists had demonstrated that psychiatric work could be completely medicalized. It was no longer necessary that it be performed in separate facilities by distinct occupational groups. The psychotropic drugs made it possible to produce manageable patients in the same facilities and with the same occupational division of labour used in other branches of medicine. On the basis of these findings McKerracher began to advocate that all psychiatric patients requiring hospitalization be treated by GPs in *general wards* of general hospitals with specialist psychiatrists acting as consultants. Thus, after 1960 McKerracher maintained that even specialized psychiatric wards were unnecessary.

The complete medicalization of in-patient psychiatric work was guaranteed by the medical monopoly of drug prescription. To the extent that drugs were used, and following their introduction they quickly superseded all other forms of patient management, physicians were required in the psychiatric labour process. Through their use, the longstanding ideological claim that mental illness could be medically treated in the community was transformed into a description of psychiatric practice.

The medicalization of psychiatric work, however, cannot be understood in terms of a simple technological determinism. The drugs were a necessary but not sufficient condition for this to occur. They only had the effect of medicalizing psychiatric work given the political and economic preconditions of legislative monopoly of drug prescription and government attempts to minimize medical care costs.

The medicalization of psychiatric work had a number of consequences for the social relations and forces of psychiatric work. For one thing, it rendered the large mental hospitals technologically obsolete and economically unviable. Thus, the psychotropic drugs laid the foundation for the subsequent depopulation and abandonment of the mental hospitals. Similarly, the psychotropic drugs and the medicalization of psychiatric work made the small community mental hospitals of the Saskatchewan Plan redundant.

Support for the Saskatchewan Plan, however, was based upon more than a belief in the efficacy of the small community mental hospital as a form of treatment. For PSB-employed psychiatrists the Saskatchewan Plan, with its recommendation for the construction of six new hospitals, also entailed an expanding job market, increased occupational security, influence and status. That is, the community mental hospitals, like the asylums in the nineteenth century, promised much to the occupational group which secured control of them. In Saskatchewan, there was no doubt the

PSB-employed psychiatrists would have benefitted from this situation. The medicalization of psychiatry not only ended this opportunity, it threatened to undermine their existing employment base. General hospital psychiatry, as the principal manifestation of the medicalization of psychiatric work, was thus a source of conflict. Dr. Frank Coburn stated:

> [McKerracher] demonstrated that you could treat all types of mental illness in a hospital ward. His thinking began to move away from the small hospital into the concept of a psychiatric ward integrated into a general hospital. He felt that this was better than a separate hospital because he felt that psychiatric patients had long suffered from the alienation between psychiatry and the rest of medicine. We needed to be part of the main stream . . . .
>
> [McKerracher] and [the director of PSB] became at loggerheads, because if [McKerracher] had been able to get all the hospitals to have psychiatric wards, the Psychiatric Services Branch would have withered away. So that was a threat to [the director of PSB].[64]

This conflict intensified support for the Saskatchewan Plan, which for many remained an emotionally charged symbol of progressive and humane treatment of the mentally ill. By the end of the 1950s, public support for the principles of the Saskatchewan Plan had not only been demonstrated by the CMHA, with an estimated membership of fifty thousand, but also by trade unions, chambers of commerce, women's groups, service clubs, the Saskatchewan College of Physicians and Surgeons (SCPS) and, in 1959, even the provincial Liberal party. For most of these groups, support for the Saskatchewan Plan was support for the humane treatment of the mentally ill. For others, particularly the SCPS and the Liberal party, support was based upon more mercenary political motives.

The Liberal party wanted to be identified with a popular programme that the CCF had abandoned, and thereby gain electoral support. The SCPS, involved in the early stages of a confrontation with the CCF government over the establishment of medicare, also wished to strengthen their position. It was thought this could be done by arguing that the CCF's abandonment of the Saskatchewan Plan was simply one indication of its callous disregard for the health care of the Saskatchewan people. It was argued by homology that the proposed medicare legislation would also result in a poor quality of general medical care.

Support for the Saskatchewan Plan became virtually unanimous (the only exception was the business community of Weyburn) in 1959, when the SPNA publicly endorsed the concept of small community mental hospitals for the first time. Although the SPNA had never openly opposed the Saskatchewan Plan, they felt threatened by it. Their failure to support the proposal for community mental hospitals resulted from the decision to put them under the control of local general hospital boards. It was reasoned by the provincial government that if the community mental hospitals were administered by a local general hospital board, the claim that they were really psychiatric units of general hospitals, and therefore eligible for federal money, would be easier to sustain. The concern of the psychiatric nurses was that the SRNA would be successful in exerting pressure on local hospital boards to exclude RPNs from employment within community mental hospitals, and for this reason were reluctant to endorse the plan.

Compared to the certain exclusion from employment that general hospital psychiatry promised, the community mental hospital option became more appealing. It was, however, still a second choice for the psychiatric nurses. Their preferred strategy for dealing with the development of community psychiatry was to move into the field of social work.

Arguing that no one was "better qualified to do follow-up work and to educate the home family and the community than the person who has helped the patient return to health,"[65] they had been attempting to move into social work since 1955. PSB management, however, maintained the psychiatric nurses' curriculum did not prepare them for social work, which was argued to require training to at least the baccalaureate level. Even when it was impossible to fill all the established social work positions with fully trained social workers, PSB management did not want to use psychiatric nurses in that capacity. Rather than do so, the DPH established a bursary programme to help defray the cost of social work training. This programme was successful insofar as it helped increase the contingent of social workers in PSB from none in 1944 to twenty-six in 1959. Of those twenty-six positions, eighteen were filled by MSWs and eight by persons with baccalaureate degrees. The baccalaureates were all receiving further training.

If one uses credentials and length of formal training as an indicator of skill levels, it becomes clear that the government and PSB management were not deskilling community psychiatric work. This conclusion is also supported by the fact that opposition to the incursion of psychiatric nurses into the field of social work came from PSB management, not from social workers. Thus, it cannot be argued that management was attempting to apply the Babbage Principle to community psychiatric work but was prevented from doing so by social worker opposition. At that time, social workers were in a relatively weak position, and dependent on PSB management to represent their interests.

This dependence was the product of three factors. First was the fact that the primary locus of psychiatric work was still the large mental hospitals which were dominated by psychiatrists. Community-based work was viewed by PSB management as ancillary to mental hospital psychiatry. The second factor was the relatively small number of social workers employed by PSB. The third factor was their geographic dispersion. In 1959, of the twenty-six social workers employed by PSB, five were at SHNB, ten were at SHW, and the rest were either receiving training or distributed among the various mental health clinics and psychiatric wards around the province. As the locus of psychiatric work in the province shifted from mental hospital to community throughout the 1960s, the number of social workers increased and their acceptance of an ancillary role decreased.

Compared to social workers, PSB-employed psychiatric nurses were a potent force. Their large numbers, strong organization and concentration in the large mental hospitals provided them with a degree of occupational power second only to that of psychiatrists. When this substantial power was finally thrown into the struggle for the Saskatchewan Plan, the CCF government found itself confronted with a virtual consensus of opinion in support of the plan for small community mental hospitals and it was deemed that the political costs of not proceeding with the Saskatchewan Plan exceeded the financial costs of so doing. As a result, the government announced in the 1960 Speech from the Throne that construction would begin on a 148-bed regional mental hospital at Yorkton. This decision, although certainly influenced by the SPNA's public support, cannot fully be understood without looking at the broader political context within which it occurred.

It will be recalled that the CCF was elected in 1944 on a political platform that promised the creation of a complete system of socialized medicine. Sixteen years later, this promise had not been fulfilled. Part of the reason for this delay was the expense involved. By the early 1960s, however, political developments within the CCF made it imperative to proceed with the implementation of a compulsory universal medical insurance scheme in the province regardless of the cost.

The CCF had always aspired to federal power and when the party reformed as the New Democratic Party (NDP) in the early 1960s, Premier Douglas contested and won the leadership of the national NDP. It was felt that electoral success at the federal level under Douglas at least partially depended upon having the long-promised medical insurance plan for Saskatchewan in place. It was recognized that not only would Medicare be financially expensive, politically it would probably cost the CCF-NDP the 1964 provincial election. On the other hand, it was thought the cost of not pursuing this path would be political extinction. As Douglas observed in 1961:

> It would be much easier to play it safe and stay where I am for I am convinced that with hard work the C.C.F. can win the next provincial election. However, a movement like ours will either go forward or deteriorate.

> There is a tide running in national affairs which calls for drastic action and commensurate sacrifice. Even if we can retain Saskatchewan indefinitely this will not resolve the fundamental problems of low farm prices, unemployment and the dangers of nuclear war. If we are to grapple with these problems effectively, then the New Party must make substantial gains in the next federal election.[66]

The major source of opposition to the proposed Medicare legislation came from the province's doctors and their political allies. Although the doctors had publicly endorsed state-run insurance in the 1940s, by 1960 they had reversed their position, probably due to the increasing urbanization of the province. The concentration of population increased the possibility for doctors to operate profitable private practices and private insurance schemes, and their opposition was fierce. Similarly the CCF-NDP, perceiving its political future to be at stake, would not back down. Tensions mounted, positions were polarized, and the conflict intensified, culminating in 1962 with the doctors' strike.[67]

Before engaging in a political life-or-death struggle, the provincial government wanted to be sure it had a strong position from which to fight. It was with this in mind, and with a June 1960 election on the horizon, that the government announced the construction of a regional psychiatric hospital in Yorkton. Speaking in the legislature on 1 March 1960 the minister of public works stated that half of the one million dollars needed for construction was included in the 1960 provincial budget. It was also made clear at the time that this did not represent full acceptance of the Saskatchewan Plan. Rather, the minister of public health suggested the Yorkton facility should be seen as a pilot project, the efficacy of which would influence future decisions. Even with this qualification the CCF won the June 1960 election. It also brought an unusual degree of harmony to the DPH and PSB. PSB management and other psychiatrists viewed the Yorkton decision as a great victory and the psychiatric nurses were greatly relieved. The nurses felt a major battle in the ongoing struggle for job security had been won, and in a letter to the minister of public health stated: "We would like to offer the services of Registered Psychiatric Nurses when you are assigning staff to this hospital."[68]

The SPNA, however, did not rest content. Remembering that their attempts to move into the field of social work had been blocked by the DPH and PSB management, they petitioned the minister of public health to create the position of psychiatric nursing consultant. As envisaged by the SPNA, this was to be a management position which would

> provide expert advice to the Director and his Deputy, and as required to other members of the Branch office staff, on matters dealing with Psychiatric Nursing, e.g. he will draw up a plan for the staffing of the new Community Psychiatric Centres with nurses.[69]

It was also suggested that the consultant could assist PSB management in "improving training programs for Psychiatric Nursing"[70] the objective being to offset management's objections to employing RPNs in the community labour process. Although economic considerations postponed the creation of this position, it was finally established in 1963, as the Co-ordinator of Psychiatric Nursing Programs.

The jubilation surrounding the announcement of construction of the community mental hospital at Yorkton in 1960 soured when construction had not yet begun by the summer of 1961. The most vituperative of the critics was the director of PSB. Not surprisingly the government, enmeshed in a bitter battle with the doctors over Medicare, was highly sensitive to public criticism from its own medical employees. This sensitivity became intolerance when the director of PSB, before a meeting of the SCPS, accused the government of duplicity and immorality:

> After six years of effort and frustration there has not been any acceptance by the government of the plan nor has even one unit been constructed. When dealing with the politician we find that they have an entirely different sense of values from what we have. To them the vote is all important.[71]

The government's response was swift and harsh:

> the vicious and unwarranted public criticism of Government policy which [the director of PSB] saw fit to deliver at the recent meeting of the College of Physicians and Surgeons has gone beyond all limits of conduct that can be tolerated, and necessitates that his services be dispensed with.[72]

Given the political agenda of Premier Douglas and the national CCF-NDP, it was deemed inexpedient to fire the director immediately since this would "open up the whole mental hospital situation to criticism and provide a field day for the opposition."[73] In an attempt to avoid a political scandal, the minister of public health decided that "action in this matter should await the conclusion of the current session of the Legislature. I shall deal with the termination of [the director's] services at that time."[74]

Meanwhile, struggles over the enactment of the proposed Medicare legislation continued to escalate. Ironically, one of the political casualties of this growing crisis was the minister of public health. Within four weeks of deciding to dismiss the director of PSB, he resigned his portfolio and ultimately crossed the floor of the legislature. The director of PSB retained his postition until 1965.

Given this general political context, two factors endemic to the psychiatric labour process in Saskatchewan combined to protect the director of PSB from his employer. First, he was personally identified with the proposals of the Saskatchewan Plan, which in turn were identified with the progressive modern approach to psychiatry and the mentally ill. This was the case not only in the province, but all across North America and Europe.[75] In fact, it was largely the prospect of being able to work within a progressive psychiatric programme that enticed many psychiatrists to work in Saskatchewan. As a result, psychiatrists employed by PSB were united in their support of the Saskatchewan Plan and the director of PSB, and they let the government know it.[76] The threat implicit within the expressions of occupational solidarity was that dismissal of the director of PSB would result in the loss of other PSB psychiatrists. Given the chronic shortage of fully licensed psychiatrists, the prospect of losing those already employed was almost as intolerable to the government as the public criticism generated by the director's attacks. The second factor protecting the director's job was really an extension of this tight labour market — if there were few fully qualified psychiatrists, psychiatrists with demonstrated administrative qualities were virtually non-existent. Commenting on this, a professor of psychiatry from the University of Saskatchewan, who was a CCF supporter, asked the minister of public health:

> Whom could we replace him with? I can think of no one in the Province at present or in recent years who would do and recruitment from Canada, United States or abroad seems difficult to the point of impossibility.[77]

Given that it was assumed the director of PSB would be a fully qualified psychiatrist, the incumbent enjoyed an unusual degree of job security. The government was aware of this, as the following memo from the minister of public health to the premier indicates:

> his awareness of the acute shortage of professional personnel with comparable qualifications led him to assume that he was irreplaceable, and that, accordingly, he could be a law unto himself. Admittedly, the difficulty in being able to secure a suitable replacement contributed to the degree of leniency which was extended to him, even though in many instances the provocation was extreme.[78]

Primarily as a result of these factors, Lawson stayed on as the director of PSB and continued to bring pressure to bear on the government to implement the Saskatchewan Plan. Construction on the 148-bed mental hospital at Yorkton began in 1963, and it was finally opened in October of that year.

# Chapter Five

# The Medicalization of Psychiatry and the Depopulation of the Mental Hospitals, 1963-1971

The transformation of the forces of psychiatric production, in particular the use of psychotropic drugs and the growth of general hospital psychiatry upon which the medicalization of psychiatric work was based, was a precondition for the depopulation of the mental hospitals and the rapid expansion of community psychiatry. It is suggested that the rapid expansion of the community psychiatric labour process was a necessary condition for an emergent de-medicalization of public sector community psychiatry. This chapter examines the social, political and economic context within which these developments occurred, as well as the consequences they had for the social relations of the psychiatric labour process.

Although the depopulation of the mental hospitals had a technical base in the form of psychotropic drugs, it would not have been possible without organizational and operational changes to PSB. In an unpublished paper entitled "Reducing the Population of a Mental Hospital," written by a number of PSB psychiatrists, four changes were identified as responsible for reducing inmate populations:

1. Controlled admission policy.
2. The integration of admission units to regional psychiatric facilities.
3. An active psychogeriatric program for patients aged 65 and over.
4. An active rehabilitation program for patients under 65 years of age suffering from functional psychosis with a long term detention in a mental hospital.[1]

These changes were facilitated by the 1961 Mental Health Act,[2] which was an adaptation of the 1959 British Mental Health Act. Both acts legislatively recognized the medicalization of psychiatric work and established the legal basis for making psychiatric treatment more similar to non-psychiatric medical treatment. McKerracher noted in his report on psychiatric services to the 1964 Royal Commission on Health Services in Canada:

> In a recent revision of its legislation for dealing with the mentally disordered, Saskatchewan has moved well ahead of the other nine provinces. As in the 1959 legislation in Britain, the recently passed Mental Health Act in Saskatchewan has made admission of psychiatric patients very much like the admission of any other patient to any hospital.[3]

These changes were generally welcomed by PSB management-psychiatrists, partly because it was thought it would help them achieve status parity with other medical specialists.

The lack of status accorded to psychiatrists, however, was only partly a product of the differential mode of psychiatric treatment. Equally as important was the fact that psychiatrists, especially in North America, were traditionally state employees. Although they experienced a degree of autonomy within that relationship uncharacteristic of most occupational groups, they were less autonomous than their counterparts in private practice. To the extent that occupational autonomy and self-control are core elements in the ideology of professionalism, the mediation of these characteristics contributed to the lack of professional status accorded psychiatrists by other medical practitioners. This interpretation seems to be supported in a memo to the minister of public health, in which the deputy minister discussed the problem of labour relations with PSB-employed physicians:

> Physicians generally do not like to be considered in the same category as civil servants. For the majority it may well be desirable to work out a contractual relationship. This will give them a special status and alleviate their position in the eyes of their counterparts in private practice.[4]

According physicians a special status was particularly important after 1963. In that year the comprehensive medical care insurance scheme established by the CCF became fully operational. Since the plan included payment for psychiatric services, private practice became a viable option for an increased number of psychiatrists. Employment with PSB consequently became less appealing for fully licensed psychiatrists primarily interested in clinical work. It must be pointed out, however, that in 1964 there were still only three private practice psychiatrists in the province. PSB management's attempts to make public sector employment more attractive for psychiatrists were handicapped by decreasing budgets, which were a manifestation of the Liberal government's least-cost approach to social services.

## The Liberal Government and PSB

The Liberals, under the leadership of Ross Thatcher, defeated the CCF-NDP at the polls in May 1964, ending twenty years of CCF rule. Ross Thatcher, who had become party leader in 1959, was a dynamic and autocratic leader who personally determined party policy until his death in 1971.[5] He was also described as a conservative ideologue[6] who had two political goals: the defeat of the socialist CCF-NDP, and the promotion of private enterprise.[7]

Following electoral victory in 1964, Liberal policy consisted of the promotion of private enterprise. This took the form of various government subsidies to the private sector. This strategy required substantial revenues; revenues which were to come, in part, from savings made in the operation of government services and enterprises. Thatcher realized a wholesale dismantling of CCF welfare programmes was politically inexpedient.[8] He therefore undertook to reduce the costs of service production without reducing the level of service provision. In July 1964, less than eight weeks after the Liberal rise to power, a three-man provincial Royal Commission on Government Administration was established to provide guidelines to achieve that objective.

The report of the Royal Commission, published in 1965, stated its main objective was "to endeavour to bring to government administration in Saskatchewan the understanding and the application of the techniques of modern management science."[9] It asserted that these techniques, "deliberately and consciously applied in an environment of responsible management, will result in least cost solutions to the requirements of government."[10] The "key to government productivity" was seen to reside in the "effective and efficient utilization of the human resource."[11]

The effective and efficient utilization of the human resource was of special concern for the DPH which, with 2,670 employees, was the largest and fastest growing government department. PSB alone employed 2,140 workers in 1964 — over 17 percent of all provincial government employees.[12] Furthermore, these workers were unionized, a situation with which the Liberals were unhappy. This dissatisfaction was derived from the feeling that the union contracts impinged upon management rights.[13]

The unions under the CCF-NDP had achieved a degree of power, *vis-à-vis* the government as employer, that was unusual in Canada. In fact, in 1964 Saskatchewan had the only unionized provincial civil service in Canada. This power had been used to establish a measure of control of the psychiatric labour process, which proved problematic from the point of view of some in-hospital management. The unions and the CCF government, however, had developed a basically cooperative working relationship so that, prior to

1964, the CCF government deemed it unnecessary, and indeed politically unwise, to attempt to curtail union power. Howard A. Scarrow, the executive secretary of the Commonwealth Studies Centre of Duke University, made a similar observation regarding public sector employer-employee relations under the CCF. Referring to the unionization of the civil service he stated:

> There is little doubt that the experiment in Saskatchewan has been eminently successful in providing a sound basis for a generally harmonious employer-employee relationship. The Government, though, like most employers reluctant to grant salary increases and other concessions, has shown no disposition to abandon the scheme . . . .[14]

The Liberals, however, had no political commitment to the unions. In fact, they felt strong unions were a problem, the root of which was the PSC:

> The Public Service Commission, as the agent of management in the government, has been the source of erosion of government management rights. The Commission has placed great emphasis on a mechanistic approach to employer-employee relationships covering everything from hours of work to compensation. Virtually no emphasis has been placed upon the development of the individual employee into a more responsible and successful human being.[15]

This paternalistic concern for the development of the individual employee was an ideological device to legitimate the Liberals' anti-union policies. For example, it was suggested that the most effective way to make an employee more responsible and successful was to revise management-worker relations in two respects: first by inserting a management rights clause into all union contracts, and second, by reducing the number of employees covered by collective agreements. The second objective was achieved by expanding the definition of management to include all supervisory personnel. The 1965 Royal Commission on Government Administration expressed these objectives as follows:

> First, the government must re-establish its right to manage its programs. Nowhere in any of the contracts does there exist a clause which specifies the retention of all rights of management not specifically bargained to the union. The lack of a 'management rights' clause is not typical of progressive union-management contracts.
>
> Second, most contracts between unions and organizations, specifically exclude individuals in management and confidential positions. . . . The wording of *The Trade Union Act* tends to define management as those having the authority to hire or fire. . . .
>
> It would . . . appear that the definition of a manager as one who achieves his organization's goals through the direction of the work of others would be more practical for the government service.[16]

The consequence of classifying all supervisory positions as out of scope allowed for the circumvention of union seniority rights in appointments, promotions and transfers, a goal PSB management had been trying to achieve for some time.

It was also recommended that "strong labour relations and bargaining skills be established within the Central Personnel Services Branch,"[17] in an attempt to offset union power. In addition, guidelines for a salary policy were recommended. The commission suggested that the government establish competitive pay scales, but added,

> *Your Commissioners do not believe that the government should be the leader in establishing salary levels but that it must be prepared to offer competitive salaries.*[18] [emphasis in original]

The Liberal government apparently heeded only the first half of this suggestion. Consequently, the chronic labour power shortages characteristic of PSB worsened throughout the 1960s. Even in the early part of the decade the shortage of adequate labour power was critical, especially at the senior level:

> It is clear that the problem of senior level classification and compensation is reaching *crisis* proportions in the Public Service of Saskatchewan. Unless appropriate adjustments to senior level salaries are made, there is

> indication that the public service will be unable to attract a continuing supply of competent individuals to maintain present and projected programs. Pressures generated by heavy market demand for highly competent, highly skilled personnel has bid away some of these people from the Saskatchewan Public Service. Intensified industrialization within the province, especially by national and international companies, will exert additional pressures.[19] [emphasis in original]

These fears were based upon the expectation that development of the provincial potash industry would have a multiplier effect on the economy and thereby lead to the diversification and increased industrialization of the province promised by the Liberals. This, however, did not happen, at least partially because the cycles of demand for potash roughly correspond to the demand for cereals. The industrialization of the provincial economy was therefore ephemeral. The shortage of labour power was not. Although labour power shortages were not caused by the Liberal government's antagonistic industrial relations policy and aggressive cost-cutting, they were certainly worsened by these, especially after 1966.

The Liberals denied they were hostile to trade unions but, as Smith has pointed out in his history of the provincial Liberal Party, "their record in labour legislation, highlighted by the passage in 1966 of legislation forcing striking workers in essential services back to work, persuaded few of Liberal sincerity on this score."[20]

The public sector unions, which had developed under the political umbrella of the pro-labour CCF, were naturally taken aback by these attacks on their power and autonomy. They soon found that without political backing, union power and rights were greatly curtailed. The unions were not prepared, either organizationally or politically, for these sustained attacks. Their negotiation and bargaining strategy had developed within a generally supportive political context created by the CCF. Consequently the unions undertook to persuade the government, through discussions and published articles, of "the need for fair and impartial procedures for settling disputes."[21]

The Liberal government interpreted this approach as a sign of weakness and further curtailed union power, a move for which the unions were again unprepared. Referring to a 1969 government decision to deny a union request for a conciliation board, the Saskatchewan Government Employees' Association was only able to express surprise and anger over the government's action: "we did not expect that the government's reply to our appeal for improved disputes procedures would be the suppression of the little that was available."[22]

Although the same article suggested union goals could be pursued via militant tactics, many were fearful of the consequences of such actions:

> if a peaceful request for a Conciliation Board is denied at the cost of setting the clock back 25 years [ie., to pre-1944 management-labour relations], what sort of repressive action would be visited on employees who, for example, withheld services or committed some lesser acts of protest which annoyed the government?[23]

The unions responded to this new tenor of management-union relations not by taking a militant stand butby developing a sophisticated approach to contract bargaining and negotiations. However, weakened as they were by the Liberal government, the unions were forced into a purely defensive role throughout the 1960s.

The Liberal government weakened the unions as part of an attempt to minimize resistance to its various cost-cutting measures. These included the implementation of a hiring freeze and the reduction of public sector salary ranges from fifty-five to twenty-five, as recommended by the 1965 royal commission.[24] The government also undertook to reduce the size of the total civil service by 2 percent. Some departments and branches, however, were harder hit than others. Between 1964 and 1971, for example, PSB had its total establishment reduced from 2,140 to 2,070, a reduction of 3.27 percent.

Even within PSB, however, these layoffs were not evenly distributed across occupational groups. There was a 49 percent increase in the number of psychiatrists and a 51 percent increase in the number of social workers employed by PSB throughout that period. Psychologists, however, were reduced by 11 percent, and psychiatric nurses by 16 percent. The new occupation of community psychiatric nursing, created in 1964, had fifty members by 1971 (see Table 6). This changing occupational structure corresponds to the continued transition from mental hospital to community psychiatry, a process which was greatly speeded by the aggressive pursuit of least-cost solutions. In particular, the depopulation of the mental hospitals received added impetus (see Table 7).

**Table 6**
**Changes in Selected PBS Staffing Levels, 1964 and 1971**

| Year | Total Positions | Psychiatrists | Social Workers | Psychologists | CPNS | Nursing Staff* |
|---|---|---|---|---|---|---|
| 1964 | 2,140 | 30 | 36 | 18 | 6 | 1,303 |
| 1971 | 2,070 | 59 | 73 | 16 | 50 | 1,086 |

*Includes nursing staff at the provincial institutions for the mentally retarded.
*Source:* Saskatchewan Department of Public Health, Annual Reports.

**Table 7**
**Reduction of Inmate Population, SHW, 1962-1966**

| Year | Total Inmate Population | Percentage Change |
|---|---|---|
| 1962 | 1,478 | 18.67 |
| 1963 | 1,202 | 33.78 |
| 1964 | 796 | 30.53 |
| 1965 | 553 | 9.40 |
| 1966 | 501 | |

*Source:* Saskatchewan Department of Public Health, Annual Reports.

**Depopulation and Protest**

The principle underlying depopulation was described by PSB management as the "resettlement in the community of institutionalized patients not requiring active in-patient psychiatric care."[25] This move to get chronic psychotics and geriatric patients out of the mental hospitals was done in one of three ways: patients were either discharged, placed on trial leave or boarded-out. The ideal for PSB management, both ideologically and financially, was to discharge the patients outright, since PSB had no financial responsibility for discharged patients. Responsibility for their care and maintenance devolved onto their families or some other government department, usually the Department of Social Services.

To the extent that it was not possible to discharge patients outright, PSB released them into approved homes. Under Section 28 of the 1961 Mental Health Act, PSB was authorized to pay a sum not exceeding sixty dollars per month to the operators of approved homes, for basic care and maintenance; for special care and maintenance, authorization was provided to pay an additional sum not exceeding forty dollars per month. Necessary drugs and clothing were also supplied and, in addition, five dollars per month could be paid to the patient for "comfort money."[26] In the case of patients returned to the community on trial leave while remaining on the register of the institution, PSB only assumed responsibility for their medical or psychiatric care, which consisted primarily of drugs. There was thus a financial incentive to discharge as many patients as possible, even if only for short periods.

The extent of the savings can be seen by comparing per diem costs for patients in SHW and approved homes. In 1969, for example, the cost of care and treatment at SHW was in excess of twenty dollars per day[27] while the daily cost per patient in an approved home was only about six dollars. An examination of the years 1964-67 (see Figure 18) indicates the potential cost savings were being realized. However, although the government was saving money, there were political costs incurred by the policy of rapid depopulation.

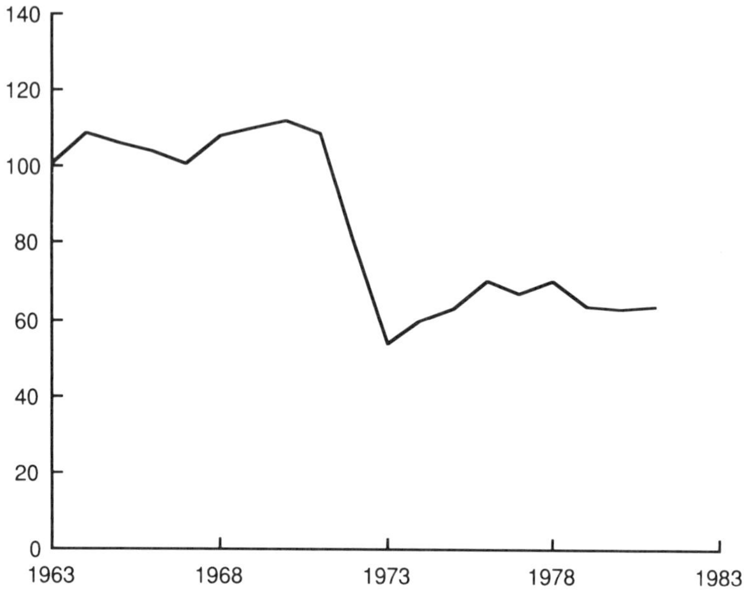


*Figure 18*
*Changes in PSB Budget Controlled for Inflation, 1963 to 1981*
*(Base 1963 Equals 100)*

*Source: Saskatchewan Department of Public Health Annual Reports; and Saskatchewan Public Accounts Committee Annual Report. Indexing to Inflation from Statistics Canada, Consumer Price Index.*

In the early stages these took the form of public criticisms of the programme.

The government responded by coopting the complainants. In early 1966, an eight-member Ad Hoc Committee on the Re-settlement of Mental Hospital Patients was established; four members of this committee were appointed by the minister of public health and four by the mayor of Weyburn.[28]

The establishment of this committee entailed a certain amount of political risk, especially given the strong representation of opponents to DPH policy and PSB practices, and concern to this effect was expressed within the cabinet. The minister of public health, however, thought the worst of the public criticism could be laid at the door of the CCF. Writing in 1966 to the minister of industry and commerce, the minister of public health stated: "We should . . . not be embarrassed that a look is being taken at the program since it has not materially changed since we became the government."[29] In addition, it was thought the political risks could be minimized by establishing the terms of reference for the committee.

The terms of reference were "to examine and make recommendations to [the minister of public health] with respect to the efficacy of the practical application of the admission and discharge policies of mental hospitals in Saskatchewan and in particular the Saskatchewan Hospital Weyburn. . . ."[30] By participating in the committee under these terms, some of the most vocal critics of the depopulation policy had been coopted into providing suggestions on how to improve the administration of that very policy.

The DPH further outmaneuvered the appointees from Weyburn by including two PSB-employed psychiatrists on the committee. These psychiatrists, one of whom was soon to become the director of PSB, preempted much substantive criticism of the depopulation policy by asserting that decisions regarding community placement were medical decisions, made on the basis of what was best for the patient. The effectiveness of this tactic is evident in the following comments taken from the report of the ad hoc committee:

> In presenting our findings we emphasize that, as a laybody, we do not feel competent to judge a professional program, but we feel obliged and privileged under the Terms of Reference to comment on our impressions of the various aspects of the program, both in its objectives and application. Where our opinions usurp professional prerogatives, we apologize.[31]

The PSB psychiatrists, by asserting depopulation was a medical prerogative, effectively precluded consideration of the two issues of major concern: fears for community safety, and the economic impact on the community of declining inpatient populations. Neither of these issues figured prominently in the committee's report, although both were clearly expressed in the submission of the Weyburn chamber of commerce to the committee. The chamber of commerce submission added:

> We are concerned too, with the impact this program is having on our commerce. We understand the hospital staff has been reduced by some 60 persons in the last year. This means a payroll loss of some $21,000 monthly, or $250,000 annually. And as the hospital patient load is reduced, certainly further drastic cuts can be expected in the staff.
>
> We of Weyburn fear history is repeating itself. Ten years ago, the Department of Public Health moved the training school out of Weyburn to Moose Jaw, taking some 300 workers out of our city. In terms of dollars and cents, our community lost a three-quarter million dollar payroll. In addition, about 1,000 persons left our community by way of staff members and their families.[32]

Given this as the principal concern and base of opposition, the efficacy of the DPH's cooptation strategy is seen in the final report of the ad hoc committee, which recommended "the Saskatchewan Plan . . . be fully and enthusiastically endorsed by the Government of Saskatchewan."[33]

The committee was endorsing the original plan for complete regionalization of psychiatric services. Depopulation, of course, had always been a part of that plan, but so had the continued existence of both mental hospitals. The enthusiasm of the Weyburn business community for the Saskatchewan Plan quickly dissipated when it was discovered that the Liberal government transformed it into a policy of complete depopulation and abandonment of the mental hospitals, starting with SHW. The decision to do this was based partly on experience gained at the Yorkton Psychiatric Centre.

## Community Psychiatry and the Yorkton Psychiatric Centre

The Yorkton Psychiatric Centre (YPC) became fully operational in 1964. When construction began in 1961, it was estimated that an additional 148 psychiatric beds would be required to serve the Yorkton region (1.8 beds per thousand population). This was a major downward revision from the 1957 Saskatchewan Plan estimate of five beds per thousand. This revised estimate was based on experience gained from the 1959 Swift Current mental health clinic pilot project. This pilot project, under the direction of Dr. Grunberg, "showed that many severely mentally ill patients could be cared for in the community if adequate follow-up services and community services could be provided, thus reducing the need and/ or the length of hospitalization."[34]

There were not enough trained community workers to provide adequate follow-up and community services. The shortage of trained labour power for the expanding community programmes, however, corresponded to the contraction of demand for in-hospital psychiatric labour power, particularly psychiatric nurses. The SPNA and the new coordinator of psychiatric nursing services used this opportunity to lobby successfully for the employment of psychiatric nurses in the community programmes. Partly as a result of this agitation, the occupation of community psychiatric nurse (CPN) was created in 1964.

One of the factors leading to the successful transition of psychiatric nurses from the mental hospitals to the community was the threat of political opposition. It has already been seen that the Weyburn and district business community were opposed to the depopulation of SHW. The psychiatric nurses were also opposed to this process because of the unemployment it brought in its wake (see Table 8). The Liberal government did not want these oppositional forces to coalesce. In order to silence opposition from the psychiatric nurses, it was decided to assuage their anxiety about job security by employing them to provide follow-up services to the mental patients placed in the community. The cost-conscious government not only thought this would quell criticism of the in-hospital psychiatric nurses, but also that it would provide cheap social workers for the community labour process and reduce underemployment in the mental hospitals. This process was described by a psychiatric nurse working at SHW at the time:

**Table 8**
**Staffing Levels for Psychiatric Nurses, SHW, 1964-1968**

| Year | Approved Positions | Number on Staff |
|---|---|---|
| 1964 | 643 | 621 |
| 1965 | 620 | 610 |
| 1966 | 600 | 571 |
| 1967 | 535 | 510 |
| 1968 | 479 | 464 |

*Source:* Memorandum, Administrative Assistant, to Minister of Public Health, Province of Saskatchewan, 1 October 1969, SAB, R-45, 98a (9-16). Grant Papers: Psychiatric Services, Weyburn Mental Hospital.

> what happened was, the re-admission rate . . . was fairly high, in the meantime, they are still pushing more and more chronics out, but they don't want to lay-off any nurses because the government . . . had enough bad publicity for doing this [ie., depopulating the mental hospitals], so they didn't want the nurses starting to scream they were losing their jobs because of the programs. Eventually, they had some good senior nurses that were sitting on their ass [*sic*] with literally nothing to do. So [the deputy minister of public health] said, "You people have nothing to do. Give those two nurses a car and tell them to go out and visit some of these chronics we are placing out there." And this is what happened. [It was] quickly realized that the re-admission rate on the hundred or two hundred that they were visiting quickly dropped compared to the general population. Consequently that sort of cemented their role. The same thing happened at Yorkton.[35]

The Yorkton psychiatric region was divided into five districts, each of which was assigned a community psychiatric team. These teams, consisting of a psychiatrist, a social worker and a CPN, provided follow-up services within a given district, and it was found that the number of people rehospitalized decreased, as did the duration of hospitalization and the number of patients being transferred from the Yorkton region to SHW.

By 1966 these findings further solidified the role of the CPN, and the community psychiatric team was established in all of the PSB facilities in southern Saskatchewan. "As a result," it was reported, "admissions to Saskatchewan Hospital Weyburn [were] drastically cut,"[36] from 833 in 1962 to about 350 in 1966. The establishment and expansion of employment opportunities for psychiatric nurses in the community not only helped to quiet the opposition from the SPNA, it also showed that the government was acting on the ad hoc committee's recommendations on mental patient resettlement. The acting director of PSB in 1966 commented to the deputy minister of public health that the committee's recommendation

> that there be more intensive follow-up and that more use be made of psychiatric nurses is . . . very well taken. We have already created 14 positions of community psychiatric nurses and we hope to increase this number as our needs in in-patient facilities diminish. As a matter of fact, the standard district psychiatric team should consist of a psychiatrist, a social worker and a community nurse.[37]

These district psychiatric teams also staffed the mental hygiene clinics. This was a change from the psychiatrist-social worker-psychologist division of labour recommended by Sigerist and Hincks. The CPNs were not, however, employed as substitutes for psychologists. Rather, they were employed as inexpensive social workers. That is, they were used to deskill psychiatric social work by providing follow-up services, domiciliary visits and so forth. The minimum educational requirement for social service workers, the lowest position in the social worker classification, was a baccalaureate. The training required to become a CPN was a three-week orientation course for RPNs. Thus there was a degradation of credentials. In addition, there was a clear difference in incomes. Although at the lower end of the social worker and CPN scales this only amounted to 5 percent, at the top end of the scales it was about 67 percent.[38]

The creation and employment of CPNs in this capacity slowed the rate at which psychologists were incorporated into the community psychiatric division of labour. As a result, it was not until the 1970s that the number of psychologists increased, and their influence was felt within PSB.

By 1966 it had been found that the community psychiatric team, working within the context of a boarding-out programme, could keep the in-hospital population at YPC well below the rated capacity of 148 patients. In fact, in the two years between 1964 and 1966, there had never been more than fifty in-patients at any one time. This fortuitous development led the DPH to change the rated bed capacity from 148 to sixty, and resulted in two buildings being abandoned as psychiatric facilities. One was subsequently used as the School of General Nursing for Yorkton Union Hospital, and the other converted to a geriatric unit operated by the Yorkton Union Hospital.[39]

Although the depopulation of the mental hospitals was a goal of the DPH, it had a negative effect on the per diem costs of the remaining psychiatric in-patients. These were commented on in a DPH report to the minister in August 1966. This report noted that if the rate of discharge from the two mental hospitals remained unchanged, as seemed likely given the effective removal of the two major sources of opposition,

> by 1970, 200 patients will be accommodated in Weyburn and 600 or less in North Battleford [and the] cost of providing in-patient care to the mentally ill in the mental hospitals, especially in Weyburn, will become prohibitive. . . . The whole costs for the care of the mentally ill in the mental hospitals are borne by the province. The federal government will only cost share in psychiatric units in general hospitals under the Hospital Insurance and Diagnostic Services Act.[40]

It was noted, however, that the federal government would also cost-share "if patients are on public assistance in special care or nursing homes under the Canada Assistance Plan."[41] Under the 1966 Canada Assistance Plan (CAP) the federal government agreed to pay half the cost of a number of services for which the provinces had previously been solely responsible, including health services, counselling, referral and assessment, daycare, homemaker services, care of persons in homes for the aged, nursing homes and many other kinds of special needs care.[42]

This was added incentive for the provincial government to develop community psychiatry; not only was it less expensive per service per patient than in-hospital treatment, but following the establishment of CAP many community-based facilities were eligible for 50 percent federal cost sharing. In particular, CAP provided a solution to the perpetual problem of chronic geriatric patients filling the large hospitals. They could be discharged into nursing homes and homes for the aged where, according to one provincial psychiatrist, they were often a welcome addition: "Many quiet schizophrenic patients were almost a boon to a nursing home. . . . so easy to look after."[43]

The owner and president of the Sherbrooke Nursing Home, Ltd. in Saskatoon echoed this view in a 1966 letter to the minister of public health: "I wholeheartily [*sic*] endorse your program of discharging these individuals into surroundings where they at least have a chance to recuperate and once again lead a normal life."[44] Although it is not clear that a highly tranquilized, chronic schizophrenic living in a nursing home would recuperate and lead a normal life, it is certain that a large number of drugged and docile mental patients were good for business.

However, the solution to one problem brings new ones in its wake. It was noted in 1966 that even if the mental hospital populations were greatly reduced, maintaining the institutions in any form would continue to be a non-shareable expense to the province. Referring specifically to SHW, for example, it was stated:

> Although with the reduction of patients, the direct variable operating costs can be reduced, the fixed costs will remain disproportionately high. It is estimated that by 1970 the budget of Weyburn can only be reduced from the present $3,698,000 to $2,382,000.[45]

The Liberal government, committed as it was to least-cost solutions, drew the logical conclusion: "There are, therefore, strong financial arguments for abandoning the mental hospitals replacing them by psychiatric units in general hospitals and reinforcing community psychiatric services."[46]

The creation of psychiatric units in general hospitals and the development of community psychiatric services had, of course, been an objective of the CCF between 1944 and 1964. Prior to August 1966, however, there had never been any intention of abandoning the large mental hospitals. It is true PSB management had from time to time mused about the possible disappearance of the large mental hospitals in their traditional form, but the basic goal of the Saskatchewan Plan had been to reduce inmate populations in the mental hospitals to rated bed capacities — 950 at SHW and 1,000 at SHNB — and then to utilize the physical facilities as medium-sized in-patient and regional psychiatric centres. Even given a concerted effort to reduce inmate populations, it had been thought that "the very large residue of chronic patients"[47] would necessitate the continued use of both hospitals.

The efficacy of the psychotropic drugs in producing manageable patients, combined with the existence of the CAP programme, made the complete depopulation of the mental hospitals financially irresistible. This, combined with the experience gained at YPC, led the provincial government to conclude in 1966 that "the 'Saskatchewan Plan' can work on the basis of .5 to .7 beds per thousand . . . probably the lowest ratio of psychiatric beds in North America and Western Europe."[48]

Within ten years the estimated psychiatric bed requirements had been reduced from five per thousand to .5 to .7 per thousand population. This marked the end of the plan to construct community mental hospitals contained in the original Saskatchewan Plan. It also created what private sector psychiatrists experienced as a shortage of psychiatric beds. Bitter conflicts between the private and public (PSB) sector psychiatry developed around this issue.

The decision to abandon SHW cannot be considered as part of a long-term plan or strategy for the development of psychiatric services. It was based on the principle of least-cost solutions, and in that sense it was indicative of the Liberals' approach to social services in general, and PSB in particular. Decisions concerning programme development or abandonment, staffing and training depended upon which option appeared to have greatest cost-saving potential at the time. This anarchy of cost-cutting resulted in PSB stumbling from one crisis to another throughout the 1960s. In the latter part of that decade, following their evaluation of PSB, Frazier and Pokorny stated:

> We failed to find evidence of long-range plans or projections. Despite lip service to the 'Saskatchewan Plan' it was clear that this plan has never been fully implemented. . . . Instead there has . . . evolved a makeshift transitional program [which] accounts for much of the confusion, conflict and disagreement about patient flow, admissions, discharges, and responsibilities.[49]

This is significant in terms of Wood and Kelly's observation that the existence of a management strategy, that is, a clear sighted statement of ends and means, cannot be assumed, but is an empirical question requiring demonstration.

Although the Liberal government did not have a detailed plan for psychiatry, the transition was unquestionably towards the contraction of mental hospital psychiatry and the further expansion of community psychiatry. This was also accompanied by the expansion of the provincial boarding-out programme and the creation of a system of approved homes. Between 1963 and 1971 these facilities increased in number from zero to 496. In 1971, 976 persons were accommodated in approved homes. Prior to 1966 "approved home" was something of a misnomer inasmuch as there were no criteria of approval. In light of the criticisms of the system of approved homes contained in the 1966 report of the Ad Hoc Committee on Mental Patient Resettlement, the DPH, in conjunction with the Department of Social Services, established limits on the number of occupants, minimum space requirements, and specified the requisite physical characteristics of the approved homes. There was no specification of minimum credentials for approved home operators, however, and no training provided by the DPH. As a result, no specialized psychiatric care and treatment was provided to resident mental patients.

Although the size and shape of facilities had changed, it is interesting to note that the ad hoc committee, having reviewed the approved home system, concluded that "in reality [these homes are] long-term custodial institutions."[50] It is ironic that the transformation of the mental hospital labour process from custody and care to therapeutic treatment resulted in a significant number of mental patients being discharged to new community-based, long-term custodial institutions where the primary care-givers were often unskilled and untrained guardians. It seems the transformation and skilling of the mental hospital labour process corresponded to a deskilling of part of the community psychiatric labour process; the substitution of the unskilled and inexpensive labour power of approved home operators for the relatively skilled and expensive labour power of mental hospital-based psychiatric nurses.

The fact that the approved homes were run on a commercial basis occasionally meant the quality of services provided was minimal. Operators, attempting to reduce costs, sometimes reduced services. Thus the quality of life for some mental patients in community placements was lower than it had been in the mental hospitals.[51] This tendency was noted and criticized by the CMHA:

> it appears that in certain communities where commercial enterprises are started to provide accommodation for former patients that some of these give adequate services, while others are exploiting the former patient by providing inadequate services while charging the full boarding rate.[52]

It is interesting to note that the development of approved homes marked the emergence of a twentieth-century variant of the private madhouses which had been prevalent in England throughout the eighteenth and nineteenth centuries.[53] The twentieth-century madhouses were not, however, particularly lucrative. The monthly rate for an approved home operator in 1971, for example, was $149.84 per person. This included room and board, drugs, transportation and other miscellaneous costs. Of the total number of persons placed in approved homes, PSB was only responsible for the costs of 7 percent; 62 percent were supported through the Saskatchewan Assistance Plan,[54] and 21 percent from their own resources. The remaining 10 percent were not psychiatric patients.[55] In addition, half the cost of the 7 percent for which PSB was responsible was paid by the federal government. Thus there was a clear financial incentive to expand community psychiatry.

The rapid growth in the number of approved homes, combined with the growth in the number of general hospital psychiatric in-patients (see Figure 19) belies Scull's continued insistence that decarceration entails a process of replacing institutional treatment with nothing.[56] When one adds to this the psychiatric patients in other community-based facilities,[57] such as group homes, nursing homes and geriatric centres, the simple empirical inaccuracy of his assertion becomes evident, and the *a priori* nature of his account clear. This is not to suggest the community facilities are necessarily adequate or effective, but that is quite distinct from the insistence that they do not exist.

The expansion of general hospital psychiatry, as part of the medicalization of psychiatric work, had a number of consequences for PSB-employed occupational groups, consequences which became evident to the psychiatric nurses first.

## Community Psychiatry and the Education of Psychiatric Nurses

The SPNA had endorsed the original Saskatchewan Plan in 1959 because the proposal to construct small community mental hospitals throughout the province appeared to provide the basis for expanded employment and job security. By the mid-1960s, however, it had become clear that the transmutation of the Saskatchewan Plan and the shift toward general hospital psychiatry could be accompanied by a decline in the demand for psychiatric nurses. It is ironic that psychiatric nursing, to the extent it contributed to the transformation of the psychiatric labour process and the development of community psychiatry, produced the conditions for its own possible demise.

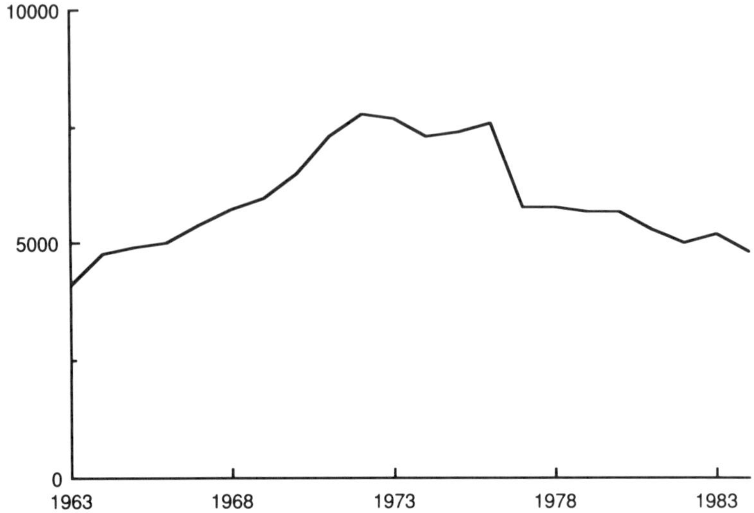


*Figure 19*
*Estimate of Volume of Hospitalization for All Psychiatric Diagnoses in General and Psychiatric Wards of General Hospitals, Saskatchewan, 1963 to 1984*
*Source: Saskatchewan Department of Public Health Annual Reports; Saskatchewan Hospital Plan Annual Reports*

The comments of the 1964 royal commission inquiry into nursing education in Canada heralded this demise: "In reviewing the 'psychiatric nurse' programme, and the function of the graduate, the perpetuation of such courses is questioned."[58] Referring to the shift to general hospital psychiatry, the report also stated:

> recent and proposed changes in the mental health field indicate the necessity for re-examination of the method of preparing practitioners in the area. One proposal for this group is that selected "psychiatric nurses" be given additional preparation through a formal education programme to qualify them as graduate registered nurses.[59]

Less than twenty years after their creation, the in-hospital training schools for psychiatric nurses were being declared obsolete. Furthermore, it was being suggested that following a period of extra training, psychiatric nurses could become registered nurses. It appeared the general nurses were close to eliminating psychiatric nurses as a distinct occupation. In fact, the SRNA had already established a supplementary training programme for RPNs in Saskatchewan, the birthplace of psychiatric nursing in Canada. Senior matriculation was required for admission to the programme, which lasted from twelve to fifteen months "depending upon the individual applicant's record."[60]

Although 80 percent of the province's psychiatric nurses were eligible for admission to this programme, the prospect of an additional year of unpaid training at their own expense was unappealing, or infeasible, for most psychiatric nurses. Many had chosen to enter the occupation for financial reasons. Prior to 1965, when the first of the major changes to the psychiatric nursing training programme took place, student nurses were paid about two hundred dollars per month and received subsidized room and board. It had thus been an attractive programme for those interested in nursing and/or the behavioural sciences but who, for financial or academic reasons, could not manage other forms of training.[61]

RPNs could also become certified nursing assistants within the general hospitals without taking a complementary course to be eligible for certification. However, this was not an appealing option for many psychiatric nurses, although it was noted that in 1965 "several have become certified as nursing assistants and are nursing in the general hospitals."[62] It appears employment as a certified nursing assistant was preferable to unemployment as an RPN.

Although a few psychiatric nurses made the transition to general hospital psychiatry, most did not. Thus, for most psychiatric nurses, conditions of work were characterized by a growing insecurity which was manifested in several ways, one of which was the emergence of a debate within the SPNA about dropping the term "nurse" from the occupational name.

As early as March 1964, the possibility of changing the occupational name to psychiatric therapist was suggested in the *Saskatchewan Psychiatric Nurse Newsletter* "as an aid to determining a professional role,"[63] an indication that the SPNA itself was beginning to address the issue. Dr.

McKerracher, the "father" of psychiatric nursing, had always opposed the appellation:

> It is to emphasize the importance of the mental hospital task and its difference from the present day requirements in the general hospital setting that I have always felt it would have been better if the ward staff in a mental hospital were called by some other name than "nurse". . . .[64]

Dr. McKerracher knew that the SRNA would not tolerate the independent existence of a nonaffiliated occupation using the title "nurse." In the mid-1940s, however, the psychiatric nurses were adamant, feeling the title bestowed status and prestige upon an occupation that had previously been shunned and vilified. For this reason many psychiatric nurses remained committed to the term:

> We must never forget that it is not our individual ideas of professionalism which determine our professional role, but it is the view and opinion of the public at large which determines the amount of respect given to any professional group as well as the role which the group is able to play in the professional world.[65]

Others, ostensibly not opposed to a name change, argued the timing was wrong: "wait until we get our Dominion Charter or even further an International Association of Psychiatric Nurses before we even think of changing our title. . . . the word Nurse is a passport to employment."[66] There were also those who had a clearer analysis and more accurately perceived the advantage of a name change:

> a change of name would very likely aid us in more easily identifying ourselves as a distinct profession, and consequently engender more professional pride and professional responsibilities. Many problems of the past and present have centred around arguments regarding the term Nurse; the R.N.'s have resented this as we would resent our own name being used by some new group.[67]

The name remained unchanged. As far as psychiatric nursing was concerned, however, it was the only thing which did. This internal debate was only one manifestation of the occupational insecurity confronting psychiatric nurses. The transition from mental hospital to community psychiatry had the effect of constricting the traditional job market. The rapid depopulation of SHW between 1964 and 1968, for example, corresponded to a reduction of RPN positions from 621 to 424.[68] The shrinking job market was accentuated by the fact that SPNA had not been able to establish reciprocity agreements with the four other provincial psychiatric nursing associations. Psychiatric nursing, as a distinct occupation, only existed in Manitoba, Saskatchewan, Alberta and British Columbia. As a result, significant employment opportunities did not exist in the rest of Canada. This restricted occupational mobility, and resulted in a degree of dependence which further heightened insecurity among psychiatric nurses and psychiatric nursing students, a fact noted in the final report of the 1964 Royal Commission on Health Services in Canada:

> Students who graduate from these programmes have a preparation limited to psychiatric nursing, and although they may be licensed in one of the four western provinces, they are essentially immobile. Students complain of this immobility and are bitter.[69]

In response to this dependence and the resultant dissatisfaction, the SPNA and the Co-ordinator of Psychiatric Nursing Programs at PSB headquarters began to restructure the psychiatric nursing curriculum. This was fully supported by PSB management and the DPH for two reasons: first, it was thought that making changes would reduce the widespread anxiety among psychiatric nurses and increase worker morale; and second, it was thought it might reduce the number of student dropouts and thereby ease the perennial shortage of labour power.

The first attempt to achieve these objectives was made in September 1965. At that time the 513-hour, thirty-six-month in-hospital training programme, originally established in 1946-47, was replaced by a pilot twenty-seven-month training programme. This programme was still provided in the mental hospitals and, although it was of shorter duration, it had been intensified by the inclusion of an additional ninety-five hours of lecture time. Student psychiatric nurses also became supernumerary to the PSB nursing service for a preclinical period of twelve weeks, and thus were not on payroll for the initial three-month period. Upon successful completion of the preclinical course work, however, they were employed as student psychiatric nurses for twenty-four months of clinical experience and further classroom instruction, at the rate of fifty dollars per month. This resulted in a substantial reduction in wage costs to the DPH. There was a further cost saving to the DPH insofar as the programme eliminated, within the initial three-month period, "those students who would fail later on academic grounds."[70] This was a significant consideration. Between 1958 and 1964 the average attrition rate was 60.1 percent. From the point of view of the DPH and PSB management, this represented a significant waste of resources.

Thus, to the PSB management and the DPH, there were real financial benefits to be gained from the restructuring of the psychiatric nurses training programme. For the SPNA, these changes were thought to be essential in order to help protect and extend employment opportunities for psychiatric nurses in the developing community programmes. This objective was made explicit in a brief presented to the 1965 Ad Hoc Committee on Nursing Education by the Coordinator of Psychiatric Nursing Programs at PSB:

> The recent trend to shift psychiatric patient services from the hospital base to the community base has placed new service demands on the psychiatric nurse. The educational programme now appears inadequate in the areas of the social sciences and community nursing, especially community nursing field experience.[71]

The committee had been established in November 1965 by the provincial minister of public health, in response to the recommendation of the 1964 Royal Commission on Health Services in Canada that "there be established in each province a Nursing Education Planning Committee."[72]

The committee was principally concerned with transforming the nature of general nursing education but, like the 1964 royal commission which preceded it, and out of which it arose, the committee critically scrutinized the psychiatric nursing training programmes as one of a number of training programmes for ancillary nursing personnel.

The ten-member ad hoc committee had three representatives from the SRNA and none from SPNA. This did not bode well for psychiatric nursing. The SRNA had opposed the existence of the occupation of psychiatric nursing since its inception. The committee provided the mechanism whereby the SRNA could strike at the source of its existence; the form and content of the psychiatric nurse training programme.

The committee's recommendation that a board of nursing education be established which would be responsible for all nursing programmes in the province was endorsed by the DPH. In 1966 the board of nursing education began to examine the feasibility of merging the psychiatric nursing education programme with the general nursing education programme, which was the financial responsibility of the Department of Education.

Although generally supportive of this transfer, the DPH and PSB management wished to ensure a continuous and adequate supply of psychiatric nurses until the mental hospitals were phased out, and this provided the psychiatric nurses with a respite:

> Since the Committee cannot assure the Minister of Public Health with absolute certainty that these conditions [i.e., an adequate number of psychiatric nurses] will be obtained in the new nursing education program in the immediate future . . . it is reluctant to unequivocally recommend the merging of the psychiatric nurse education program into the stream of general nursing education. . . . However, there is reason to believe that this merging might reasonably be accomplished in a few years.[73]

This increased the fear among psychiatric nurses that their existence was threatened, and they reacted accordingly. In 1967 the SPNA recommended to the minister of public health that, rather than coring psychiatric and general nursing education programmes, a committee on psychiatric nursing education programmes be established.

This proposed committee was to be made up of the co-ordinator of psychiatric nursing programmes, the supervisors of the schools of psychiatric nursing education, and three superintendents of nursing from psychiatric facilities. It was suggested the establishment of such a committee "would necessarily remove from the Board of Nursing Education jurisdiction to deal with matters pertaining to the education of psychiatric nurses."[74]

It was also suggested that this committee would have a number of advantages, including the guarantee of an adequate and continuing supply of psychiatric nurses. But, perhaps most important from the point of view of the SPNA, it was thought the formation of such a committee would

> provide the Psychiatric Nursing Profession and persons contemplating entering the profession with some degree of assurance of the continued existence of the Psychiatric Nurse as a distinct and specialized health worker. Such an assurance would, in our opinion, do much to restore morale among Psychiatric Nurses, who are naturally apprehensive about the future of psychiatric nursing.[75]

The DPH remained committed to its original position and the proposed committee on psychiatric nursing education programmes was not formed. The transfer and coring of the education programmes was finally completed in 1973.

In addition to the insecurity produced by the depopulation of the mental hospitals and exclusion from the rapidly expanding field of general hospital psychiatry, psychiatric nurses were confronted with the fact that PSB management, in the post-1964 period, had begun to deskill on-ward psychiatric nursing work. This was a reversal of policy. As has been seen, in 1961 the director of PSB had reported that no more than 10 percent of the on-ward staff were to be composed of untrained psychiatric aides. By 1969, however, psychiatric aides comprised at least 44 percent of the total nursing establishment at SHW.[76] This proportion of untrained to trained nursing personnel was slightly higher when the total number of PSB nursing establishments was considered, amounting to slightly more than 46 percent.

The implications of this were clearly seen by the SPNA. A 1969 submission to the minister of public health stated: "The purpose of this submission is to bring to the attention of the Department certain problems which have arisen with regard to the employment of Psychiatric Nurses Aides."[77] It went on to state that the merits of employing aides were recognized

> since they are able to perform certain unskilled, though important, duties which would otherwise have to be performed by a trained psychiatric nurse. Thus, the trained nurse is relieved of certain routine tasks and is able to devote his whole time and attention to the performance of those tasks for which he has been specifically trained.[78]

Qualified support was given for the principle of deskilling in-hospital psychiatric nursing in certain circumstances. What was of serious concern, however, was "the fact that aides are now performing on a regular basis, work which can only be safely and competently done by a trained psychiatric nurse."[79] These appeals had little impact.

PSB management and the DPH were not only deskilling on-ward work in the large mental hospitals, the same policy was being implemented in all PSB-run facilities. This produced a mutuality of interests between the SPNA and the SRNA. By the late 1960s the general nurses were employed alongside psychiatric nurses within all PSB facilities. Because of this, the SRNA was concerned about the deskilling of on-ward work. Thus the SRNA, in a 1967 submission to the minister of public health, stated that the

> ratio of professional (Registered Psychiatric Nurses and Registered Nurses) to non-professional should be 60 to 40 percent. As conditions permit, any change in this proportion should be in the direction of an increase in the professional staff.[80]

PSB management acknowledged receipt of the submission and continued the policy of deskilling. The tenuous alliance between psychiatric and general nurses failed to have any significant impact since the issue was of marginal importance to the SRNA membership, and therefore they were unwilling to pursue it with sufficient vigour to influence PSB management.

For the SPNA, on the other hand, it was a major issue, but due to an eroding power base and internal cleavages they were unable to mount an effective oppositional campaign. Ironically, the internal cleavage was a product of the success they had in gaining access to PSB's community psychiatric programmes. Thus, for CPNs, a small but expanding and influential segment of the SPNA, employment prospects were encouraging and job security looked assured.

The decision to employ psychiatric nurses in the community psychiatric labour process in 1964 was also a reversal of policy for PSB management and the DPH. The major factor underlying this reversal was the Liberal government's single-minded pursuit of least-cost solutions. Employing psychiatric nurses on the community mental health teams contributed to this cost reduction objective in two ways: first, it contributed to a reduction in the readmission rate, and thus increased the efficacy of depopulation as a cost-saving measure, and second, it contributed to an overall reduction in PSB's wage bill by deskilling psychiatric social work.

## Depopulation and Psychiatric Social Work

In the 1960s fully qualified social workers were a scarce commodity. Expanding community programmes throughout Canada and the United States resulted in a strong market position for MSWs; a situation they attempted to turn into a position of strength within PSB. The occupational power of MSWs was mediated by a number of factors, including small numbers, geographical dispersion and lack of occupational identity among non-MSW social workers. This last factor was the product of diverse educational backgrounds of psychiatric service workers — the fastest growing category of PSB-employed social workers throughout the 1960s (see Table 9). This group, which had no specific social work training, was composed of people trained to the baccalaureate level with various backgrounds in the social sciences. Commenting on his experience in 1968, for example, one PSB-employed social worker stated:

**Table 9**
**Psychiatric Services Branch, Psychiatric Social Work Staff, 1962-1971**

| Year | Number of Psychiatric Service Workers | Number of BSW Social Workers | Number of MSW Social Workers | Total Number Employed | Number of Est. Pos. | Year End Vacancies |
|---|---|---|---|---|---|---|
| 1962 | 8 | 3 | 13 | 24 | 32 | 8 |
| 1963 | 10 | 4 | 16 | 30 | 36 | 6 |
| 1964 | 9 | 4 | 17 | 30 | 39 | 9 |
| 1965 | 9 | 6 | 22 | 37 | 38 | 1 |
| 1966 | 13 | 5 | 20 | 38 | 42 | 4 |
| 1967 | 16 | 6 | 14 | 36 | 47 | 11 |
| 1968 | 28 | 6 | 19 | 53 | 60 | 7 |
| 1969 | – | – | – | – | 73 | – |
| 1970 | – | – | – | – | – | – |
| 1971 | 29 | 4 | 29 | 62 | 75 | 13 |

*Source:* Memorandum, Director, Psychiatric Services Branch, Province of Saskatchewan, to Minister of Public Health, Province of Saskatchewan, 27 January 1969, SAB, R-45, 87b. Grant Papers: Psychiatric Services Staff; and Saskatchewan Department of Public Health Annual Reports.

> I got a job with the [Psychiatric Services] Branch because I didn't know what else to do with a BA in sociology and psychology — you know, you are a misfit in the world . . . anyway I sent out several applications with my BA, and someone suggested that I apply to [the Department of Public] Health — I didn't know about Health, I didn't know about social workers — I didn't know what a social worker was! It certainly wasn't a life-long design that I always had . . . to become a social worker. . . . It wasn't until five years after I was in the service I even knew what a social worker was I suppose.[81]

Within the context of rapidly expanding community programmes (see Figure 20), this lack of occupational identity also contributed to a degree of interoccupational cooperation between CPNs and social workers that lasted until the end of the decade. Even though CPNs were being employed as inexpensive substitutes for social workers, they were not

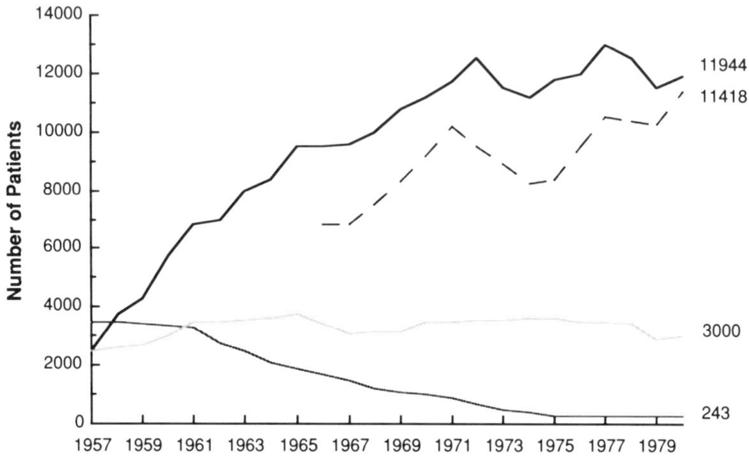


*Figure 20*
*Changes in Psychiatric Service Patterns Between 1957 and 1980 in Saskatchewan**

*Code:*

- *Total Community Clients**
- *Number of Patients in Mental Hospitals*
- *Total Admissions to All Psychiatric Facilities**
- *Community Client Contacts (divided by 10)*

**Includes University Hospital (1957-1977)*
*Source: Saskatchewan Health Annual Report 1980-81*

initially perceived as a threat to job security. In fact, social workers generally welcomed CPNs as a much needed source of help, especially given their knowledge of the effects of psychotropic drugs. A PSB-employed social worker stated: "I don't know, looking back, how it [Social Work within PSB] was a whole lot different than Psychiatric Nursing . . . except that Psychiatric Nurses knew more about medications and they could anticipate what certain behaviours might be caused by, something which we didn't know."[82]

By the end of the decade this interoccupational harmony was beginning to dissipate. Management, in an attempt to rationalize PSB, was forcing the various occupational groups to clarify their roles and functions. Social workers were particularly concerned to distinguish, and protect, themselves from CPNs and psychiatrists.[83]

In 1969, for example, a paper presented to the Chief Social Workers annual meeting pointed out:

> our profession is now being challenged to define its role; especially since lately the term 'Social Psychiatry' has become in vogue, first with the doctors and through them with the Community Nurses. The doctors have had enough of being prescription writers and the Nurses of mothering hopeless chronics, and who can blame them? *But in the meantime we find ourselves sandwiched between two disciplines who are both vying for half our pie.*[84] [emphasis added]

The author went on to express concern for the continued viability of social work within PSB, unless a new strategy in the battle for position was adopted. Interestingly, the strategy proffered was the voluntary deskilling of social work. This was to be accompanied, however, by an increase in the control and autonomy of MSWs. The system proposed was, in fact, similar to the internal contractor system prevalent in many British industries before the turn of the century.[85]

The social workers suggested there should only be two MSWs per region. This, it was argued, would allow for the reclassification of "the many vacant M.S.W. positions to service worker positions."[86] The money thus saved could then be transferred to the remaining MSW positions in order to "attract and maintain the best M.S.W.s."[87]

This was thought to be a viable solution due to the fact that at the time the schools of social work around the country were beginning to turn out students with Bachelors of Social Work (BSW) who were "purported to be super clinicians. . . ."[88] Thus, PSB-employed MSWs suggested BSWs could be hired to perform clinical work as effectively, but less expensively than MSWs. Elaborating upon the implications of this, it was stated:

> This means that the role for M.S.W. (which I have foreseen for sometime now) will be: to design new programs, test their effectiveness, design new ways to train non-M.S.W.s for these programs, train the non-M.S.W.s and then turn the job over to them; something

> like a 'responsible social work officer' delegating his work to others.[89]

It was recognized, however, that delegating one's work to others could be dangerous. First, it might result in a further dilution of occupational identity and solidarity, thereby reducing occupational power, and second, effective substitution threatens the position of the more expensive occupation. As a solution to the first potential problem, it was suggested that a new management position be created and filled by an MSW. The proposed provincial training and research officer was to have as one function the task of ensuring that all

> non-M.S.W.s . . . acquire at least enough training in psychiatric social work to know what social work is all about in the framework of psychiatry, and to ensure that their loyalty to our profession as distinct from being confused [*sic*] with Nursing, Psychology or Psychiatry.[90]

The proposed solution to the second problem was to secure complete control over the practice of social work. Thus, it was suggested that "each Chief Social Worker should have the power to hire and dismiss non-M.S.W.s from his or her department."[91] These powers, which clearly usurped traditional management prerogatives, were thought to be necessary for two interrelated reasons:

> (1) the M.S.W. must remain in control and as any businessman or orientation course in management will tell, the authority to dismiss staff is an essential factor in maintaining control.
> (2) the Civil Service is a notorious resting place for accumulating dead wood, and without the authority to dismiss we may get ourselves into hopeless situations of incompetency and ineptness.[92]

It was precisely for these reasons, however, that the DPH would not concede the right to hire and fire to the social workers. It is ironic the social workers were suggesting to the Liberal government that they be given the right to self-management. It was the Liberal government which, only a few years earlier, had inserted a management rights clause into all collective agreements. Moreover, the other PSB-employed occupations would be unlikely to support self-management for social workers unless they too were granted similar powers, the effect of which would have been the elimination of PSB management in its traditional form. PSB management and medically trained psychiatrists were, of course, opposed to these suggestions and they were not implemented.

As the struggles for autonomy and job security continued, the occupational solidarity of the social workers increased and, within the context of expanding community programmes, resulted in an increase in occupational power. The continuing struggles of social workers for occupational autonomy, especially from domination by medically trained psychiatrists, produced a crisis of management which had significant consequences for the organization of psychiatric work. By the early 1970s these struggles for autonomy and security had turned into a conscious attempt to de-medicalize community psychiatric work.

## Community Psychiatry and Psychiatrists

Accompanying the expansion of community psychiatry was a reduction of psychiatric in-patient beds. In a further attempt to reduce costs, in-patient staff were cut and wages were frozen for all public sector employees, including psychiatrists. This aggravated the problem of recruitment and retention for all categories of labour power, but especially psychiatrists. Those psychiatrists who were employed complained bitterly about working conditions and salaries. One of the vehicles for this discontent was the SPA.

In a September 1967 memorandum to the minister of public health, the deputy minister discussed the timing and content of a proposed meeting with the SPA:

> I am sure that their major concern will be the number of vacancies in the Psychiatric Services and that they will argue that this can only be rectified by making working conditions more comparable [to those in other provinces]. Certainly, Saskatchewan has gone backwards when compared with other provinces over the last three or four years.[93]

The extent and implications of this backsliding were made known to the premier in a November 1967 memo from the minister of public health. Included with this memo was a copy of an Ontario government advertisement which offered a certified specialist in psychiatry an annual income of $18,000 to $22,000 with four weeks holiday per year. In Saskatchewan the salary range was $15,260 to $18,550 with three weeks annual vacation. The minister of public health concluded: "I can assure you that this difference makes it next to impossible to recruit anyone."[94]

The few fully qualified psychiatrists who were employed became increasingly critical of DPH's management of the community psychiatric programmes. The following submission to the DPH from a psychiatrist who had just resigned describes the working conditions at the YPC, once considered the crown jewel of the Saskatchewan Plan and community psychiatry:

> we are practicing conveyor belt psychiatry with overloaded staff offering only minimal support and treatment. Patients and staff are becoming quite dissatisfied and risks are being taken because of the impossibility of arranging follow-up of patients.[95]

The shortage of labour power was so serious the director of PSB expressed the fear that it might be necessary to close several community psychiatric facilities, including YPC:

> Troubles of the Psychiatric Services Branch are coming to a head and it would be well to point out to the Minister the likelihood of having to close facilities. The most pressing problem is the shortage of psychiatrists; who can get better conditions of service elsewhere. What the reaction of the public will be to closing such facilities as Yorkton [Psychiatric Centre], I do not know, but it would be well if the Minister were to consider this possibility now before the decision is actually forced upon us.[96]

It must be recognized these dire predictions were part of a bargaining strategy on the part of PSB-employed psychiatrists to improve incomes and conditions of employment. The fact that no PSB facilities closed is indicative of this. On the other hand, income levels and conditions of employment which resulted from Liberal policy had produced a real personnel crisis. Contributing to this crisis was the fact that by the mid-1960s private practice psychiatry had become not only possible but quite lucrative.

## Private Sector Psychiatry

The increased urbanization of the province and the establishment of the Medical Care Insurance Commission (MCIC) by the CCF in 1962 created the material base upon which private sector psychiatry developed.[97] With the inclusion of psychiatric services in the insured service structure, private practice physicians became increasingly interested in the organization and management of psychiatric facilities throughout the 1960s.

One issue of particular concern was the admission and discharge policies in place at PSB-operated facilities, to which private practitioners were experiencing considerable difficulty in having their patients admitted. This was due not only to the decision to reduce drastically the number of psychiatric beds, but also to the rigid admissions policy which had been implemented as part of the strategy to depopulate and close the two provincial mental hospitals. There was also some concern expressed by private sector psychiatrists that they were not being consulted regarding the discharge of their patients, many of whom, when released, were described as grossly psychotic and physically violent.[98]

Those in private practice considered this lack of communication regarding the release of patients, and the difficulty of having patients admitted to PSB facilities, as government interference and usurpation of professional prerogatives. Private practitioners thus attempted to pressure the DPH to change its admissions and discharge policies. This lobbying was pursued through the SCPS, which suggested that better communication be established between the public and private sectors.[99] The minister of public health responded that he would welcome such a development, but he added he was aware "that until very recently the medical profession showed very little interest in mental illness, and considered emotional disorders as a nuisance rather than a disease in the real sense of the word."[100] He was referring to the pre-medicare days when many physicians dumped troublesome psychiatric patients into the large mental hospitals, and his tone did little to relieve tensions, especially given the steadfast commitment of the DPH to the prevailing admissions and discharge policies. Thus the conflict between the DPH and the private psychiatrists escalated.

As part of the struggle for access to psychiatric beds, the SCPS threatened to discontinue issuing temporary permits to practice to unlicensed PSB psychiatrists. These two-year permits were granted to psychiatrists with credentials not recognized by the SCPS. The permit holders were allowed to practice psychiatry as employees of PSB, but they could not enter private practice. The DPH had become almost completely dependent on unlicensed psychiatrists; in 1969, only six of sixty-nine psychiatrist positions were filled by fully licensed psychiatrists. Had the SCPS stopped granting permits, PSB undoubtedly would have collapsed. For political reasons the government could not allow this and consequently began to negotiate over the concerns of the private sector regarding admissions and discharge procedures.

PSB management-psychiatrists attempted to transform this pressure from the private sector on the DPH to their own advantage. In the late 1960s PSB management-psychiatrists and the SPA (most of whose members were still PSB psychiatrists) argued that the only way to deal with this conflict was to increase public sector psychiatrists' incomes substantially and otherwise improve their working conditions. This would supposedly solve the problem of recruitment and retention of fully qualified psychiatrists and reduce DPH reliance on the SCPS for temporary permits to practice, thereby eliminating private sector leverage. PSB management made a number of specific recommendations for improving working conditions. Among these were the creation of a better superannuation plan, the extension of the annual vacation period to four weeks, and permission to allow part-time private practice outside working hours.[101] With regard to this last recommendation, it was pointed out that "this would only really be attractive to fully licensed and fully qualified psychiatrists and would provide them with a great incentive to stay."[102]

Only Alberta and Saskatchewan did not allow private practice privileges for provincially employed psychiatrists.[103] The director of PSB argued to the DPH that the granting of part-time private practice privileges to provincially employed psychiatrists was unlikely to result in a conflict of interest, and that "with proper controls it can work successfully and more service from existing qualified personnel can be obtained. . . . [and] physicians like it because it makes them similar to their colleagues in private practice."[104]

It was thought that the extension of part-time private practice privileges to PSB-employed psychiatrists would help to solve the labour power shortage, and would also result in increased overall productivity in the private sector. This in turn would reduce the number of patients treated in the public sector and thereby the cost incurred by PSB. The director of PSB, as a psychiatrist, fully endorsed the suggestion, although in his capacity as a manager he expressed some concern regarding the possibility of a negative response from the growing number of already disgruntled psychiatrists in private practice.

Another worry of PSB management was that the extension of the right to part-time private practice to psychiatrists would set a precedent which could then be used by other occupational groups to achieve the same rights. Due to the struggles for occupational autonomy which were beginning to take place, it was particularly feared that social workers would make similar demands. Management's fears were assuaged by the response to a 1969 nationwide survey of all provincial psychiatric services systems, which revealed no private psychiatry opposition in provinces where part-time private practice was allowed. Similarly, it reportedly had no "effect on other government professionals."[105] The positive results of the survey, and the fact that there was no private sector opposition, led PSB management to endorse the proposal. DPH officials, however, opposed it.

It has been seen that management is not a unified monolith characterized by a consensus on all issues.[106] Thus, the DPH recommended that the provincial Budget Bureau reject the part-time private practice proposal for PSB psychiatrists, not because they did not believe it would provide an inducement to attract more qualified staff, but because they feared "it would dilute the total effort directed to the Department's main objective."[107] The main objective was cost reduction, which was to be achieved by depopulation and prevention of hospitalization. The mounting demand of private sector psychiatrists for more and easier access to psychiatric beds was in conflict with this objective. The DPH, fearing a conflict of interests, was therefore disinclined to encourage this growing demand by allowing part-time private practice privileges for their own employees.

Also, to the extent that part-time private practice would have attracted more qualified staff, it would have resulted in additional salary costs. Since the main objective was cost reduction, there was little incentive for the DPH to adopt the part-time practice proposal. The rejection of this recommendation resulted in an escalation of intramanagement tensions and conflicts.

Added to these conflicts was the reemergence of public criticism of the psychiatric programmes. The most damning criticisms came from Weyburn, particularly from former members of the 1966 Ad Hoc Committee on Mental Patient Resettlement, who felt they had been duped into supporting the Liberals' transmogrified version of the Saskatchewan Plan.

One of the Weyburn appointees, the editor of the local newspaper, attacked the Liberal government. One editorial, entitled "And don't blame the CCF," suggested the Liberals' version of the Saskatchewan Plan, and especially the decision to close SHW, was based on crass financial and careerist considerations:

> The provincial government . . . has taken advantage of the psychiatrist's zeal to prove a point in order to save a few million dollars by closing an institution which had become renowned for its treatment of the mentally ill.[108]

The editorial compared acceptance of the new Saskatchewan Plan to the social and personal tragedy produced by the "premature release of thalidomide. . . . You might say that the Thatcher government has committed social thalidomide — not to mention political suicide when the people of this province discover how monstrous is the deed that has been done."[109] The editorial also provided pointed criticisms of the actual operation of community psychiatry:

> mental patients are pumped full of drugs which keep them from becoming violent, handed a supply of medicine for future use, and dumped into private homes where, in most cases, they have no trained supervision, no recreation, and in many instances, inadequate facilities.[110]

In mid-1967, the mass murder of a family of nine at Shell Lake by a recently released mental patient generated widespread fear and galvanized the oppositional forces. The government could no longer dismiss criticisms as the self-seeking wailings of sectional interests. Forced to react, the government instituted an independent investigation of PSB and its policies. To that end, Dr. Shervert H. Frazier of Texas, assisted by his associate, Dr. Alex D. Pokorny, conducted a series of public and private meetings throughout the province in October and November 1967.

## The Frazier Report

The terms of reference for the Frazier inquiry were:

1. To review the program of the Psychiatric Services Branch of the Saskatchewan Department of Public Health with particular reference to:
   (a) Admission and discharge criteria of the inpatient facilities.
   (b) The quality of psychiatric treatments.
   (c) The adequacy of outpatient care provided by the facilities, with particular reference to the follow-up of discharged patients.
   (d) Any undesirable practice, occurring within the context of the specific objectives of the program.

2. To make any other relevant observation and recommendations.[111]

Although supportive of the principles of community psychiatry, the Frazier Report was extremely critical of many of the specifics of the Saskatchewan programme. In particular, the report was critical of the lack of management planning and objectives, underfunding, understaffing and the failure to encourage community participation.

Understaffing was considered the most serious problem, especially with regard to the community programmes:

> It was in this area that we found the most serious problem. In our opinion, the Psychiatric Services Branch is in the midst of a *personnel crisis.* Many staff people have already left the program and others are considering leaving. This problem is the most severe with psychiatrists, psychologists, and social workers, but also involves psychiatric nurses and other categories. It should be stressed that emphasis on home placement, depends on a certain irreducible number of field personnel to carry out, direct, and supervise the program. If the available staff drops below this number, the whole system will break down, patients will have to be returned to large institutions, etc. Unfortunately it is possible to operate a large institution with substandard staffing; the resulting conditions may be terrible but the entire operation is out of sight and may therefore be tolerated. When patients are living in the community and widely dispersed, the system will not function without sufficient staff, and the resulting deterioration in patient condition will be so visible to the community that it will no doubt be intolerable.[112] [emphasis in original]

Frazier also suggested that the "low morale due to staff shortages, and lack of definite goals"[113] was contributing to the high rates of turnover and attrition among PSB workers. In 1967, for example, seventeen senior psychiatrists and several junior psychiatrists quit, the number of MSWs dropped from twenty-six to thirteen, and there was a net loss of psychologists.

Frazier was unequivocal concerning the responsibility for this situation:

> One of the most recent influences [leading to the personnel crisis] has been a gradual financial squeeze on the Branch. Salaries have fallen behind, and the leaders of the program began to leave. Furthermore, community psychiatry began to catch on in other provinces and the U.S., so that veterans of the Saskatchewan program were in increasing demand. The Province has gradually drifted into a situation in which it is trying to run a first-rate program on a second rate budget, and this simply will not work. As a result, quality of care is slipping, duties are being reassigned to less qualified personnel, caseloads are increasing, and work days are becoming longer, all contributing to demoralization. At the present time the personnel situation is of crisis proportions and must be given first priority.[114]

Thus, the deskilling and intensification of the psychiatric labour process was contributing to the high rates of staff turnover and attrition which was threatening the capacity of PSB to continue to produce psychiatric services.

Frazier made a number of specific recommendations for dealing with this crisis. These included a 25 percent salary increase for psychiatrists, about 20 percent for social workers, 15 percent for psychologists and 10-15 percent for psychiatric nurses. In addition, it was recommended that the ceiling be removed from the pension plan and an "additional rural differential . . . be paid to those working away from urban centres."[115]

Frazier was also critical of the lack of in-patient facilities: "Despite lip service to the 'Saskatchewan Plan,' it was clear this plan has never been fully implemented."[116] As has been seen, the original Saskatchewan Plan had been abandoned by the CCF government by 1958, when it was found that community mental hospitals would not be eligible for federal funds under the terms of the Hospital Insurance and Diagnostic Services Act. As an alternative, the CCF had opted for psychiatric units in general hospitals which were eligible for federal cost sharing. This alternative was still referred to, however, as the Saskatchewan Plan. Under the Liberals, the search for least-cost solutions led to the abandonment of psychiatric units in favour of having private practice GPs provide psychiatric services for those requiring hospitalization in general wards of general hospitals. This was the approach advocated by McKerracher after 1960. It amounted to a plan for the complete privatization and medicalization of psychiatry in the province. From the point of view of a cost-conscious government, McKerracher's plan had obvious advantages; it eliminated the cost of constructing separate psychiatric facilities, but more importantly it eliminated the on-going expense of staffing and managing those facilities. Thus even psychiatric units which had been constructed, such as the Prince Albert Psychiatric Centre (PAPC), were not opened right away.

As has been seen, general ward GP psychiatry was opposed by private practice psychiatrists because it resulted in a shortage of psychiatric beds. It was also opposed by psychiatric nurses who feared unemployment, and by PSB management-psychiatrists who feared it would eventually result in PSB (and their careers) withering away.

PSB management, therefore, enthusiastically embraced Frazier's suggestion that in-patient psychiatric services "should be centered in psychiatric units of General Hospitals."[117] Commenting on this recommendation and its relationship to McKerracher's plan, the director of PSB stated in a February 1968 memo to the minister of public health:

> If costs are to be kept down, then the urban system [of psychiatric services] must be controlled by the Department of Public Health. If the philosophy of private enterprise in psychiatry is preferred then the plan suggested by Dr. McKerracher should be adopted. The main problem with it is the very considerable expense and the fact that it is most improbable that the plan will take care of the whole psychiatric population. What is likely to happen if the McKerracher Plan is adopted is that there will be a growth in the private sector of psychiatrists dealing mainly with the milder neuroses while the more severe cases will still be taken care by the government units. *This means that the cost of*

> *psychiatric care is likely to sharply rise.*[118] [emphasis in original]

Thus it was clear to PSB management that the complete medicalization and privatization of psychiatry had to be opposed since it would reduce public sector in-patient facilities to expensive psychiatric warehouses for chronic psychotics, basically what they had been in the pre-World War II period.

Prior to 1968 the Liberal government had no specific plan for psychiatric in-patient facilities. Cost-reduction was the only guiding principle. In that year, however, the federal government implemented a medical care insurance programme which provided for fifty-fifty cost sharing of all medical costs.[119] For Saskatchewan, this meant the cost of private practice psychiatric services had been halved. With this economic incentive, private practice psychiatry became a growth industry (see Figure 21). In fact, psychotherapy was the fastest growing category of service provided by private sector medical practitioners.

After 1968, therefore, the Liberal government finally had a plan for psychiatry: complete privatization of psychiatric in-patient services and a further cheapening of out-patient community services.

With this in mind, the government turned its attention to Frazier's criticism of the lack of community involvement in the community psychiatric programmes. With regard to this, the DPH thought the CMHA could be usefully involved through the operation of an expanded system of White Cross centres. These were drop-in social and recreational centres for ex-mental patients which the CMHA had been operating since 1955. Relations between the government and the CMHA had become strained, however, largely due to CMHA criticism of PSB. As a result, there was little coordination of activities between PSB and the CMHA. Commenting on this in a memo to the minister of public health, the deputy minister observed "I am afraid the Department for some years has encouraged this state of affairs by taking somewhat of a hostile attitude towards the Association."[120] Although the government wanted to change that, it was felt a satisfactory

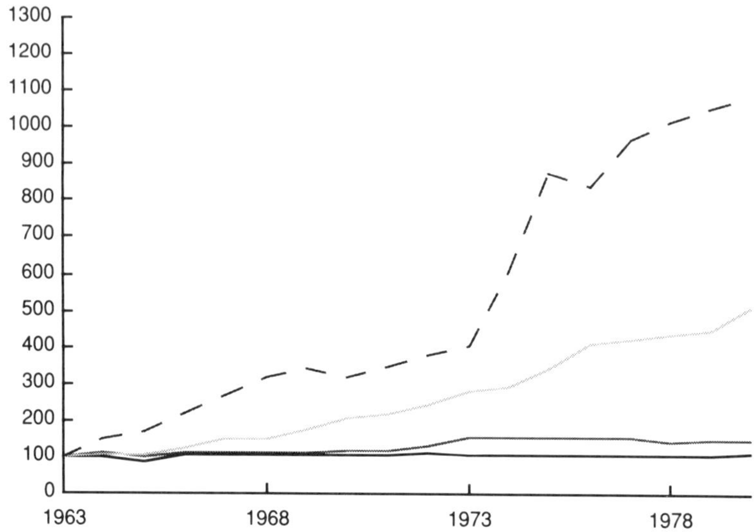


*Figure 21*
*Annual Percentage Change in Services Per 1000 Beneficiaries for Selected Types of Services Provided by Private Practice Physicians (Base 1963 Equals 100)*

*Code:*

——— *Psychotherapy**
……… *Consultations*
═══ *Office Visits*
— — — *Home and Emergency*

**1975 increase in services is in part due to the fact that effective 1 May 1975 the method of counting these services by Family Practitioners was revised to fifteen minute units from thirty minute units.*
*Source: Saskatchewan MCIC Annual Reports*

working arrangement was impossible so long as the incumbent executive director, a salaried employee of the CMHA, retained his position. However, it was noted that

> Because of the financial independence of this agency [it had been agreed at a meeting of DPH officials] it would be imprudent to take too aggressive a stand [on the issue of replacing the incumbent Executive Director] since we very much desire their assistance and support in developing White Cross Centres across the province.[121]

The financial independence of CMHA had derived from its large membership, but by the late 1960s two factors combined to undermine this membership base and hence the CMHA's autonomy. The first was the success of the CMHA in achieving its initial goal of improving conditions in the provincial mental hospitals. It had been relatively easy to mobilize public support for the cleaning up of the snake pits. By 1968 the depopulation policy had successfully eliminated the problem of overcrowding and with it the highly emotive issue upon which the CMHA had built its membership and financial autonomy. The second contributing factor to the reduction of the financial autonomy of the CMHA was its involvement in the direct provision of psychiatric services in the form of White Cross centres. Although the first White Cross centre opened in Regina in November 1955, the number rapidly expanded as the rate of discharge from the mental hospitals increased. As a result, the CMHA was operating on a deficit budget by the late 1960s.

It was at this Achilles heel that the DPH struck. The deputy minister of public health suggested that the CMHA be offered a dollar-for-dollar matching grant for the expansion of its White Cross centre programme if the executive director was replaced.

It was recognized that this kind of direct interference in the internal affairs of a non-government association could have negative political consequences. The deputy minister therefore suggested the executive director could be hired by PSB if he was dismissed from the CMHA. It was felt that this would remove him as an obstacle to the government's plans, and would reduce the chances of his dismissal becoming a public issue:

> I believe that the [executive director of CMHA] is a qualified social worker and we could possibly absorb him into the service. This would undoubtedly cause difficulties but these would be minor compared to the difficulties he is presently creating.[122]

In order to get the matching grants, the executive officers of the CMHA board of directors decided to fire the "troublesome" employee, but did so somewhat clumsily. Commenting on this to the minister of public health, the deputy minister stated:

> While I am not surprised that they made the decision to dismiss him, I was very surprised that they went about it the way they did, especially since I gave them every opportunity to consult with us so that a satisfactory resolution could be reached if they decided to dismiss him.[123]

The executive director was angry about losing his job, especially when he was told the reason was partly due to "situations for which no one was to blame,"[124] and partly due to the fact "the government was annoyed with him."[125] He requested that the government establish an impartial inquiry into the operation of the CMHA. He suggested this would not only "help settle the many difficulties and conflicts that the Saskatchewan Division appears to be encountering" but it would also "absolve the CMHA staff and officers of the suggestion of poor administration . . . and most likely give some recommendation to avoid undue influence by government officials."[126]

The government refused this request and, although displeased with the lack of finesse displayed by the CMHA board of directors, remained committed to its original position:

> I think that an action like this had to come if the CMHA is going to operate in a businesslike fashion. My only regret is that CMHA were unable to carry out the housekeeping change without the trauma and backbiting that is obviously going to follow.[127]

Through the manipulation of the CMHA's board of directors, the DPH came to exert considerable influence in the development and operation of social and recreational centres for ex-mental patients in the province without incurring major operational or administrative expenses.

This coordination and integration of CMHA volunteer work into PSB's programme of community psychiatry can also be interpreted as a further deskilling of community psychiatric work. Under this arrangement volunteer workers rather than PSB employees organized and supervised social and recreational activities, thus effectively reducing the cost of producing psychiatric services.

The government's domination of the CMHA increased throughout the first half of the 1970s as the CMHA increasingly came to rely on government grants for its operations. As a consequence, the CMHA ceased to be a major force shaping the development of psychiatric services in the province and instead became an inexpensive provider of community psychiatric services. This situation began to turn around by the late 1970s. By the early 1980s the CMHA, under new leadership, was again effectively lobbying the government and giving directions for the development of the provincial psychiatric services system.

From the point of view of the DPH, the takeover of CMHA in the late 1960s was a success in two ways: first, at minimal expense the community programme had been expanded, and second, the expanding system of White Cross centres was seen as evidence that positive action was being taken on the recommendations of the Frazier report. The more expensive of Frazier's recommendations, such as increased numbers of community workers and wage increases, were not acted upon so quickly. Faced with continued opposition, however, the DPH did not want to appear inactive. Therefore another study was commissioned.

### The Rationalization of PSB

MDT Associates of Winnipeg, Manitoba, were retained for an initial fee of ten thousand dollars to perform an operational audit of PSB, the result of which, according to a letter from MDT Associates to the deputy minister of public health, would be "a detailed plan of operational evolution, with a specific set of recommendations in the policy, organizational, systems and administrative sectors which are fully compatible with provincial goals and priorities, and which can be implemented by your own staff."[128]

The director of PSB was much more concise. In a memorandum to the minister of public health, he stated that

MDT Associates had been retained to specify how some of Frazier's "most important recommendations [could] be implemented by *better organization* of existing resources."[129] [emphasis in original]

It was generally recognized that a significant reallocation of PSB resources was necessary in order to sustain and expand community psychiatric services. MDT Associates claimed in 1968, for example, that "although the emphasis of the Saskatchewan program had swung from institution to regionalization and care in the community, . . . 80% of the budget was still spent on institutions as against 20% on the community aspects."[130]

The reduction of inmate populations, especially at SHW, had significantly contributed to this imbalance. With declining inmate populations, the cost per patient had correspondingly increased so that by 1968 the per diem costs at SHW were twice as high as at SHNB.[131] This simply reaffirmed the government's decision to abandon SHW, although it was decided that the physical plant would be converted to other uses in an attempt to minimize the economic impact on the community and political opposition. Out of a range of options considered, it was decided a nursing home would be the most acceptable alternative, not only because it would be eligible for federal cost sharing under CAP, but also because it would result in the least worker dislocation and "give the city a fairly large volume of business."[132]

Although the government apparently had already decided to abandon SHW, MDT Associates suggested that having this come in the form of a recommendation from an outside consultant had certain political advantages:

> It puts you in a position, regarding the phasing-over of Weyburn, to indicate that this is simply the recommendation of your consultant, and that detailed implications will be carefully studied by your staff before major decisions are implemented. It allows you to test response without becoming over-committed.[133]

Another aspect of the strategy to reduce opposition to decisions that had already been made was to co-opt the oppositional forces into assisting in the process of planning the transition from mental hospital to community. The involvement of the oppositional groups, including unions, staff and town councils, can be understood as cooptation rather than equal participation since they were not allowed to participate in discussions until after the various management committees established by MDT Associates had produced detailed plans. The MDT consultant suggested to the minister of public health that

> the unions be involved through attendance at meetings of [selected committees] . . . when these committees feel their work has advanced sufficiently to permit such consultations. . . .
>
> I believe that the above represents the most positive and least traumatic way of proceeding with this essential work. It provides for a developing dialogue at different levels, rather than abrupt announcements to town councils, unions or staff.[134]

The process of coopting opposition worked as well for the DPH in 1968 as it had in 1966, and as it had for Dr. MacNeill in the pre-war period. Opposition from the Weyburn business community dissipated with the promise of a continuing flow of government money, and the SPNA was mollified with the promise of continued employment in the proposed nursing home.

The closure of the mental hospitals, although a major undertaking, was only part of the plan to privatize all psychiatric in-patient facilities. For those not closed, this was to be achieved by transferring control and financial responsibility to local hospital boards. The MDT consultant correctly anticipated this would generate intense opposition, not only from within PSB, but also from the local hospital boards which would resist the added financial burden entailed in such a transfer. Thus, he informed the government:

> It seems clear to me that, at the present time, the government cannot delegate its overall responsibility for psychiatric services to local hospital boards. At the same time, a gradual integration should be provided for, to the extent that the overall integrity of the program does

> not suffer. We must be careful here that vested interests of individuals in the Branch and in the local hospitals do not over-ride general goals and objectives.[135]

As the first step in the plan to transfer control of psychiatric in-patient facilities to local hospital boards, the MDT consultant suggested that the PAPC be opened. He anticipated this would reduce opposition from psychiatric nurses and private sector psychiatrists, as well as serving as a bellwether for privatization:

> I have suggested to [the director of PSB] that a two or three year plan be developed to gradually phase the regional centre over to the hospital board, with the Branch assuming a less directive and more coordinating role. This allows the Branch to establish a solid program initially, as part of its overall provincial plan. Should difficulties with the hospital develop during the two or three year phasing over period, the process of integration can be slowed down or even reversed.[136]

The DPH agreed to open the sixty-bed PAPC primarily to serve as a test case of the transfer of control of in-patient facilities to local hospital boards. They remained unwilling, however, to construct any new beds, therefore pressure from private practice psychiatrists continued to mount. In an attempt to reduce this pressure, as well as pressure from the SPNA, the DPH offered to provide "more ancillary help [to] physicians of all kinds (and not only psychiatrists) [to enable them] to follow-up and treat more patients in the community."[137]

The opening of PAPC and this commitment to community psychiatry required increased expenditures. Thus, following the recommendations of both Frazier and MDT Associates, the government announced an 11.3 percent increase in PSB's budget to be administered over a two-year period. This increase was described as "the largest percentage and absolute increase in [PSB's] history."[138] It amounted to just over 1.5 million dollars, and was used to finance a 10 percent increase in psychiatrists' salaries and expand the number of community psychiatric positions. This led to a 66 percent increase in physicians with psychiatric specialty qualifications, a 73 percent increase in social workers with MSW qualifications and the creation of twenty-five new community positions.[139]

Although this budget increase was announced, not all the money was spent. The Liberal government attempted to finance the salary increases and expanded community programmes by raising the per diem charge at the provincial mental hospitals and by reducing the possibility of exemption from those charges.

The CCF government had passed legislation in 1944 which provided for "free" treatment in provincial mental hospitals during a person's lifetime. If upon death the person left an estate, however, the province could file a claim against it at the per diem rate of $3.50. This was raised to $5.00 per day in 1959. This legislation, however, had an important proviso; any portion of the estate passing to the father, mother, husband, wife, children, or siblings of a former patient residing in Saskatchewan was exempt from these charges.

In 1968 the Liberal government retroactively amended the Mental Health Act so that the list of surviving relatives who might benefit was reduced to the widow or widower. In addition, the widow or widower of a former patient was only entitled to the first ten thousand dollars of the estate, anything above that being subject to the per diem charge.

The amount collected from estates, although it increased slightly in fiscal year 1968-69, actually decreased in subsequent years (see Table 10). Ironically, this decrease was largely the consequence of the community psychiatric programmes and the depopulation policy. Thus, revenues from estates decreased because the number of long-stay patients in hospitals had diminished, the duration of stay had decreased (see Figure 22) and hence the number of people that died in hospital decreased,[140] and funds of former patients were used to pay for their support in nursing homes and approved homes, thus decreasing the size of the estates.

The effects of the 1968 amendments in terms of increased revenues were not all that had been hoped for by the Liberal government. The NDP, however, effectively used this issue to gain political support by arguing that the Liberals were not concerned about the well-being of the people of the prov-

**Table 10**
**Amount Collected for Care of Former Mental Hospital Patients, 1963-1971**

| Year | SHNB | SHW | Amount Received from Estates Only | Total Amount Received* |
|---|---|---|---|---|
| 1963-64 | 374,481 | 256,086 | – | 630,567 |
| 1964-65 | 303,491 | 248,988 | – | 552,479 |
| 1965-66 | 288,290 | 166,655 | – | 454,945 |
| 1966-67 | 342,888 | 187,709 | 410,987 | 530,597 |
| 1967-68 | 349,274 | 209,801 | 425,575 | 559,075 |
| 1968-69 | 478,951 | 393,863 | 480,747 | 842,814 |
| 1969-70 | 461,177 | 173,426 | 382,832 | 634,603 |
| 1970-71 | 332,264 | 122,261 | 365,360 | 454,525 |

*Most of the non-estate revenues came from charges to the federal government which is responsible for certain categories of patient. These included war veterans, inmates of penetentiaries, refugees and, until 31 March 1969, native peoples.

*Source:* Constructed from information provided in "Historical Review of the Mental Health Legislation as it Applies to Collections for the Cost of Care and Treatment of Former Patients," SAB, R-565,326. Blakeney Papers: Public Health: Mental Health Act.

ince but were simply concerned with saving a few dollars. Upon its election in 1971 the NDP immediately rescinded the 1968 amendment, as well as the 1966 Essential Services Emergency Act, the most regressive of the Liberals' labour legislation.

The shift to community psychiatry had other implications for the DPH and PSB management. In particular, the extensive changes wrought in both the social relations and forces of production necessitated the development and application of new technologies and techniques of management. This took the form of a more extensive use of computers. Thus, in January 1966, the Electronic Data Processing (EDP) system was introduced into PSB in part to allow management to monitor worker productivity and control the community psychiatric work force.

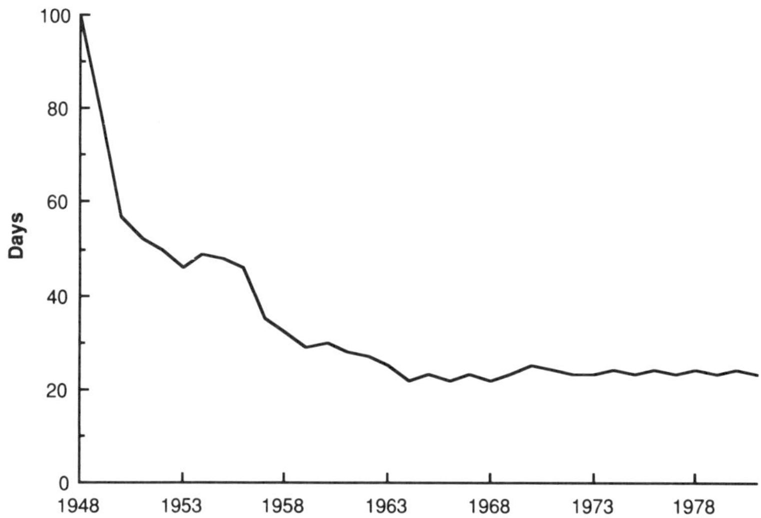


*Figure 22*
*Median Length of Stay in Designated Psychiatric Facilities, 1948 to 1981*

*Source: Adults Working Paper: Task Force on Mental Health in Saskatchewan; and Statistics Canada, Mental Health Statistics, vol. 1 (Annual)*

The non-medical community psychiatric occupations felt that the input categories employed by EDP were biased in favour of psychiatrists. They argued the input data was based upon the specific nature and organization of the psychiatrist's work, and therefore did not accurately reflect the workloads of the non-medical staff. Within the context of developing struggles against medical domination, EDP contributed to an escalation rather than a resolution of the problems of managing the community psychiatric labour force. Ironically, one of the things that focussed community worker discontent was the MDT Associates study which attempted to contribute to the development of a more effective management system through the precise definition of occupational roles and functions. It was largely the interoccupation struggles of the community psychiatric labour process which shaped the development of psychiatry in Saskatchewan throughout the 1970s and into the 1980s.

# Chapter Six

# The De-Medicalization of Community Psychiatric Work

The early 1970s saw the NDP government complete a number of cost-cutting measures initiated by the Liberals. These included the depopulation of SHW and its conversion to a regional psychiatric centre, transfer of psychiatric nursing education programmes to the Department of Education and the further specialization of service delivery. The specialization of service delivery was achieved by the transfer of programmes for mentally retarded and geriatric psychiatric patients to Core Services and the Department of Social Services respectively. Primarily as a result of these changes, PSB's total budget declined from $16.7 million in fiscal year 1971-72 to $9.3 million in fiscal year 1973-74.

The NDP government also made a number of changes to Liberal policy. The decision to abandon SHNB, for example, was reversed, and a programme of constructing psychiatric in-patient beds was undertaken. The decision not to abandon SHNB was made largely at the instigation of PSB management and pressure from SHNB psychiatric nurses. The construction of psychiatric in-patient beds was partially the product of pressure from private practice psychiatrists. Both developments slowed the trend towards complete privatization of psychiatric in-patient services begun by the Liberals.

The most significant development of the 1970s, however, was the appointment of the first non-medical director of a psychiatric facility. This was the product of various struggles which took place between the community-based occupations, primarily social workers, and mental hospital-based psychiatrists. These centred around the attempts of the community occupations to gain control of their own work and autonomy from medical domination. The appointment of the first non-medical director of SHNB in 1973 paved the way for a similar appointment at PSB in 1979. Both these developments are indicative of a de-medicalization of public sector psychiatric work. The catalyst for these developments was the depopulation and conversion of SHNB to a medium-sized mental hospital and a regional psychiatric centre.

## The Conversion of SHNB

In 1968, MDT Associates had recommended that both mental hospitals be phased out: SHW within five years, and SHNB within fifteen. The conversion of SHW was completed by 1971, but the DPH decided against phasing out SHNB. This decision was made largely at the urging of PSB management, who successfully argued that the province required a mental hospital for the foreseeable future. It was, therefore, decided to convert SHNB to a regional psychiatric centre and a medium-sized hospital.

To facilitate the depopulation and conversion of SHNB the Liberals in 1970 had replaced the in-hospital management, including the executive director, the administrator and the director of nursing. The decision to reduce the population of SHNB was motivated by more than the desire to reduce costs. It was also part of an attempt to reduce the shortage of psychiatrists. It was hoped the reduction in patient numbers would result in an improvement in both staff-patient ratios and general conditions of patient accommodation to a level which would allow SHNB to be accredited as a teaching institution. SHNB had lost its previous accreditation in the 1960s. Accreditation would permit the province to provide medical graduates with specialty training in psychiatry. The DPH and PSB management thought this would make it possible to recruit local medical graduates who might be more inclined to stay in the province, and perhaps with PSB.

Although the NDP had decided not to abandon SHNB, the reduction of patient numbers, the specialization of service delivery and a basic mistrust of the DPH and PSB management resulted in much anxiety and low morale among in-hospital psychiatric nurses. One social worker stated that throughout the late 1960s and early 1970s

> there was an 'illness' in the institution [SHNB]; the staff called it 'Weyburnitis' — they were afraid that what happened at Weyburn would happen at North Battleford, and they would lose their jobs.[1]

The rapid reduction of in-patient numbers (from 1,619 in 1963 to 541 at the beginning of 1971), combined with ward integration at SHNB, also resulted in a worsening of working conditions for in-hospital psychiatric nurses. Commenting on the effect of reduced in-patient numbers on working conditions, a confidential 1971 report to the minister of public health from the deputy minister, the director of PSB, and a university psychiatrist stated:

> This has led to a need for a smaller staff and reduced opportunities for promotion, relief from shift work, higher pay, etc. Many of the employees have been with the hospital for 25 years or more and have limited vocational mobility in view of present unemployment and their ages. Other provinces are now training their own psychiatric personnel, so that employment opportunities in the psychiatric field outside the province is [*sic*] also limited.[2]

In-hospital psychiatric nurses responded to this deterioration of market position and working conditions by opposing the depopulation of SHNB. This resulted in much conflict between on-ward psychiatric nurses and in-hospital management. The DPH, of course, remained committed to reducing in-patient populations, although they did attempt to soften the impact of these changes for the psychiatric nurses. The above-quoted report, for example, observed that

> Nothing can and should be done to retard the shrinking population of the hospital, but some provision needs to be made to help the workers displaced. This is a technological change in the delivery of psychiatric services and the workers should not be made to pay for it.[3]

It is interesting to note that the transformation of SHNB from a large custodial facility to a small treatment facility is referred to as a technological change. This supports the conceptualization of physical facilities as an element of the means of psychiatric production. It also supports the claim that changes in the elements of the forces of production (FP) influence the social relations of production (SRP), particularly the nature and organization of work (i.e., the occupational division of labour). As a response to the suggestion that workers not be made to bear the full brunt of technological changes, the DPH instituted a policy of early retirement with full pension for psychiatric nurses.

This did not address the source of anxiety, worker-management relations remained tense, and conflicts continued to escalate. The legislative secretary to the minister of public health, following a personal investigation of union complaints at SHNB in late 1971, reported to the minister:

> The basic criticism is that senior administrators act arbitrarily, ignore criticism and suggestions, are uncommunicative, and treat staff unfairly in punishing critics and practising favoritism. In many cases the decisions taken by [the director of nursing] and [the executive director, SHNB] appear rational and progressive, but they have been taken with little or no involvement of the staff. Accordingly . . . the staff, both professional and non-professional, the progressive and more conservative are equally alienated.[4]

The conflicts between in-hospital nurses and management in themselves would probably not have been particularly significant. They were taking place, however, against a backdrop of expanding community programmes and intense struggles of community psychiatric workers against medical domination. As a consequence, the in-hospital conflicts contributed to an imminent crisis of management, the resolution of which would mark a major step toward the de-medicalization of public sector psychiatric work. Before considering this, however, attention will be turned to a brief examination of the private sector community psychiatric labour process and some of the dominant trends characteristic of it.

### De-medicalization and Private Sector Psychiatry

As has been seen, the involvement of private practice GPs in the provision of psychiatric services had long been advocated as a way to reduce the rate of mental hospitalization. It was argued that out-patient treatment was cheaper than in-patient treatment and the involvement of GPs would therefore be a cost-cutting preventive measure. This had great appeal to legislators charged with responsibility for the provision of psychiatric services. Thus, in the early 1960s, government successfully encouraged provincial GPs to become involved in psychiatric practice through the inclusion of psychotherapy as an insured service within the MCIC service structure (see Figure 23). This trend received added impetus in the post-1968 period with the establishment of a federal medicare insurance plan. Under the terms of this plan medical care, including psychiatric, services were cost shared. This halved the costs to the province on a per service basis.

As a result of these financial incentives, the private sector produced most of the psychiatric services in the province; between 1969 and 1971, 85 percent of psychiatric diagnoses of all kinds were provided solely by the private sector, including both GPs and specialist psychiatrists. In the same period, however, the private sector "accounted for only one-third of all psychiatric health care costs."[5] In addition, over 70 percent of all private sector patients receiving a psychiatric diagnosis were seen only by a GP; the major form of treatment being chemo/psychotherapy.[6] On the other hand, the public sector accounted for 66 percent of total psychiatric costs, although it treated only 14 percent of all individuals

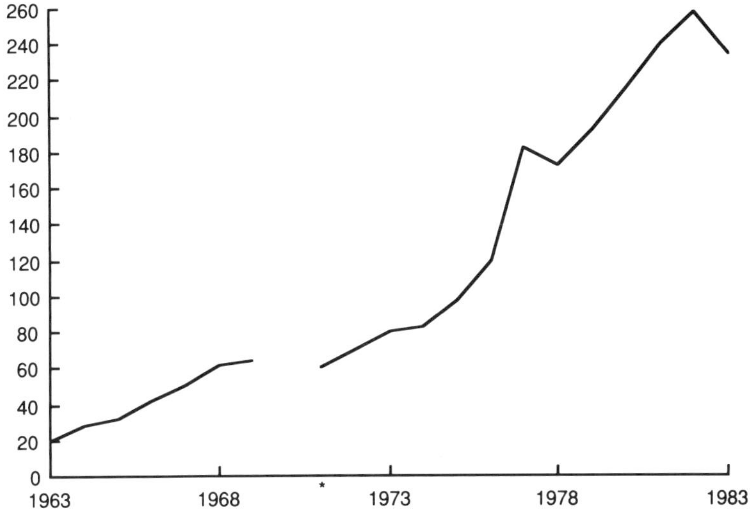


*Figure 23*
*Estimate of the Rate of Psychiatric Services Provided by Fee-for-Service Practitioners, 1963 to 1981 (Services Per 1000 Population)*

**Change in definition from: "Visit services, consultations and hospital care rendered in connection with psychiatry or counselling as well as special procedures by a psychiatrist" to "treatment interviews, group therapy, and counselling."*
*Source: Saskatchewan MCIC Annual Reports*

given a psychiatric diagnosis.[7] A 1979 DPH report on psychiatric services pointed out that "in terms of average treatment cost per patient, public inpatients cost most to treat, followed by private inpatients, public outpatients and private outpatients."[8]

The government, which was bearing the costs in both sectors, clearly had an interest in trying to shift the treatment load to the private sector, and especially to the nonspecialist private outpatient sector. In order to achieve this objective, in 1975 MCIC revised the physician fee schedule so that the method of counting GP psychiatric services was reduced to fifteen-minute units from thirty-minute units.[9] This meant that GPs could produce twice as many psychiatric services per time period. This resulted in a dramatic increase in the number of psychotherapeutic services provided. In return for this concession the provincial GPs had to agree to a reduced fee per service (see Table 11) but this was easily offset by the expansion in the number of psychotherapeutic services provided (see Table 12). Therefore, even though the cost per service was lowest for private sector GPs, the growth in the volume of services contributed to rapidly rising costs.

As well, the nature of the psychiatric disorders treated by private sector GPs raised doubts that early medical intervention results in overall cost-savings. Between 1969 and 1974, for example, 70 percent of the patients receiving primary psychiatric diagnoses from GPs were reported to have had only a neurosis diagnosis, "indicating the relatively minor nature of the illness involved."[10] The PSB asked if those cases would have resulted in hospitalization without medical intervention, and if medical intervention was necessary for their effective treatment. The answer in both cases was probably not.

The final report of the Service Interface Study suggested there were two

> distinct types of patients who differ significantly in terms of severity and duration of their respective illnesses. . . . rather than there being a continuum where less severe problems may develop into more severe problems, if left untreated, there may in fact be distinct types of patients whose problems arise from diverse combinations of genetic and biological determinants and social and cultural environments. If so, a substantial re-ordering of programme activities and priorities may be necessary. . . .[11]

The reordering of programme activities is thought to be especially important because of the projected increase in the aged population. This demographic shift, which is common to all advanced industrial countries, is expected to be accompanied by a "high utilization of medical services for psychiatric disorders."[12] This is of particular concern to policy makers in Saskatchewan not only because the province has the highest proportion of people aged sixty-five years and over in Canada, but also because the Saskatchewan aged have the greatest longevity in the country. The sixty-five and

**Table 11**
**Average Payment for Psychotherapy and Proportion of Services Provided by Type of Practitioner, 1963-1982**

| Year | Type of Service | GP | | Specialist | |
|---|---|---|---|---|---|
| | Psychotherapy | Payment | Proportion of Total | Payment | Proportion of Total |
| 1963 | | | 53.2 | | 46.8 |
| 1964 | | | 52.0 | | 48.0 |
| 1965 | | | 51.3 | | 48.7 |
| 1966 | | | 42.1 | | 57.9 |
| 1967 | | | 41.6 | | 58.4 |
| 1968 | | | 34.9 | | 65.1 |
| 1969 | | | 40.6 | | 59.4 |
| 1970 | | | 53.7 | | 46.3 |
| 1971 | | | 48.9 | | 51.1 |
| 1972 | | | 50.1 | | 49.9 |
| 1973 | | 9.67* | 49.4 | 10.38* | 50.6 |
| 1974 | | 9.79 | 40.4 | 9.72 | 59.6 |
| 1975 | | 7.07 | 62.4 | 11.16 | 37.6 |
| 1976 | | 6.59 | 71.84 | 12.13 | 28.16 |
| 1977 | | 6.80 | 75.51 | 12.71 | 24.49 |
| 1978 | | 7.15 | 72.51 | 14.29 | 27.49 |
| 1979 | | 7.13 | 75.33 | 15.11 | 24.67 |
| 1980 | | 7.84 | 73.03 | 16.60 | 26.97 |
| 1981-82 | | 8.99 | 75.31 | 19.06 | 24.69 |

*This data was not available prior to 1973.
*Source:* Saskatchewan MCIC Annual Reports.

over age group is the largest consumer of health and social services, including psychiatric services.[13] The anticipated increase in demand is likely to be accompanied by an increase in costs.

In response to this, the state has undertaken a number of initiatives directed towards reducing the fiscal burden of escalating health care costs. These have included attempts "to reverse the trend toward increasing medicalization of living by encouraging personal responsibility for mental health,"[14] as well as attempts to transform the nature and organization of medical work.

**Table 12**
**Number and Rate of Psychiatric Services Provided by Fee-for-Service Physicians in Saskatchewan by Type of Practitioner, 1963-1982**

| Year | Type of Service Psychotherapy | Number of Services (thousands) | Rate per 1000 | Percentage of Total by Type of Practitioner | |
|---|---|---|---|---|---|
| | | | | GP | Specialist Psychiatrist |
| 1963 | | 15.9 | 19.6 | 53.2 | 46.8 |
| 1964 | | 23.6 | 28.6 | 52.0 | 48.0 |
| 1965 | | 26.9 | 32.3 | 51.3 | 48.7 |
| 1966 | | 39.0 | 45.1 | 42.1 | 57.9 |
| 1967 | | 47.6 | 54.0 | 41.6 | 58.4 |
| 1968 | | 55.4 | 63.0 | 34.0 | 65.1 |
| 1969 | | 59.2 | 65.0 | 40.6 | 59.4 |
| 1970 | | 56.1 | 63.0 | 53.7 | 46.3 |
| 1971 | | 63.4 | 71.0 | 48.9 | 51.1 |
| 1972 | | 72.4 | 81.0 | 50.1 | 49.9 |
| 1973 | | 76.2 | 86.0 | 49.4 | 50.6 |
| 1974 | | 90.5 | 103.0 | 40.4 | 59.6 |
| 1975 | | 108.6 | 122.0 | 62.4 | 37.6 |
| 1976 | | 163.5 | 180.0 | 71.84 | 28.16 |
| 1977 | | 162.1 | 176.0 | 75.51 | 24.49 |
| 1978 | | 181.0 | 195.0 | 72.51 | 27.49 |
| 1979 | | 199.1 | 213.0 | 75.33 | 24.67 |
| 1980 | | 224.9 | 239.0 | 73.03 | 26.97 |
| 1981-82 | | 246.2 | 249.0 | 75.31 | 24.69 |

*Source:* Saskatchewan MCIC Annual Reports.

## The Transformation of Medical Work

Saskatchewan governments have been in the vanguard of reorganizing medical-psychiatric work in Canada largely because of the ground-breaking involvement of the CCF in state-sponsored medical insurance.[15] At the same time that the CCF was establishing a comprehensive and compulsory system of medical insurance in 1962, it also undertook to transform the medical FP. This took the form of a system of community clinics as an alternative to general hospital and private practice medicine.

The community clinics, which are managed by local non-medical boards, offer a full spectrum of diagnostic and treatment services, including psychiatric services. Private practice physicians have generally opposed the creation and operation of these clinics because of the threat they pose to incomes and autonomy.[16] Following the creation of a national system of medical insurance in 1968, however, the federal and other provincial governments became increasingly concerned about "the accelerating rate of spending in health services."[17] In 1970 the Hastings committee was established and two years later submitted a report to the conference of health ministers.

Largely as a result of the Saskatchewan experience with community-managed clinics,[18] the Hastings Report recommended the creation of a system of community health centres for Canada. Physicians throughout Canada opposed these proposals for the same reasons they had opposed the creation of the Saskatchewan community clinics ten years earlier. These were, of course, legitimate concerns: the Regina Community Clinic, for example, had successfully deskilled psychiatric work through "the use of a medical social worker to provide psychotherapeutic services in lieu of a psychiatrist."[19] The Hastings Report suggested the proposed community health centres could also contribute to the demedicalization of psychiatric work:

> The community health centres by involving the public and using the interdisciplinary team, including the clinical psychologist and other mental health personnel, provide a setting in which there can be a greater emphasis on the psycho-social aspects of care.[20]

These threats to autonomy and income were viewed with increasing trepidation by private practice physicians across Canada. The situation became intolerable to physicians in the early 1970s, however, when the non-medical management board of the Regina Community Clinic petitioned the NDP government for increased power to manage the clinic. This was granted in the form of a new budgeting procedure. As a result, early in 1974, the fourteen physicians on the medical staff resigned en masse.[21]

Opponents of the Hastings Report were jubilant: they could point to the developments in Regina as proof that the community clinic system was not a viable alternative to private practice or medically managed group practice. Legislators, always wary of becoming enmeshed in an unpopular confrontation with the doctors, backed down and the community health centre largely has remained in political limbo.

The issue of community control, however, will not likely disappear because physicians claim it violates their "professional" prerogatives. Consumers, and consumer advocacy groups, are increasingly demanding a role in decision-making in the area of health-care delivery. With regard to psychiatric services, it has already been seen that the CMHA, among other things, has long been an advocate for mental patients. There are, however, other groups, whose membership is mostly psychiatric patients and ex-psychiatric patients, which are also beginning to perform this function. In Saskatoon, for example, there are currently two such groups, Newstart and Crocus Co-op. Both groups attempt to secure the resources which will allow their constituents to manage their own affairs and live as independently as possible.

The principle of patient self-management was established in the 1950s and 1960s in the form of the "therapeutic community." These attempts at individual behaviour modification and social skills training were instigated as part of the process of depopulating the mental hospitals. The emphasis on behaviour modification as a form of psychiatric treatment not only helped to empty the mental hospitals; by expanding the number of community placements, it laid the foundation for the growth in numbers of non-medical community psychiatric workers.

Throughout the 1970s, as non-medical community psychiatric workers struggled for occupational autonomy, and mental patients began to struggle for legal rights, an alliance against medical domination developed between some community-based occupations and mental patients. It is interesting that the successful transformation of insanity into mental illness produced the conditions for the emergence of the patient rights movement and the establishment of an anti-psychiatrist alliance. It is maintained that if persons diagnosed as mentally ill are in fact ill, they should be protected from any negative consequences of their treatment, and have the right to refuse treatment. This issue is now being resolved not only in Saskatchewan,[22] but throughout Canada. A 26 April 1984 story in the *Globe and Mail,* entitled "When Therapy Becomes Assault," argued for the legal right of an Ontario mental patient to refuse electro-convulsive therapy (ECT), a right which the Ontario Supreme Court decided the patient did not have. The article, written by a Toronto lawyer, argued that forced medical treatment effectively constitutes an assault upon the patient and that making such assault legal only serves to bring disrepute to both medicine and law. In the last instance, the author concluded, the only judge concerning the requirement for treatment must be the patient.[23]

Whether that is always true or not, psychiatric patients are increasingly using the courts to establish and formalize their rights. As a result, the nature and organization of psychiatric work is being influenced by judicial decisions. A good example of this was cited in the 1981 report of the provincial Thrust Working Party entitled *Community Based Alternatives for Mental Health Care.* It was reported that as a result of a class action suit brought against the State of Massachusetts in the early 1970s, by lawyers acting on behalf of patients in a state mental hospital, a "comprehensive set of community alternatives [to the mental hospital] was prescribed" for the state. According to an attorney handling the patients' case, the judgement was the first

> to both establish a broad right to treatment in the *least restrictive* alternative and to compel the state government to provide such alternatives, including a detailed design of the type, number and cost of these programs and services.[24] [emphasis in original]

Three distinct components were specified as necessary for a comprehensive community mental health system:

> (1) residential environments that are the least restrictive and most normal settings appropriate for each resident or client; (2) non-residential treatment, training and support programs which are geographically separate from community residences . . .; and (3) management services

> to adequately develop, co-ordinate, administer, monitor, and evaluate this network of environments and programs.[25]

The Massachusetts decision had a real impact on the development of community psychiatry in Saskatchewan. PSB's description of its Child-Youth Services, for example, echoes the first requirement specified above:

> The Psychiatric Services Branch provides services to children and youth to enhance the mental health of both the child and family, to prevent handicapping through early detection and structured intervention, to remediate the impact of emotional and mental disorder through direct treatment and family support, and where necessary, *to provide the least restrictive residential alternative in conjunction with other services.* Coordination and consultation with other organizations serving children, youth and families are emphasized to strengthen the response of communities.[26] [emphasis added]

The specification of a management system as a requirement for the network of community facilities returns attention to the issue of community management boards. Although it is a moribund issue in the private sector at this time, it is a growing reality in public sector psychiatry.

It appears that the first proposal for community control of psychiatric facilities in Saskatchewan was made in 1969 by a psychologist who also recommended that the boards have a full-time paid executive director.[27] The government rejected the specifics of this proposal due to opposition from PSB management and the costs involved. The DPH supported the principle of community management boards, however, and stated that it would "encourage the co-ordination of services . . . by a voluntary group using existing resources."[28] The non-medical community occupations also supported the establishment of community boards, because they saw them as a mechanism for challenging medical domination of the community psychiatric labour process.

The first non-medical director of a PSB facility, a clinical psychologist, wrote in 1972:

> the concept of community control of . . . mental health programs appears to be a rational and democratic way of helping to sort out the priorities as the community sees them. Obviously professionals cannot just turn their problems over to elected representatives and hope that they will be solved since they have not been able to solve them themselves. However, at least some of the [interoccupation] conflicts . . . can be viewed in the light of what the community wants and not what some professional apologist feels.[29]

Community management boards became a reality in 1976-77. In that year it was announced that an alternative to the "approved home" was being developed:

> For the past year or more this branch has given serious consideration to the development of group homes in an attempt to develop a more complete continuum of non-institutional residential options which would provide viable alternatives to large special care facilities and acute treatment hospitals.[30]

The group homes differed from ordinary boarding houses and approved homes in that they had guaranteed funding, salaried non-medical operators, and most important for present purposes, they were managed by a volunteer community board. The first of the provincial group homes opened in Swift Current in 1976, and by the beginning of the 1980s there was a group home in all eight psychiatric regions.

It is also interesting to note that the group homes were designed as a residential alternative to acute treatment hospitals. By the mid-1970s, most psychiatric in-patient services were produced in general hospitals. The group homes, conceptualized as part of the FP of psychiatric production, constitute a material basis for the de-medicalization of psychiatric work. The fact that they are managed by non-medical community boards and staffed by non-medical occupations confirms this tendency.

It is ironic that the medicalization of psychiatric work, by asserting the isomorphism of mental and physical illness, provided the basis for the relegalization of the therapeutic relation in the form of a struggle to guarantee the legal rights of mental patients. It was this legal protection of patient rights which, as Skultans has shown, was opposed by nineteenth-century proponents of the medicalization of psychiatry because of the obstruction it created to early treatment.

In the second half of the twentieth century the growth of the patient rights movement has also corresponded to an emphasis on personal responsibility for mental health. The emphasis on this, through the advocacy of a self-care and lifestyles ideology, has been one of the ways governments have attempted to reverse the trend towards an increased medicalization of living. The reorganization and de-medicalization of psychiatric work is closely related to, and justified by, this ideology.

## De-medicalization and the Self-Care and Lifestyles Ideology

The emphasis on self-care and lifestyles is one aspect of a developing ideology which maintains many psychiatric disorders are not mental illnesses, but rather psycho-social problems with living. This ideology found expression in a 1974 working paper of the federal minister of health and welfare entitled *A New Perspective on the Health of Canadians*:

> individual blame must be accepted by many for the deleterious effect on health of their respective lifestyles. Sedentary living, smoking, over-eating, driving while impaired by alcohol, drug abuse and failure to wear seat belts are among the many contributors to physical or mental illness for which the individual must accept some responsibility and for which he should seek correction.[31]

Although these observations are true, it is equally true that individual lifestyles do not occur in a vacuum. Thus Bolaria has argued that this ideology diverts attention from the social etiology of disease and illness and by so doing "promotes a course of action oriented toward individual behavior modification rather than changing the existing social, economic and political institutions and the health sector."[32] Certainly the primary objective of the widely disseminated lifestyles ideology[33] is individual behaviour modification. In contrast to Bolaria's contention that this prevents changes in the health sector I maintain that it is accompanied by, and achieved through, the transformation of health care work. With regard to psychiatric services, it is accompanied by the de-medicalization of psychiatric work.

The expected effect of the widespread dissemination of this ideology, or more precisely the advantages to be had from the application of this ideology to individual health care practices, was clearly expressed in the final report of the Services Interface Study. Referring to the increased demand for psychiatric services expected as a result of the previously mentioned demographic shift, the report observed: "The effects [i.e., costs] of increased utilization may be lessened somewhat by individuals taking more personal responsibility for their health and social support."[34] However, even if the state and other interested parties are completely successful in having individuals take more personal responsibility for their health and social support, the demand for some kind of professional services likely will increase. It is on this basis that the non-medical psychiatric occupations appear to be developing their occupational strategies. Their main argument is that non-medical psychiatric services are as effective, but less expensive, than medically provided services.

Simply making these arguments, or even demonstrating their veracity, is no guarantee that the shift toward the de-medicalization of community psychiatric services will occur. The medical profession has a strong interest in maintaining the hard-won status quo. The executive director of SPNA stated that there may be political disincentives for the government to de-medicalize psychiatric work:

> there is a tremendous amount of incentive on the part of the government to maintain the status quo .... Look at all the people it keeps happy. What other non-program keeps so many people happy? Think about it! Keeping the people happy because they don't have to go to those threatening clinics — you don't have to tell them

> [non-medical psychotherapists] that you are beating up your wife, or throwing your kids against the wall, or that you are in a drunken stupor every Friday night — you just have to tell the doctor that you are feeling kind of lousy and you get a quick fix. The physician is as happy as hell, Lord only knows the druggist is thrilled and look at all the people you have appeased by not doing anything. It would be political suicide for somebody to come up and say "We are no longer going to pay physicians for prescribing the psychotropics and for seeing people with those kinds of problems."[35]

Thus there are countervailing forces to the de-medicalization of both private and public sector psychiatric work. In Saskatchewan PSB-employed psychiatrists and private sector psychiatrists have engaged in protracted struggles to defend their occupational interests. Throughout the 1960s and 1970s these struggles often took the form of conflicts *between* private sector psychiatrists, the DPH and PSB management-psychiatrists. In the early part of the 1970s these struggles were primarily over control of psychiatric in-patient beds.

## Public-Private Sector Conflict

As has been seen, the greatest proportion of psychiatric services are produced by private practice physicians. The public and private sectors, however, do not exist in isolation. Private practice psychiatrists require access to psychiatric beds which are controlled by PSB. PSB requires temporary permits for unlicensed psychiatrists, which are controlled by private sector practitioners through their domination of the SCPS. Conflicts developed between the public and private sectors over these issues, and resulted in changes to licensing procedures and the number of psychiatric in-patient beds by the mid-1970s.

The poor relations between PSB and private practice psychiatrists were complicated by the relatively autonomous position of the Department of Psychiatry, University of Saskatchewan. University-employed psychiatrists felt the in-patient beds in the psychiatric ward of the University Hospital were required for their own work, and therefore refused admitting privileges to all but one of Saskatoon's seven private practice psychiatrists, who was allowed access to only two beds.

The other private practice psychiatrists had access only to the eight psychiatric beds in Saskatoon City Hospital.[36] They argued that because they saw more patients per year than either the university or PSB-employed psychiatrists they required access to more psychiatric beds and follow-up services and made this point in a 1972 letter to the minister of public health:

> It does seem grossly unfair that those psychiatrists providing the greatest amount of service to their community, and therefore their patients, are prevented from making use of the largest, and in fact the only . . . recognized . . . psychiatric in-patient facility in this city and its ancilliary services such as its Department of Psychology, Psychiatric Social Work, etc.[37]

While it was acknowledged that private practice psychiatrists saw more patients than PSB and university psychiatrists, it was also pointed out that "private psychiatrists working on a fee-for-service basis tend to treat the least sick members of the psychiatric population."[38] PSB management also suggested that if more psychiatric beds were added "most psychiatrists would be attracted into fee-for-service work which would . . . become more profitable."[39] The DPH, confronted with the chronic shortage of psychiatric labour power, was not inclined to produce the conditions whereby even more psychiatrists would leave for private practice.

It was also argued by the director of PSB that "in the private sector beds mean money,"[40] therefore, allowing private practice psychiatrists unrestricted access to provincially financed psychiatric beds would result in an increased rate of utilization and a rapid escalation of costs.[41] The fact that expanding the number and allowing easier access to psychiatric beds would increase costs precluded the DPH from undertaking an extensive construction programme or changing the admissions policy. The fact that private sector incomes were partly dependent upon access to in-patient beds guaranteed they would be tenacious in their demands.

Bitter conflicts ensued which were not resolved until the mid-1970s when the DPH undertook an extensive programme of constructing psychiatric in-patient beds throughout the province.

In the early 1970s, however, the private sector psychiatrists felt PSB's policy regarding in-patient beds was so detrimental to their incomes that they began to proclaim that the DPH was attempting to drive them out of existence. A March 1972 article in the *Regina Leader-Post*, entitled "Psychiatrist Slams Mental Health Plans," opened with a statement by a Regina psychiatrist, who charged that the provincial government was "trying to squeeze out private psychiatry in the city because the private sector is showing up the defects in psychiatric care provided under the government-operated mental services plan."[42]

In fact, it was the public sector that had just avoided extinction. PSB management, with a vivid memory of the Liberals' plan to privatize in-patient services, still feared for its continued existence, and took every opportunity to convince the government that public sector psychiatry was effective, efficient and necessary.

The private sector used more than public criticism in its attempt to pressure the government into providing more and easier access to psychiatric beds. At one point, Dr. Abram Hoffer, a former PSB employee who had moved into private practice in Saskatoon, requested he be allowed to open a private hospital which would specialize in the orthomolecular treatment of schizophrenia. This particular treatment had been pioneered by Drs. Hoffer and Osmond in the mid-1950s. The fact that orthomolecular therapy had never been widely adopted by other PSB psychiatrists greatly annoyed Dr. Hoffer, who persistently tried to persuade PSB management of the superiority of his approach. His proposal to open a private psychiatric hospital in the province was supported on the grounds that

> A private hospital using the latest orthomolecular approach would (1) greatly reduce costs of operation, especially if the Department did not insist on overstaffing the hospital with social workers, psychologists,

> and nurses. (2) greatly reduce the relapse and readmission rate.[43]

The DPH refused and the idea of a private psychiatric hospital died.[44] The struggle for in-patient beds, however, continued.

The fact that PSB had long been unable to recruit and retain adequate quantities of fully licensed psychiatrists was a major source of leverage for the private practice psychiatrists. As has been seen, PSB had come to rely on unlicensed psychiatrists working on temporary permits issued by the SCPS. The SCPS, dominated by private practice physicians and politically and ideologically committed to private practice, threatened to make it more difficult for PSB to get or extend permits if private sector demands were not met. The denial of temporary permits would have resulted in the collapse of PSB, and PSB management therefore recommended that medical licensing laws be changed to ease their dependence on the SCPS:

> The present time limit built into the permit to practice must be abandoned. . . . This would require a change in legislation. The College would not like it. On the other hand it does not interfere with private practice. It is also better from their point of view than widening the conditions for full registration, e.g. by including graduates on the commonwealth list of the United Kingdom.[45]

The CCF had threatened to change medical licensing laws during the dispute with the provincial doctors over the establishment of Medicare in the early 1960s.[46] Recalling its defeat, the SCPS was not willing to become enmeshed in a full-blown confrontation with the NDP over the issue of temporary permits. Similarly, the NDP government did not wish to see a political crisis created by another confrontation with the province's doctors. The shortage of psychiatric labour power, however, was jeopardizing the capacity of the DPH to provide adequate services, which was also a potential political crisis. Through a series of negotiations between the DPH and the SCPS,[47] the tensions were kept in check and the SCPS softened its hard-line stance on issuing and renewing permits.

The crisis of medical labour power, however, remained. A previous proposal to allow part-time private practice for fully licensed PSB psychiatrists in an attempt to make public sector employment more attractive had been rejected. PSB management, therefore, suggested an increase in the use of private psychiatrists on a contractual basis. This would not only help alleviate PSB's shortage of labour power, it would also help convince private practice psychiatrists that PSB was not trying to drive them out of existence, and thereby help reduce tensions. Since poor relations guaranteed that there would not be a major influx of private sector psychiatrists, this option did not solve the immediate problem.

As another proposed solution PSB management suggested the number of established positions for psychiatrists be reduced. This is somewhat surprising given that the major problem was supposedly a shortage of psychiatrists. The director of PSB suggested, however, that the money saved could be used to increase psychiatrists' salaries and improve their fringe benefits, which would make public sector psychiatry more attractive to fully licensed psychiatrists. The reduced number of psychiatrists would probably be unable to handle service loads, and it was recommended that they be used primarily as consultants to private practice GPs and non-medical community occupations who would provide the necessary treatment. This is precisely the role McKerracher had been advocating for psychiatrists since the mid-1940s.

In the early 1970s it finally became PSB policy. The DPH established a contractual employment option in 1974-75 and began to reduce the number of established positions for psychiatrists. Between 1973 and 1982 the number of PSB-employed psychiatrists dropped from fifty-eight to forty-two, ten of which were new contract positions. These developments are significant insofar as they are an instance of the Babbage Principle being applied to psychiatric work.

The deskilling of psychiatrists' work, although possibly a long-range solution to the labour power crisis, also failed to solve the immediate problem. To address that problem an international recruitment campaign was launched in the United Kingdom and Ireland. It was thought that this would be the most fruitful recruiting ground since the SCPS recognized psychiatric qualifications from those areas. Thus the deputy minister of public health, himself a physician, went to Saskatchewan House, London, England in April 1972.

At that time criticisms of the British experience with community psychiatry were beginning to appear in the professional journals. The lead article in the 15 May 1971 volume of the *British Medical Journal* criticized the unseemly haste with which British mental hospitals were being phased out, especially given the inadequate development of community-based alternatives.[48] This criticism of the British programme of community psychiatry was fortuitous for PSB management. In the 18 September 1971 volume of the same journal a letter from two PSB-employed psychiatrists was published. The authors opened their letter by stating they would like to comment on "the effectiveness of community mental health programs,"[49] and provided a glowing description of the provincial system of community psychiatry. Their account amounted to a free advertisement for PSB.

The private practitioners in the province were quick to respond, six of whom jointly signed a letter to the editor of the *British Medical Journal* which was published 20 November 1971. This letter opened with the comment: "We find it necessary to challenge some of the claims made . . . about psychiatric services in Saskatchewan . . . despite the repeated and numerous claims emanating from Saskatchewan we cannot agree that the effectiveness of so-called community care in the province has been substantiated."[50]

The initial reaction of PSB management was to refute the critics. The director of PSB thought this was necessary for two reasons: "(a) the bad effect within the service of morale if I don't; and (b) the letter by [the six private practice psychiatrists] is liable to have a very damaging effect on recruitment."[51] Given relations between PSB and the private sector, this may well have been the intent. Upon further reflection, however, the wisdom of responding to the criticisms in public was doubted:

> a letter by the Director of the service will be very apt to be looked on as a whitewash job no matter how closely

> it sticks to the incontrovertible facts. Furthermore, it will merely provide an excuse for further letters which will give the authors more publicity than they deserve.[52]

In spite of the criticisms of the private sector psychiatrists, the recruitment campaign resulted in a number of new psychiatrists coming to the province, although the attrition rate, at over 30 percent, remained high.[53] As a result, the crisis of labour power continued, as did the attacks of private sector psychiatrists. It was not until 1975, when the minister of public health announced "the initial stages of a major plan for the redistribution of psychiatric beds throughout the province to permit a more equitable allocation of in-patient services,"[54] that relations between public and private sector improved.

The initial step in this plan actually took place the preceding year when the Munroe Wing of the Regina General Hospital was relocated and expanded from thirty to forty-four beds. The plan also provided for an additional forty beds in Saskatoon; twenty to be added to the University Hospital, and twenty to be included in a new in-patient unit at City Hospital. In addition to the fourteen beds that had been added to the Munroe Wing, approval was given for the establishment of ten more at the Plains Health Centre, Regina. Swift Current Union Hospital received approval for fourteen in-patient beds, and following various renovations at SHNB, provision was made for the transfer of some beds to the Battlefords Union Hospital. This programme of psychiatric bed expansion continued into the 1980s.

While private psychiatrists were struggling for an expansion of in-patient facilities, other occupational groups were struggling for the expansion of community-based alternatives and against medical domination. Both struggles centred around the depopulation of the mental hospitals, particularly SHNB, in the early 1970s.

## Interoccupation Struggles: Social Work and Psychiatry

Interoccupational conflict had been assuming a new form within PSB since the mid-1960s. The transition to community psychiatry marked a change in the nature and the actual location of production of psychiatric services. Within the public sector in particular, psychiatric services came increasingly to be produced by non-medical labour power. As a consequence, the non-medical occupations, especially social workers, began to agitate for more autonomy. These struggles met with some initial success. In August 1971, for example, MSWs at SHW were allowed to accept direct referrals. A similar arrangement was made at SHNB in January 1972.[55]

In light of the escalating conflicts at SHNB, the director of PSB decided to end this practice. Thus, on 10 February 1972, he stated in a memo to the minister of public health that he would be going to Weyburn the following day "to rescind this policy immediately and to make all referrals come to a psychiatrist in the first instance who may assign them as he feels appropriate."[56] Rather than quelling social worker demands for autonomy, this fuelled the fire and provided the social workers with an increased sense of being oppressed by both psychiatrists and PSB management.

Not surprisingly, this further polarized the situation and united the social workers. In addition, it became clear to the social workers that if they were to get a sympathetic hearing with regard to their demands for occupational autonomy, it would be necessary to circumvent the medically dominated PSB management. Thus, the social workers took their case directly to the minister of public health, a move which annoyed PSB management. The director of PSB, writing to the minister of public health in June 1972, stated:

> I must say I am personally getting fed up in dealing with writers who by-pass all normal lines of communication. Nobody can quarrel with this in an extreme case but I do feel the mechanism is being abused and results in diminishing credibility for the whole organizational structure of Psychiatric Services.[57]

In particular, it diminished the credibility of management claims that they controlled the psychiatric labour process. It was also becoming accepted among DPH officials that the crisis of management in PSB was at least partly caused by the fact that the medically dominated PSB management was unable to distinguish between occupational and organizational interests.

The problems of exclusively employing medically trained psychiatrists as PSB management had been recognized by DPH officials for some time. In a 17 October 1966 memo, for example, it was noted by the minister of public health that

> Improving efficiency in an agency providing services which are themselves complex and difficult to measure is difficult. The Department, with limited resources at its disposal is attempting to do this in quite a vigorous way. Many definite problems exist here. Most of our managers are professionals who are poorly trained as managers and who have difficulty seeing themselves in this role. Attempts are being made to correct this by a limited in-service training program.[58]

By 1972 it had been decided that this was insufficient to deal with the situation, especially as it was developing at SHNB. In March of that year, therefore, it was decided to hire a non-medical executive director for SHNB. Although the decision was made, no action was taken at that time because the DPH wanted the incumbent executive director to complete the changes required for accreditation. By June 1972, however, conflicts between SHNB management and the non-medical community psychiatric occupations, especially the social workers, had reached the point where the DPH felt it imperative to intervene directly into the management of the hospital.[59]

The principal reason for this was that the conflicts were beginning to extend beyond PSB. The DPH did not want a crisis of management in PSB to become a more general political crisis if it were at all avoidable. Thus, when the provincial councillor for the Saskatoon Mayfair NDP became involved in the struggles on the side of the social workers, the DPH took action.

The event that instigated this chain of events was an attempt (not the first) by the executive director of SHNB to have the administrative supervisor of social work at the hospital dismissed. The preceding year the executive director of SHNB apparently had taken out of context a number of comments from the annual report of the social services department (SHNB) in an attempt to demonstrate that the department "was not well organized, was confused about its role, and needed guidance."[60] The administrative director of social work wrote the director of PSB refuting the account of the department's functioning contained in this report and requesting that PSB management intervene "to work out a policy regarding the proper role of social work."[61]

The director of PSB got involved, but not in the way the administrative director of social work had anticipated. On 1 June 1972, following a consultation with the director of PSB, the executive director of SHNB gave the administrative director of social work an unsatisfactory job rating. On the basis of this, it was recommended that he be demoted from Social Worker IV to Social Worker I, which would have precluded him from occupying his position. This information was given to the provincial councillor who pointed out in a letter to the minister of public health that, among other things, such a demotion was

> In effect . . . a dismissal, since anyone suffering a loss of position and status of this nature would find it impossible to remain on the job. Since previous ratings have been suitable, this sudden turn of events seems to hinge on his differences of opinion regarding such matters as the manner of accepting referrals from the community, the methods of treatment, supervision, staff deployment, etc. [the administrative director of social work] has . . . not been able to get any orderly discussion of his case among the doctors at the hospital, nor has he been allowed to present it to higher administration.[62]

The administrative director of social work appealed the decision, and although the director of PSB and the executive director of SHNB remained committed to their original positions, officials in the minister's office overturned the decision. This was a major blow to PSB management, although they remained undeterred in their efforts to maintain dominance of the psychiatric division of labour. Thus, on 26 June 1972, a memo addressed to "All Medical Staff and All Social Service Staff" was posted in the hospital. It proclaimed: "Effective July 1, 1972, Social Workers assigned to the various teams will be responsible to the psychiatric team leader, administratively and otherwise."[63]

This confirmed the feeling among social workers at SHNB that there was a concerted attempt underway to eliminate psychiatric social work in the North Battleford region. A letter to the minister of public health from a social worker at SHNB clearly expressed this feeling:

> A recent confrontation with the Director of psychiatric services produced the reiterated statements that this institution is to serve the needs of mental illness not mental health. This, of course, lends credence to another of his statements, which questioned the validity of the inclusion of professional social work at S.H.N.B. It is my hope . . . to indicate the legitimate concerns of the social workers as well as to indicate my support for the responsible and constructive approaches taken by [the administrative director] of the social work department.[64]

Thus social worker solidarity and resolve were being strengthened despite, or perhaps because of, attempts by PSB management to limit occupational autonomy and maintain the subordination of the community-based occupational groups.

As tensions mounted, threatening the capacity for continued service delivery, the DPH began to pressure PSB management for a resolution of the intensifying conflicts. PSB management remained committed to continued medical domination, as can be seen from the following memo from the director of PSB to the minister of public health:

> I am satisfied . . . that the social work and medical staff are not pulling together and that this is primarily because the social workers seek greater autonomy than the medical staff are prepared to give them . . . the social worker must be a member of a team and the psychiatrist the leader of the team. I don't see how anything else could work when we are dealing with severely ill patients, many of whom require medications.[65]

In a sense, the director of PSB had played directly into the hands of the social workers. It was precisely their point that within the context of community psychiatry the persons seen were not, in most cases, severely ill. They were, rather, people in need of assistance with aspects of their problems in living.

## Psychology and Anti-Psychiatry

It is interesting to note that at the height of the tensions between psychiatrists and social workers in June 1972, the Psychological Society of Saskatchewan (PSS) had Dr. Thomas Szasz as the keynote speaker for their annual institute. The chairman of the PSS wrote the minister of public health inviting him, or his representatives, to attend a half-day meeting with Dr. Szasz. It was suggested that such a meeting could "lead to the formulation of policies that would result in a substantial financial saving for the Public Health Purse."[66]

The letter quoted several paragraphs from Szasz's book *Insanity and Ideology* and concluded by stating that non-medical occupations "by reason of training and experience, could more extensively, effectively and economically be employed to address these *problems in living* now masked primarily as medical problems and as such, substantially inflating the Provincial Health Budget."[67] [emphasis in original] As a final comment it was suggested that DPH officials, if they decided to meet with Dr. Szasz, might like to pay a proportion of his per diem fee.

Although the DPH was always interested in cost-cutting proposals it was felt, given the public controversy already created by the attacks of the private psychiatrists and the internal struggles occurring throughout the system, that "it would be entirely inadvisable to consider bringing Dr. Szasz to Saskatchewan."[68] The associate director of PSB added, in support of this negative recommendation,

> I am told that [Dr. Szasz] is very anti-government services and opposes governments being involved in the delivery of psychiatric services. Furthermore, it has been suggested that he is a capitalist of the first order and this

> is perhaps borne out by the fact that his fee is $1,000 a day.[69]

Certainly this was a damning criticism for the socialist NDP government. A more germane reason for not sponsoring Szasz's trip was to demonstrate to the increasingly beleaguered PSB psychiatrists that their employer had not also joined in the attacks upon them, although this support proved more apparent than real.

Even without DPH support the PSS did sponsor Dr. Szasz's trip to the province, and he provided them with the ideological justification for seeking greater occupational autonomy. It was realized, however, that in order to be successful in their bid for occupational autonomy, a strong unified organization was needed. Thus, the Saskatchewan Psychological Association, which had already established an "Ad Hoc Committee to Investigate possible alternatives to the Registered Psychologists Act" in November 1971, began to pursue this objective with increased vigour.[70] Due to the diversity of specialty, techniques and credentials, psychology as a whole was not able to sustain the claim of occupational unity and hence the attempt to gain occupational parity with medically trained psychiatrists was ineffectual. These struggles continued throughout the 1970s and 1980s with psychologists taking an increasingly active role in the struggles against the medical domination of the public sector community psychiatric labour process. In the summer of 1972, however, social workers were in the vanguard of these struggles.

### Crisis Resolution: A Non-Medical Director for SHNB

The entry of the psychologists into the struggles for occupational independence from medical domination indicated a serious escalation of interoccupation and management-worker conflicts to DPH officials. Social workers were leaving, psychiatrists were leaving and, increasingly, the DPH was being petitioned to intervene, as in the following letter from a social worker to the minister of public health:

> Many people from the Social Work Department are making plans to leave or transfer including myself.

> Polarization of Social Workers and administration has occurred, no one is communicating now and at this point in time not much hope is left outside of direct action from your department.[71]

The DPH responded quickly. On 5 July the executive officer to the minister of public health and the director of PSB flew from Regina to North Battleford to investigate. Reporting his findings to the minister of public health on 12 July, the executive officer stated he had spoken with nurses, social workers and doctors, and although he found one MSW

> to be somewhat paranoid about the "plot" being devised by the medical staff to get rid of the social workers . . . there was undoubtedly some basis for his feeling that the medical staff in general and [the executive director of SHNB] in particular are not prepared to hear the ideas for change which the social workers are espousing.[72]

Although the executive director of SHNB and the administrative supervisor of the Social Services Department had agreed to cooperate, the executive officer to the minister of public health correctly observed that

> an accommodation between the two men will not solve the basic interdisciplinary problem between the two professions. I suspect that the problem will take a long time to resolve and will not be resolved just because relationships between the two main disputants in this case are patched up.[73]

The observation that the problem was structural rather than simply a clash of personalities was astute. The advice given to the minister of public health that "for the moment we would be better not to take sides and to make it plain to both sides . . . that it is up to them to solve the problem and find some compromise,"[74] was less than useful, and was ignored.

In mid-July, in an attempt to reduce interoccupation conflicts, the DPH decided to proceed with the plan to appoint a non-medical director of SHNB. The incumbent executive director of SHNB, although he professed agreement with "the concept of freeing physicians to do medical work [and letting] professional administrators run the hospital"[75] was opposed to the timing of the change for two reasons. First, as he stated, "I have put a tremendous amount of work into raising the standards of care in this hospital and I consider it very important to my future career to leave this hospital in an accredited status."[76] Second, as was reported by the deputy minister of public health, he felt that

> The placing of an ad for an Executive Director at this time might be construed by members of the Saskatchewan Hospital North Battleford staff as indicating that you are in effect "throwing out" [the executive director and the administrator].[77]

In fact, the minister of public health, in consultation with his deputy minister and associate deputy minister, had devised a plan for the replacement of the incumbent director of PSB by a non-medical director.[78] This plan, which was to be implemented by the end of 1973, was presented to and accepted by the premier in August 1972.[79] The minister of public health also observed in a memo to the premier that he had not "hinted to the management staff of the Branch of such a change."[80] The stage was thus set for a significant shift in occupational power.

In July 1972, however, no non-medical director was available to take over the position at SHNB. Also, because PSB management had not been informed of the plans of the DPH, the executive director of SHNB and other PSB medical staff apparently assumed that the lack of action was implicit support for the status quo and an endorsement of the continued medical domination of the psychiatric division of labour. The executive director of SHNB apparently assumed that his original position *vis-à-vis* the dismissal of the administrative supervisor of social services had received implicit endorsement. Thus, in mid-August he wrote the director of PSB that "over the past month [the administrative supervisor of social work] has made no attempt to co-operate with the Administration of this hospital. . . . He is undermining his workers, his attitude is divisive and when at times he does not wish to 'obey the rules' he indicates he would prefer to take matters 'to a higher level.'"[81] The memorandum concluded with a reiteration of the recommendation that the administrative director of social work be dismissed.[82]

His recommendation was again rejected by the DPH. Two days later, despite protests from SHNB management, the minister of public health announced the DPH would be advertising for a non-medical executive director for the hospital immediately. Soon after, the executive director and the administrator of SHNB submitted their resignations, although not before they had improved conditions at SHNB to the stage where it was possible to receive accreditation.

PSB management-psychiatrists were concerned that these developments would encourage the community occupations in their struggles for occupational autonomy. Thus the director of PSB issued a memorandum to all PSB unit heads regarding the distribution of power within the psychiatric team:

> The psychiatrist shall function as the leader of the team . . . when problems arise they should be settled at the team level whenever possible. Clear policies and guidelines regarding the functioning of the team should be drawn up in each region and the team members should be familiar with the legislation under which we operate (i.e., the Mental Health Act and its accompanying regulations).[83]

The simple assertion that psychiatrists would be team leaders was not well received. Also, by drawing attention to the legislative basis of psychiatrists' power, the director of PSB gave a specific focus to the community workers' struggles for autonomy.

The director of psychiatric social work, in a memo to the director of PSB, stated that he was disturbed by the policy that team leaders would be psychiatrists:

> I believe it is important to establish that this is not merely a "psychiatrist program" but a service that involves a conglomerate of specialties. A team system should be developed wherein all disciplines can work together on an equal plane with the team leadership being determined by the particular needs of the consumer in each case. If this is not possible within the

> present Act and Regulations then I feel that the Act should be updated.[84]

The director of PSB remained adamant; psychiatrists must have overall leadership.[85] Justifying his position to the minister of public health, he stated:

> I don't want to give the impression of molly-coddling psychiatrists but I know for a fact that a considerable number of psychiatrists are now planning to leave the province and friction with the social work group is a strong factor. A service denuded of medically trained people can only lead to personal and political tragedy and I hope and trust that everything possible will be done to decrease divisiveness between the two groups.[86]

Although little was done to reduce divisiveness immediately, the DPH did come out clearly in support of the community psychiatric programmes and occupations by appointing a clinical psychlogist as executive director of SHNB. This appointment marked a significant shift in the balance of interoccupational power away from the medically trained, in-patient-oriented psychiatrists toward the community-based, social-psychologically trained occupations. This shift was part of a conscious policy of the minister of public health, as his news release made clear:

> In making this appointment we are striking out in new directions . . . I feel that psychiatrists are needed primarily to provide clinical services to patients and consultations to other mental health professionals . . . in many cases they are overburdened with administrative duties.[87]

The new directions clearly implied that within the community psychiatric division of labour the psychiatrist was not necessarily to assume the position of leader, as had been consistently asserted by PSB management. It is interesting to note that not only had the minister used the terminology of the non-medical community-based workers, but he also endorsed the consultant role for psychiatrists.

The appointment of a clinical psychologist, although a surprise to PSB management-psychiatrists, was a logical choice for two reasons: first, it clearly demonstrated the commitment of the DPH to the further development of community psychiatry, and second, the person appointed, had been employed by PSB since 1966, and was familiar with the nature and history of the problems of Saskatchewan psychiatry. In addition, he had already addressed himself to the problems of interoccupation conflicts in a paper presented to the 1972 Canadian Psychology Association Institute on Community Psychology held in Montreal. In this paper, entitled "Role Conflicts Within a Provincial Community Mental Health Program," he argued:

> To promote interdisciplinary co-operation and development it is necessary first to recognize that all professions are claiming expertise in the same field. . . . At the unit level there needs to be more communication and sharing of decision making between the various professions . . . changes are required in mental health acts to specifically mandate the crucial areas of prevention and consultation.[88]

Not only were the various occupations claiming expertise in the same field, they were claiming expertise in the same techniques and treatments. These included various forms of individual and group psychotherapy, counselling, resocializing and other psycho-social manipulations of the patient's environment.[89]

This created problems because, as one social worker stated "everyone can do psychotherapy, no one has a patent on psychotherapy or counselling."[90] This contributed to the perpetuation of interoccupation conflicts, because no occupation was able to establish a monopoly of a particular sphere or technique of community psychiatric work in the same way that medically trained psychiatrists had secured a monopoly of drug prescription and domination of the in-hospital psychiatric labour process.

The newly appointed director of PSB's suggestion that there needed to be more communication and sharing of decision making between the various professions contributed to the DPH decision to establish the Ad Hoc Committee on Psychiatric Team Structure in 1973.

### The Ad Hoc Committee on Psychiatric Team Structure

The terms of reference for this committee were quite broad. Its mandate was to

> Examine the responsibilities of the various disciplines on the Psychiatric Services Team in terms of the Mental Health Act and its Regulations [and]. . . . Examine and comment on the role of various disciplines in the Psychiatric Team, namely, Psychiatrist, Social Worker, Psychologist and Community Psychiatric Nurse.[91]

The committee was also charged with responsibility for recommending changes in the organization of psychiatric work and the distribution of occupational power.

The committee itself consisted of eight members drawn from the four contending occupations, and a DPH executive assistant who acted as secretary. The original committee was composed of two psychiatrists, one psychologist, two social workers and three community psychiatric nurses. The first organizational meeting was held 9 February 1973 in Regina.

The committee met nine times and submitted its final report to the deputy minister of public health in May. In it were outlined twenty-five problems identified by the various occupational submissions, and twenty-five solutions.

The problems fell into three categories: (1) occupational autonomy and control; (2) management practices and decision-making; and (3) service organization and delivery. Since most management positions were occupied by psychiatrists, the criticisms of management practices and decision-making procedures had direct implications for the struggles for occupational autonomy. Similarly, demands for occupational autonomy, which were primarily struggles against the medical domination of the community psychiatric labour process, were also struggles against PSB management. The primacy of the struggles for autonomy from medical domination found clear expression in the concluding statement of the final report:

> Psychiatry must recognize the right of every professional group to define its own functions and areas of competence and to set up its own educational and training

> programs, and to establish its own standards of service. No profession should attempt to define the functions and responsibilities of any other profession.[92]

PSB-employed psychiatrists were disturbed with the general tenor of the report and its recommendations. In a three-page position paper on the final report of the committee, submitted to the director of PSB on 26 September, it was stated that "all the psychiatrists except two who communicated with us felt that psychiatrists were *NOT* adequately represented on the Ad Hoc Committee. This is a serious matter."[93] [emphasis in original] It was serious to the psychiatrists since several of the recommendations were intended to displace them from their dominant position in the psychiatric occupational division of labour.

The psychiatrists' position paper acknowledged that it was "essential that professions of various disciplines and backgrounds contribute to the assessment and treatment"[94] of the mentally ill. The problem, as the psychiatrists saw it, was "the relative status or involvement different professionals"[95] were to have in that process. The psychiatrists argued that the non-medical occupations wanted to take over work they claimed was exclusively theirs. To substantiate their claim to exclusive jurisdiction over work involved in the treatment of the mentally ill, the psychiatrists invoked Sections 65 and 69 of the Medical Profession Act. That act, it was pointed out,

> creates an offence and provides for the imposition of a penalty for any person not registered under the Act [who engages] in the practice of, professes to engage in the practice of, or advertises to give advice on medicine. . . . every person shall be deemed to practice medicine within the meaning of this Act who holds himself out as being able to diagnose, treat, operate or prescribe for any human disease, pain, injury, disability or physical condition, or who offers or undertakes by any means or methods to diagnose, treat, operate or prescribe for any human disease, pain, injury, disability or physical condition.[96]

It seemed evident to PSB psychiatrists that "the medical practitioner can be the only person responsible for diagnoses and medical treatment"[97] of *mental illness.* It was indicated, however, that there was nothing in the act to prevent "social workers from practicing social work, or nurses from practicing nursing, or psychologists from practicing psychology."[98] From the point of view of the community-based occupations, this was precisely the problem. As long as mental illness was being treated, those with medical training were legislatively guaranteed control of psychiatric work and dominance of the psychiatric division of labour.

The non-medically trained community workers were struggling for autonomy from this medical domination. The social workers and psychologists, in particular, claimed to be working with a health- (as opposed to illness-) oriented psycho-social model. They denied that all psychiatric conditions were *ipso facto* medical conditions.

The community-based occupations were quite willing to concede medical dominance and control of the in-hospital psychiatric labour process, but not of the community psychiatric labour process. PSB management-psychiatrists remained unmoved. In fact, the assault on medical dominance served to unify the psychiatrists into a powerful defensive force.

In August 1973, as a result of the recommendations of the ad hoc committee, the director of PSB issued a set of proposed guidelines on interrelationships amongst the various occupational groups. The thirteen points proposed were prefaced with the comment that "*First priority must . . . go to those who are mentally or emotionally disordered and sick patients must always receive primary consideration.*"[99] [emphasis in original]

With regard to the contentious issue of referrals, the guidelines allowed that "Direct referrals of out-patients . . . may be made by physicians and other persons and agencies approved by the Medical Officer in charge to unit psychiatrists, social workers, psychologists or community psychiatric nurses."[100] However, all referrals not made specifically to a non-medical occupation (the majority) were to be delegated by the medical officer in charge. In addition, each department head was to "make a list of the staff who may accept referrals and forward the list to the medical officer in charge of the facility for final approval."[101] The response of the community-based groups was not positive. As one social worker stated to the director of PSB, "the atmosphere conveyed by your proposed guidelines is near to being a polarized opposite of the intent of the recommendations of the report of the Ad Hoc Committee on Psychiatric Team Structure."[102]

The director responded to the social workers by stating that although he understood, and even agreed with the demands of the non-medical occupational groups for autonomy, under the regulations of the 1961 Mental Health Act there was little to be done. He also stated that he would be "interested to have suggestions . . . about how the Mental Health Act might be changed. . . . The problem now is of finding a formula which is reasonably safe, effective and satisfactory to the principal mental health professions."[103] It appeared to many that little had changed.

It was unlikely that a satisfactory formula would be found for two reasons: first, psychiatrists had become united in their own occupational defence; and second, they opposed the director of PSB's call for suggestions to change the Mental Health Act. As one PSB-employed psychiatrist wrote in 1973: "I would hate to see . . . any type of legislation on function or *definition of authority* and responsibility relating to organizational structure and I myself would strongly oppose any such changes."[104] [emphasis in original]

Psychiatrists argued that changes in the legislative specification of occupational functions and powers were unnecessary because the problems were the result of individual feelings: "I fail to see how the further definition of roles will help solve people's feelings about either each other or the circumstances in which they work."[105]

Social workers and psychologists, however, were strong supporters of legislative change, as can be seen from the following memo submitted to the ad hoc committee in March 1973: "It is my sincere hope that your committee's major recommendation will be that the Mental Health Act be totally re-written, not revised again but that it be re-written with a totally new approach taken."[106] It was perceived by social workers and psychologists that the 1961 Mental Health Act was a manifestation of struggles between the medical and legal professions for control of the definition and treatment of mental disorders. As such, it did not provide for the non-medical definition and treatment of people with living problems. Commenting on the 1961 Mental Health Act, the director of Munroe Youth Services, a psychologist, stated: "As a piece of legislation it is extremely restrictive and is based upon an entirely out-moded concept of medical-legal control of . . . the . . . mentally ill."[107] The community psychiatric occupations, therefore, continued their efforts to change the Mental Health Act. The momentum of the drive for de-medicalization, however, suddenly appeared to dwindle. There were two reasons for this: first, the threat of PSB-employed psychiatrists to leave the programme; and second, the emergence of a split in the unity of the community psychiatric occupations.

With regard to the first point, it should be noted that the threats were not idle. In March 1973, for example, all four psychiatrists at YPC quit because of "dissatisfaction with salary and working conditions."[108] The second factor was the split which developed between the psychiatric nurses and the social workers. Psychiatric nursing was the one occupation that had a stake in both the mental hospital and community-based psychiatric labour processes. The split in the solidarity of the community psychiatric occupations was a product of this. Although CPNs supported the demand for autonomy from medical domination, the hospital-based psychiatric nurses, by far the largest proportion of psychiatric nurses, perceived that their occupational interests lay with the continuation of the traditional psychiatrist-nurse relationship. It was argued that

> If psychiatric illness is a medical condition, should this not be primarily treated and managed basically by medically oriented and educated personnel? i.e. Initially Doctor-Nurse approach? Under the concept that psychiatry is a medical condition [*sic*], how does the social worker rank next in line to the psychiatrist on case involvement? To our knowledge social workers have no

> formal medical or psychiatric education in comparison to psychiatrists and psychiatric nurses.[109]

The support of the psychiatric nurses for the medical model of mental illness was based on the fact that in terms of providing community psychiatric, non-medical services, psychiatric nurses were less well prepared in formal education and credentials than were either social workers or psychologists. Therefore, as is implicit in the above quotation, there was some concern that if the psycho-social model propounded by the social workers and psychologists superseded the medical model, the relatively high status of the psychiatric nurse as the subordinate, but favoured, assistant of the psychiatrist would be jeopardized. The psychiatric nurses, however, demanded certain concessions for their support:

> regarding the psychiatrist giving up some of his menial responsibilities, we see the psychiatric nurse as being the most appropriate group [*sic*] to assume these responsibilities because of our basic medical and psychiatric training and background experience.[110]

Although the mental hospital-based psychiatric nurses thought they were the heirs apparent for some of the psychiatrists' more menial functions, they also felt they should be "appointed the *team leader* and *primary therapist* [for those patients] requiring resocialization, behavior therapy, work training, habit formation etc."[111] [emphasis in original] The psychiatrists had never been opposed to the non-medical occupations performing *appointed* therapeutic duties, so long as it was the psychiatrist who made the appointment and determined the scope of responsibility and autonomy. One PSB-employed psychiatrist, in discussing the history and position of social work and community psychiatric nursing within the psychiatric division of labour, stated that

> Initially social workers and community nurses were employed to follow-up people discharged from hospital to community. These professionals were employed as paramedical staff to relieve medical staff of jobs which

> could be done by lesser trained persons. This concept of ancilliary workers dominated the thinking. The social worker or nurse was seen as someone who carried out the doctors [*sic*] orders and helped him accomplish his goal. The doctor was seen, theoretically at any rate, as the person who understood fully the problem and knew all the answers.[112]

A clearer exposition of the Babbage Principle could not be found. However, the community psychiatric occupational groups were not *initially* employed to relieve medical staff of jobs which could be done by lesser-trained persons, because psychiatrists had never performed follow-ups and domiciliary visits.

With the in-hospital psychiatric nurses supporting the occupational status quo, PSB management-psychiatrists became more entrenched in their position, a process facilitated by the fact the psychiatric nurses also mounted their own attack on the social workers. The psychiatric nurses argued that due to high rates of attrition among both psychiatrists and social workers, there was no continuity of treatment in the community programmes originated and operated by those two occupations. It was further argued that, as a consequence of the high attrition and turnover rates among psychiatrists and social workers, and given the relative stability of psychiatric nursing, the community programmes were, in fact, being carried by the psychiatric nurses. In the experience of the psychiatric nurses, it was found, and greatly resented, that when new psychiatrists or social workers were employed in a region psychiatric nurses were relegated to a lower status than they felt they deserved. This generated antagonism which was directed mostly towards the social workers, as was evident in a recommendation made by the psychiatric nurses from the Weyburn Psychiatric Centre for changes to the team structure. It was suggested that

> Consideration [be] given to utilizing social workers on a referral basis only. As the program exists at the present time there seems to be no justification for a social worker being attached to every psychiatric team. "With due respect" the training of social workers (including

> B.A.'s and M.S.W.'s) appears non-relevant to a psychiatric program. There is little evidence to prove that their orientation and training include knowledge sufficient to prepare them for working with patients presenting psychiatric problems.[113]

The psychiatric nurses viewed the social workers as the main enemy, since they were thought to be interposing themselves in the psychiatrist-psychiatric nurse dyad and usurping psychiatric nursing work. It might be argued, however, that it was in fact the psychiatric nurses, struggling to ensure occupational survival and individual security, who were attempting to usurp traditional social work functions:

> The traditional social worker's duties such as: application to welfare, basic routine histories, checking SHSP [Saskatchewan Hospital Services Plan] coverage, etc., could be done by Community Psychiatric Nurses or ward nurses rather than a trained social worker. This would allow the social workers time to do their specialty which they have long discussed and has not yet been defined.[114]

Psychiatric nurses had coveted social work positions since the mid-1950s, and the creation of CPNs in 1964 was at least partly the result of a long battle to secure a place in the community psychiatric division of labour. It also marked a process of deskilling psychiatric social work.

Although the psychiatric nurses saw themselves in direct competition with the social workers, this was not the case with psychologists. It was thought at the time that "psychologists assume their rightful place in the treatment program."[115] There was little conflict between psychiatric nurses and psychologists because psychologists, although they did perform some therapeutic functions, were largely involved in providing psychological assessments and psychological testing as a diagnostic aid and, therefore, were not seen to be in direct competition with the psychiatric nurses.

The psychologists, however, stirred to action by the activities of the Ad Hoc Committee on Psychiatric Team Structure, became increasingly involved in the struggle against medical domination. Commenting on interoccupation relations in 1973, one PSB-employed psychologist stated:

> the dissension in the ranks does not stem from competing modes of treatment, treatment philosophies, or helper-client relationships. The issue is essentially whether psychiatrists should have the authority, power, and hence the prestige and financial reward that goes with it, while other professions serve as ancillary to psychiatry. . . . The disparity in salaries, the rights, duties, responsibilities and decision-making powers of the psychiatrist rankles those other members of the alleged "team" who feel their training, knowledge, and work to be as important, often more important, in the treatment of those we choose to designate as psychiatrically ill. . . . *The fundamental issue is power*, and the authoritarian domination of the mental health field by the medical profession.[116] [emphasis in original]

Social workers and psychologists increasingly came to be allied against psychiatrists and psychiatric nurses throughout the 1970s.

DPH officials, although generally supportive of social workers and psychologists due to the cost-saving potential of the non-medical community psychiatric labour process, were, for political reasons, unwilling to mount a direct offensive on the conservative psychiatrist-psychiatric nurse alliance. As a consequence, the 1972 plan to hire a non-medical director for PSB was not realized until 1979. Although the intensity of the interoccupational conflicts diminished following the appointment of a non-medical director of SHNB, the struggles of psychologists and social workers against medical domination continued.

In the mid-1970s PSB management attempted to defuse this interoccupational conflict by eliminating occupational coordinators at PSB head office and replacing them with programme heads. The major programmes were Child-Youth Services, Rehabilitation Services, Residential Services and Geriatric Services. One of the objectives of this programme-oriented management strategy was the replacement of occupational identification with programme identification. It was hoped that occupational interests would thus be superseded by programme objectives and result in a reduction of inter-occupational conflicts and increased efficiency in PSB operations. The desired objectives were not fully achieved, however, as the various occupations tended to claim specific programmes, or groups of programmes. The psychologists and social workers have, over the past decade, expanded the psycho-social programmes, such as Child-Youth Services, Marriage Counselling and Day-Hospital Services, to the point that they now command as many resources as the traditional medically oriented programmes, thus improving their bargaining position within PSB. Therefore the trend toward de-medicalization, although not characterized by the bitter conflicts of the early 1970s, is continuing.

As was indicated, psychologists are now spearheading the assault on the continued, but certainly reduced, medical domination of the public sector psychiatric labour process. Armed with the powerful argument of cost-effectiveness, and backed by the recommendations of the Hastings Report, they have recently begun to lobby for an expanded role within the psychiatric labour process. Between August and December 1982, for example, the Psychological Society of Saskatchewan sent letters to local MPs, and both federal and provincial ministers of health. The objective of this lobbying campaign was to influence the then proposed Canada Health Care Act to "recognize and legitimize psychologists' role in the health care field."[117] The provincial psychologists emphasized the fact that physicians in the province, who were paid 30 to 50 percent more than doctoral-level clinical psychologists, spent at least 30 percent of their time in psycho-social counselling work.[118] This is work for which, the psychologists argued, medically trained physicians were ill equipped: "As a result citizens are poorly served (medicated for psycho/social problems) and have to pay increasingly high taxes for ineffective services."[119] They see the solution as access of non-medical "health professional groups . . . to public funding."[120]

All non-medical occupations were lobbying for the inclusion of their services under the terms of Medicare. These activities met with some success, for when the Canada Health

Act received Royal Assent on 17 April 1984, it stated that non-medical health-care occupations were authorized to provide insured services when permitted to do so by a provincial government. The evidence suggests that the provincial governments, concerned with reducing expenditures, will provide for the coverage of non-medical health care services through some type of insurance scheme. One would suspect, given the experience with medically dominated fee-for-service systems presently in place, that provincial governments might opt for the coverage of these non-medical services on a capitation basis. Another option is to continue to provide these services by salaried workers, either employed directly by the government, or by some kind of community health centre. In addition, there is always the possibility for the development of some combination or permutation of the above, especially given the possibility that now exists in the province for private sector hospitals/in-patient facilities.[121]

At this point the future of community psychiatry is uncertain. There are, however, forces at work which lead one to expect an increasing tendency towards the privatization and commodification of mental health services.[122] What seems certain is that the de-medicalization of community psychiatric work will continue. The 1985 Mental Health Services Act, among other things, was an expression of this trend.

It also seems certain that there will be a continuing trend towards the use of computers in psychiatric work. The incorporation of this technology into the psychiatric labour process is likely to facilitate the continued de-medicalization and possible deskilling of psychiatric work. It is also likely computer technology will not be controlled by medically trained psychiatric workers. In fact, the further development and extension of that technology is likely to be the material base from which the de-medicalization of community psychiatric work is completed. There is a substantial body of literature which deals with the various uses of computers in the field of psychiatry. Acording to Spero, these are:

> (1) data collection; (2) objective identification of symptom clusters; (3) assignment of diagnosis, treatment form and prognosis; (4) evaluation of patient progress; (5) treatment *per se*.[123]

Spero has also pointed out that the first four spheres are related to diagnosis, and fall into the range of activities over which medically trained workers have traditionally claimed exclusive control. The fifth area, although only at an experimental stage, refers to "actual *intervention*, or what would eventually be called computerized psychotherapy."[124] [emphasis in original]

Although there seems to be a general consensus among all psychiatric occupations that computers will never be able to completely replace the living psychotherapist, there also seems to be a consensus regarding the potential of computers to automate the medical component of psychiatric work:

> I think when you are dealing with mental health issues you cannot take the therapist — the person of the therapist — totally out of it, but you can do some things to automate it so it goes quicker. I think medicine, the medical component, is one of the things that are the most vulnerable to that — the dispensing of medications and so on.[125]

The vulnerability of the medical component derives from the scienticity of medical work. That is, knowledge which can be standardized and systematized is vulnerable to automation. It is precisely this process that has been identified as the mechanism underlying the transition from the formal to the real subordination of labour. Knowledge that can be codified can be taken over by management and used to separate conception from execution in any labour process.

At present, psychologists in Saskatchewan have a *de facto* advantage with regard to the control of computer technology because, since as early as 1964, they have "devoted considerable time to studying data-gathering and analyzing processes and to the potential use of computers in the psychiatric field."[126] The provincial psychologists seem to be particularly interested in establishing a monopoly over the work of psychological assessments and testing. Currently, psychological assessments performed by physicians are covered by Medicare. Provincial psychologists think that if the cost of psychological assessments performed by psychologists can be further reduced in relation to those performed by physicians through the automation of that work, it will be to their occupational advantage. It is realized, however, that the use of technology can cut both ways, and that if computerized psychological assessment can undermine the occupational base of medical labour power, it can do the same to psychological labour power. Commenting on that point, a provincial psychologist stated:

> we will make damn sure that we will not implement that unless we have control over it! *Absolute* control and that it will be written into all kinds of things that we have to do the interpretation. But it is a threat and the easiest way is just not to do it.[127]

Working within the context of the employment-relation, however, the introduction of computer technology into the psychiatric labour process will not be determined by occupational self-interest. Rather, the management imperatives of cost reduction, increased productivity and control are likely to be the motivating forces for the computerization of psychiatric work. It must be added that occupational interests, and the struggles thereby generated, will undoubtedly influence both the rate and form in which computer technology is introduced. Additionally, if interoccupation or management-worker struggles for control of a new technology threaten to escalate into a political crisis, the rate and form of introduction and control will be further influenced. In fact, it might be argued that one of the factors encouraging the privatization of the psychiatric labour process, besides the promise of reduced costs, would be the promise of depoliticizing psychiatric work. As has been seen, public sector psychiatry in Saskatchewan has had very few years wherein it was not in the midst of, or on the verge of, a political crisis. Privatization would relieve government officials of direct responsibility for the perpetual crisis of public sector psychiatry, and for that reason alone is likely to have strong appeal. Privatization, if indeed it does occur, will undoubtedly take place through a gradual transition, as was recommended by MDT Associates in 1968. In the interim, PSB management and the DPH will be required to manage the public sector psychiatric labour process.

It has already been suggested that the programme-oriented management system was unsuccessful in reducing interoccupation conflicts. The Thrust Committee therefore proposed the elimination of occupational distinctions altogether. This is to be achieved by the creation of a new occupation called Mental Health Worker: "Many of the positions currently assigned to particular disciplines could be reclassified using such a general title and classification description."[128] At this point no move has been made to reclassify PSB positions in the proposed manner, since any such move would likely meet with significant worker opposition and a worsening of the situation it is designed to remedy.

The Thrust Committee also recommended a second strategy for achieving the same goal, the creation of another new occupation provisionally called Community Mental Health Worker, to function as a psychiatric nurse practitioner providing basic direct services in those communities that do not currently have full-time mental health staff. Besides performing psycho-social therapy and counselling, it is suggested this proposed new occupation also be legislatively empowered to prescribe drugs.[129] This suggestion therefore entails both the de-medicalization and deskilling of psychiatric work. Thus the trend towards the deskilling and de-medicalization of community psychiatric work seems to be a reality.

# Chapter Seven

# Conclusions

The nature and organization of psychiatric work has radically changed throughout this century. The most obvious manifestation of this is the post-World War II transition from asylum to community-based psychiatry. This study has been an account of that transition as it has occurred in Saskatchewan. The rate and form of the transformation of psychiatric work associated with the development of community psychiatry was the result of a conjuncture of many forces, some internal to the relations of the psychiatric labour process and some external to them, but influential in determining the nature and organization of psychiatric work.

Drawing upon the writings of Harry Braverman and Vincente Navarro, it was hypothesized that the occupational division of labour associated with the development of community psychiatry was an instance of the deskilling of psychiatric work. Concentrating on the type of deskilling which results from the application of the Babbage Principle to work, that is, the fragmentation of work into its constituent elements and the substitution of less skilled and less expensive labour power for more skilled and more expensive labour power in the performance of those fragmented tasks, the hypothesis was rejected. That is, the development of the community psychiatric division of labour cannot be understood as an instance of the deskilling of psychiatric work. It was found that the initial development of community psychiatry marked the creation of a new psychiatric labour process, characterized by new social relations and forces of production. Thus, the community psychiatric occupations were found to be performing new tasks specific to the new community psychiatric labour process, not fragmented tasks characteristic of the mental hospital labour process. The demise of the asylum and the rise of community psychiatry thus entailed a bifurcation of psychiatric practice. On the one hand there exists a physician-dominated private sector psychiatric services system that provides in-patient treatment in general hospitals. On the other hand there exists an increasingly de-medicalized public sector psychiatric services system providing psychiatric services in mental health clinics by social scentifically trained therapists.

The transformation of psychiatric work, however, is characterized by a complex of often contradictory tendencies. Although a simple deskilling hypothesis cannot be sustained, since the mid-1960s there has been a discernible trend toward the deskilling of psychiatric work. The dominant tendency during any period is the outcome of a number of forces and social practices and cannot be known *a priori*. The determination of the dominant tendency requires a conjunctural analysis such as has been presented here.

The second theme running throughout this study is the medicalization of psychiatric work, and the periodization of that process. This theme constitutes a debate with Andrew Scull, who has provided an analysis of the medicalization and professionalization of asylum psychiatry in nineteenth-century England. Scull maintains that the medicalization of psychiatric work was essentially completed by the end of the nineteenth century, and that the work of medical superintendents of asylums was professionalized by the adoption of psychoanalytic theory during the interwar years.

Following Freidson's suggestion that the issue of professionalization might be fruitfully replaced by a focus on the issues of the organization and control of work and its consequences for workers, organizations and society, the transformation of psychiatric work was analyzed in terms of a theory of the labour process. This theory, which conceptualizes a labour process as the purposive activity which occurs at the interface of the social relations and forces of production, led to a questioning of Scull's periodization of the medicalization of asylum psychiatry.

Although medically trained physicians certainly dominated the mental hospital division of labour, at the turn of the century they did not have monopoly control of the principal element of the psychiatric forces of production, the asylum. Admission to and discharge from asylums was not entirely a medical prerogative until the middle of the twentieth century. Until that time admission and discharge were either legal responsibilities or under joint medical-legal jurisdiction. Therefore, Scull's claim that medical monopoly of the asylum was achieved by the end of the nineteenth century is inaccurate. Since this imputed monopoly is the basis upon which he rests his claim regarding the medicalization of psychiatric work, it would seem that it too is inaccurate.

Even the complete medical control of admission to and discharge from the mental hospitals, however, does not necessarily correspond to the complete medicalization of psychiatric work. The work done within the mental hospitals remained largely non-medical in nature until the post-World War II period. The mental hospitals were basically custodial institutions; the little therapy which did exist consisted of "work and water." These therapies were supervised and administered by untrained ward attendants. It was not until the introduction of psychotropic drugs in the 1950s revolutionized the forces of psychiatric production that one can accurately speak of complete medicalization of psychiatric work.

Physician control of the mental hospitals and domination of the occupational division of labour, combined with the medical monopoly of drug prescription, completed the medicalization process. The introduction of the psychotropic drugs into psychiatric work corresponded to a decline in the use of other forms of restraint and treatment. This was not necessarily because the drug technology was more effective;

there is ample evidence that it was not. Rather, the almost exclusive reliance on chemotherapy can be understood as an attempt to ensure medical participation in psychiatric treatment, involvement which was guaranteed by the fact that medically trained physicians were the only ones legally empowered to prescribe drugs. In Saskatchewan this medicalization of psychiatric work was given legislative recognition in 1961 with the passage of the Mental Health Act. This legislation made mental hospital admission and discharge procedures more similar to those in general hospitals, and thus created the conditions for the rapid depopulation which began in 1963. The creation of Medicare in 1962 provided further encouragement for the medicalization of psychiatric work and formed the basis for the development of private sector psychiatry in Saskatchewan.

Medicare, by ensuring payment to physicians who provided psychotherapy on an out-patient basis, brought about the realization of the mental hygienist's long-standing ambition to convince GPs that mental illnesses were no different from physical illnesses and could, therefore, be treated in the community. Guaranteed payment, combined with the speed and ease of chemotherapy, were apparently more effective than forty years of educational efforts in bringing about these changes. Since the mid-1960s the largest proportion of psychiatric services has been produced by private practice GPs on an out-patient basis. If hospitalization is deemed necessary, a person is most likely to be admitted to a psychiatric ward of a general hospital, or even a general ward of a general hospital, not to a mental hospital. Admission to, and discharge from, general hospitals is controlled by physicians. Thus, all aspects of this brand of psychiatric work have been medicalized.

Medical superintendents of the mental hospitals, and other PSB-employed psychiatrists, although vociferous advocates of community psychiatry and the medicalization of psychiatric work in general, opposed the expansion of general hospital psychiatry. The reason for this opposition was that general hospital psychiatry eroded the employment base of PSB psychiatrists and managers. Their avid support of the

Saskatchewan Plan, particularly the establishment of small regional mental hospitals, can be partially understood in terms of the struggle for expanded employment opportunities, job security and career development. The proponents of the regional community mental hospital plan, however, also believed in the efficacy of the proposed style of building for the treatment of mental disorders. In this regard, there is an interesting historical parallel between the claims of the nineteenth-century proponents of the original asylum system and those of the twentieth-century proponents of the small regional community mental hospital system. In the latter case, however, the battle for the construction and control of the new treatment technology was largely unsuccessful.

It seems ironic that the medicalization of psychiatric work contained the seed of an incipient de-medicalization of community psychiatry. That is, the depopulation of the mental hospitals, partly the result of the medicalization of psychiatric work and more general political and economic considerations, led to the rapid expansion of the community psychiatric labour process, particularly of both the types and numbers of non-medical community psychiatric workers. The community psychiatric occupations, especially community psychiatric nurses, psychiatric social workers and psychologists, were originally employed to provide various follow-up and support services to discharged mental hospital patients. The objective of this type of work was to reduce the rate and duration of hospitalization. Arguing that such work is not medical, the community occupations, particularly social work and psychology, have been struggling against medical domination of the community psychiatric division of labour since the 1960s.

Drawing on the work of Szasz and the anti-psychiatrists for ideological justification, they claim many of the clients seen in community settings are not mentally ill but simply people with various problems in living. Therefore, it is argued that medical intervention is not only unnecessary in many cases, it may even contribute to the creation and/or perpetuation of certain problems in living. Addiction to tranquilizers and various side effects associated with the use of psychotropic drugs are cited as evidence of this claim.

Increasingly patient rights groups and other self-help groups are becoming actively involved in the search for alternatives to chemotherapy and the medical domination of community psychiatric treatment. An alliance is developing between these groups, interested community agencies and the non-medical community psychiatric occupational groups, based on the belief that appropriate non-medical intervention at an early stage can prevent an incipient problem in living from developing into a more serious condition requiring extensive, and expensive, medical intervention. The non-medical community psychiatric occupations maintain that their special expertise with psychotherapy and behaviour modification techniques ideally suits them for the performance of this preventive function. This emphasis on prevention, early intervention and mobilization of community resources is the same public health ideology used by medically trained psychiatrists to justify the transformation of insanity into mental illness throughout the first half of this century. By the 1960s and 1970s it was being used by the non-medical community psychiatric occupations to justify their attempts to transform mental illness into problems in living. The advocates of the de-medicalization of community psychiatry argue that their approach is more humane, more effective and less expensive than the medical alternative. Whether or not these claims are substantiated, they are appealing to legislators and the tax-paying public and, therefore, are likely to generate political support.

The emphasis on prevention leads to the ever-wider casting of occupational nets. Thus one sees the rapid expansion of various community psychiatric programmes, such as family and marriage counselling, child-youth services and so on. Although it is often assumed that the development of these programmes is indicative of medical imperialism and the medicalization of life, the empirical evidence from Saskatchewan indicates that these programmes are more likely to be initiated and dominated by non-medical occupational groups.

Thus, it appears that there has been a bifurcation of psychiatric service delivery. On the one hand there has emerged a physician-dominated, "private" sector psychiatric services system with chemotherapy as the primary form of outpatient treatment and inpatient services being provided when necessary in general hospitals. On the other hand, there also has developed a mental health clinic-based, public sector psychiatric services system which is increasingly dominated by non-medical therapists with social science backgrounds. Although there is some overlap between these two psychiatries, it is quite clear that there exist two distinct labour processes characterized by distinct forces and relations of production. It appears, on the basis of the analysis presented here, that this institutional bifurcation is grounded in the various attempts of different occupational groups to gain autonomy and control over certain aspects of their work. These struggles for autonomy and control are themselves based upon two competing conceptions of mental illness/disorders which appear to have both biochemical and socio-psychological causes.

As we have seen, the demise of the asylum and the rise of community psychiatry is often "explained" as a result of the triumph of the forces of enlightenment and humanitarian concern over the forces of ignorance and repression. This explanation has been shown to be inadequate. Foucault, for example, shows that the birth of the asylum in the eighteenth century, although most often presented in the above terms, can be more adequately understood as the replacement of a system of physical constraint of the insane with a system of self-control achieved through "moral treatment."[1] Foucault argues that the system of self-control cannot necessarily be viewed as more humane than the system of physical constraint because self-control produced via psychological manipulation is more insidious and repressive precisely because it is less visible. Although Foucault's observation concerning the transformation of patterns of managing the insane in the eighteenth century provide an important insight into the history of psychiatry, his announcement of the victory of socio-psychological notions of insanity and patterns of treatment was premature. Scull, for example, has shown that throughout the nineteenth century medically trained physicians attempted to discredit the claims of the proponents of "moral treatment," and to demonstrate that insanity was really mental illness requiring medical care and treatment.[2] Although physicians were willing to acknowledge that psychological treatments were effective in helping control behaviour, they remained adamant that mental illness had a somatic cause that required a somatic cure. Thus, contrary to what Foucault claims about the rise of the asylum and the rise to dominance of socio-psychological modes of treatment, Scull has shown that in the nineteenth century asylums came to be dominated by physicians who provided a wide range of somatic treatments along with various "moral" or psychological treatments. Scull has argued that the medicalization of insanity was completed by the end of the nineteenth century although I have tried to show that the process was not completed until the middle of the twentieth century. I have also tried to show that as long as the asylums remained the principal locus and form of treatment and as long as they were dominated and run by those with medical training and interests, the socio-psychological view of cause and treatment remained subordinate. By the mid-twentieth century those conditions no longer prevailed, and as has been shown, a radical transformation of the organization of psychiatric service delivery occurred.

Using a theory of the labour process this study has examined some of the factors and forces which contributed to the transformation of psychiatric work in Saskatchewan in the twentieth century. Although this approach is useful in explaining certain aspects of the form and consequences of the mental health system it leaves a number of important questions unanswered. For example, if the observed tendency towards the deskilling of public sector psychiatric work continues what will be the consequences for service consumers? Also, if the trend towards the de-medicalization of public sector services continues, or if it becomes generalized throughout the psychiatric services systems, will consumers be better off, or will they simply be replacing domination by one professional group with domination by another? More generally this study raises questions about the nature and organization of social reproduction in general. A growing body of research seems to suggest that the process of preparing people to perform structurally determined social, economic and political functions is increasingly being subjected to a process of rationalized professional control and direction. If this is the case one might well ask what the implications and consequences of this for the individual, and our liberal democratic form of society, will be.

# Appendix
# Labour Process Theory and Psychiatry

Labour process theory was revived from a somewhat somnolent state in 1974 with the publication of Harry Braverman's book *Labor and Monopoly Capital.* Although Marx was interested in the analysis of the capitalist labour process and devoted part of *Capital* to this task, subsequent generations of Marxists have addressed other issues. As a result, little work in this tradition existed, and that which did was exclusively concerned with the industrial labour process. Most Marxists thought nonindustrial labour processes were of little productive or political significance. Indeed, Marx suggested that the production of services was of such "microscopic significance when compared to the mass of capitalist production," that they could "be entirely neglected."[1] The post-World War II boom in service industries has made this somewhat offhanded dismissal of service work unacceptable.

## Braverman and the Theory of the Labour Process

Braverman, working within the Marxist tradition, but also drawing on the work of Adam Smith and Charles Babbage, has suggested that within capitalist societies the development of the occupational division of labour is based upon the principle of fragmenting work processes into their constituent elements and substituting less expensive for more expensive labour power in the execution of those fragmented tasks. This method of deskilling work is referred to as the Babbage Principle.

The Babbage Principle, first enunciated in 1832, was an addendum to Adam Smith's discussion of the sources of productivity increases achieved by the extension of the occupational division of labour. Smith argued that the three main sources of increased productivity were: (1) increased dexterity which workers develop when they perform only one, or at most a few, tasks; (2) the time saving achieved by not having workers change types of work; and (3) the invention and application of "labour saving" technology which is facilitated by specialization, and which allows one worker to do the work of many.

Although Babbage agreed that the above were important for explaining productivity increases, he added that the explanation would be incomplete if it were not stated that the employer,

> by dividing the work to be executed into different processes, each requiring different degrees of skill or force, can purchase exactly that precise quantity of both which is necessary for each process; whereas if the whole work were executed by one workman, that person must possess sufficient skill to perform the most difficult, and sufficient strength to execute the most laborious, of the operations into which the art is divided.[2]

Braverman has subsequently argued that the Babbage Principle, although first applied to "the handicrafts and then to the mechanical crafts . . . eventually becomes the underlying force governing all forms of work in capitalist society, no matter in what setting or at what hierarchical level. This might even be called the general law of the capitalist division of labour."[3]

Although many have agreed that there is a tendency for work involved in the production of material products to be deskilled, some have suggested that the work of producing "human" or "social" services, such as medical care and education, is intrinsically immune to that process. Navarro has opposed this position, arguing that there is a tendency towards the deskilling of social services work, and that it occurs both through the application of "labour-saving" technology and the Babbage Principle to that work:

> The introduction of new technologies and new organization of work occurs in *all* areas of social production. There are no areas or sectors that are intrinsically labor intensive. This point needs emphasis in view of the widely held belief that social and personal services are by definition labor intensive. . . . This position should be questioned on both theoretical and empirical grounds. The overall trend of the labor process under capitalism is the deskilling of labor and the substitution of living labor (workers) with dead labor (machines).[4]

Following this line of thought, the principal hypothesis of this book is that the occupational division of labour associated with the post-World War II emergence of community psychiatry is an instance of the deskilling of psychiatric work. The historical and empirical evidence used to test this hypothesis comes from an examination of the development of community psychiatry in Saskatchewan.

Before turning to an elaboration of the concepts and relations specific to the labour process, the relationship between the production and consumption of psychiatric services will be briefly examined.

## The Production and Consumption of Psychiatric Services

Within the Marxist theoretical tradition there are three basic elements constitutive of any labour process: (1) purposive activity, or the work itself; (2) the object upon which that work is performed; and (3) the instruments of that work.[5] In the production of psychiatric services, the purposive activity (psychiatric work itself) is directed towards the production of cures, symptom-free behaviour and/or manageable patients. Although a cure is the most desirable product, psychiatric practitioners, as well as others, are often content simply to produce manageable patients. As Crane has pointed out with reference to the use of neuroleptic drugs, many doctors, health care workers and family members who are resentful of

> the patient's behavior and are threatened by potential acts of violence fail to distinguish between manifestations of illness and reactions to frustrations. Hence, drugs are prescribed to solve all types of management problems, and failure to achieve the desired results causes an escalation of dosage, changes of drugs, and polypharmacy.[6]

Following a similar line of reasoning, Andrew Scull has suggested that the true clients of the asylum doctors in nineteenth-century England were the families of the insane and various parish officials, who used the asylum as "a convenient institution in which to dump the undesirable."[7] Although this view has a certain appeal, it is not adopted for the purposes of this study. Rather, the family of a person diagnosed as mentally ill, and other interested individuals and groups in the community, are viewed as constituting part of the public opinion and political climate which influences, but is external to, the constituent relations of the psychiatric labour process.

The consumer is thus the person actually receiving psychiatric treatment. This conceptualization is in keeping with the work of Gelvin Stevenson, who has suggested the production of human services, including medical and psychiatric services, consists of an "interaction designed to change the characteristics or condition of one of the people involved in the interaction, ie., the consumer."[8]

It is evident from this that the production of psychiatric services cannot occur independently of their immediate consumption. As Marx noted, production and consumption are to be considered as mutually determining "moments of one process."[9] Within this dialectical relationship, however, "production is the real point of departure and hence also the predominant moment."[10] Elaborating on this, Marx stated that "production thus produces not only the object but also the manner of consumption, not only objectively but subjectively. Production thus creates the consumer."[11] Following this line of reasoning, it becomes clear that in order to understand the effect of psychiatric treatment on the consumer, one must start with an analysis of the nature and organization of the psychiatric production (labour) process. A similar observation was made by Freidson, who suggested that it is the work process and perspective of the dominant profession and the ways in which these structure the activities of the other occupations in the health care division of labour that determines the experiences of those who receive medical services, especially in hospitals.[12]

The analytical distinction between production and consumption, however, is difficult to sustain, since the production of human services takes place within and through social interaction. This results in a tendency for the consumer to become actively incorporated into the production process through the supervision of medical regimes, including the administration of drugs, monitoring of diet, exercise, and so on. Weinbaum and Bridges commented upon the transformation of consumer into producer within the general medical labour process. Developing the theme of consumption as work, especially as this is performed by housewives, they noted that within modern hospitals and clinics "the housewife is little more than a detail laborer, lacking access to expertise to judge what she gets, power to choose what she will purchase, or the ability to replace the service with a self organized counter-part."[13]

The active involvement of the consumer in the psychiatric production process emerged in the 1950s with the establishment of the "therapeutic community."[14] Throughout the 1960s, and especially in the early 1970s, it became a major trend, finding widespread expression in an emphasis on self-care and the development of various self-help groups.[15]

At this point the major concepts and analytical methods of labour process theory will be briefly and schematically introduced. Within this theoretical tradition, the labour process is conceptualized as the purposive activity which occurs at the interface of the social relations and forces of production.

### Social Relations of Production

In general, social relations of production (SRP) consist of the relatively enduring relations between people, and between people and things, which result from the functions to be fulfilled in the performance of work. Thus, the SRP include: relations of ownership, hiring, and supervision; the leasing of labour power or things; relations of working with others; and the relations of working within a given setting with a given technology to produce products or services.[16] It is evident that the SRP cannot be reduced to class relations. This study is not concerned with class relations as such. This is somewhat unusual inasmuch as most Marxist literature has tried to link the changing class structure produced by the processes of capital accumulation to the prospect of revolutionary political praxis.[17] That is to say, the principal focus has been on the social (class) division of labour, and not the technical (occupational) division of labour. This study, however, focusses exclusively on the changing nature of psychiatric work and the transformation of the occupational division of labour. This follows the lead of Freidson, who has maintained that class as an analytical concept is "simply too gross to analyze the division of labour and the institutions of production in society."[18] He also suggested that

> To understand better the division of labour and . . . the crucial differences *among* occupations . . . requires . . . an emphasis on the degree to which they, as occupations rather than classes, have gained organized power to control themselves the terms, conditions and content of their work in the settings where they perform their work.[19] [emphasis in original]

A better understanding of the processes by which occupations have (or have not) gained organized power to control the terms, conditions and content of their work minimally requires an examination of a subset of four SRP. These are:

(1) employer-employee, or management-worker relations; (2) intramanagement relations, that is, relations between the various strata of management; (3) interoccupational relations, that is, the relations between the various occupational groups constitutive of a technical division of labour; and (4) intraoccupational relations. It should be pointed out that within the historical materialist tradition, all social relations are viewed as a unity of opposites. Specifically for present purposes, this refers to a unity of the opposites of cooperation and conflict.

*Employer-Employee Relations*

The central relation of the labour process is the relationship between employer and employee. The employment relation develops when one category of people sells its labour power (i.e., the actual physical and intellectual capacity to work) to another category of people in order to secure an income. Within the employment relation, the employer and/or the employer's representatives (i.e., management) have considerable power to determine what, where, when, how, and for how much an employee does the work for which he/she is hired. The employer-manager thus has a considerable degree of control over the labour process. As the interactionist literature has demonstrated, however, workplace relations, and power and autonomy within those relations, are variable and subject to negotiation. Thus, management's power to control a labour process is not complete or unproblematic.

Within the context of the employment relation, the employer attempts to control the labour power of others in order to reduce the costs of production and/or increase worker productivity, the achievement of which is never permanent. Employees may oppose attempts at management control because labour power cannot be separated from the physical existence of the person selling it. Thus, control of labour power means control of people.

The seller of labour power (the employee) has a vital interest in both the price received for his/her capacity to work and the conditions under which that capacity is realized. Herein lies the basis for a conflict of interests. Whereas the employer-manager has an interest in establishing and maintaining control of the labour power of employees in order to increase worker productivity and decrease the costs of producing a good or service, the employee has an interest in controlling the conditions and the manner in which his/her labour power is expended. In addition, employees are interested in obtaining as high a price as possible for their labour power.

This conflict is only one aspect of the total employment relation. Not only is there a structural basis for management-worker conflict inherent in the employment relation, there also exists a basis for cooperation. That is to say, because employees must sell their labour power in order to attain the means (an income) of subsistence (the goods and services required to ensure individual and extended reproduction at a culturally established standard of living), they have a real interest in the perpetuation of their own employment. More succinctly put, employees are interested in job security. In fact, Blauner has pointed out that job security is consistently reported as the most important factor in empirical studies of workers' job evaluations.[20]

In certain circumstances, because the production of goods and services depends upon the recruitment and retention of adequate quantities of appropriately skilled labour power, employers also have an interest in providing stable conditions of employment. The process of creating conditions of job security and workforce stability has been referred to as the creation of an internal labour market.[21]

The internal labour market literature, however, is characterized by a number of conceptual problems, the most significant of which is a tendency to conflate labour process relations with labour market relations. This is inappropriate because market relations fundamentally differ from production relations. Market relations are exchange relations between the owners of commodities which take place on the basis of legal equality. The owner of labour power and the owner of the means of production, for example, meet as equals in the labour market and effect an exchange on that basis. Within the sphere of production, however, such equality does not exist. After having purchased a person's labour power, the employer 'owns' that labour power and sets it to work in an attempt to achieve his/her own objectives. The employer is thus in a position of dominance *vis-à-vis* the bearer of labour power. The equality which characterizes the social relations of the market is superseded by the domination of the employee by the employer within the social relations of production. Ironically, Edwards has claimed that the concept of the internal labour market is an attempt to

> break open the "black box" of the neo-classical firm by viewing the social relations at the workplace in part as a system of labor exchange within the firm, regulating promotion, job placement, the setting of wage rates, and so forth.[22]

Job placement, the setting of wage rates, and the regulation of promotion take place within the sphere of production, which is characterized by relations of inequality and, therefore, cannot properly be analyzed as labour market, or exchange relations between equals. The conflation of these two distinct types of social relationships, in an attempt to clarify the social relations of the workplace, is therefore misguided. When one looks at the inconsistency characterizing different accounts of the development and functions of an internal labour market, the limited analytical utility of the concept becomes evident.

Doeringer and Piore have suggested that the creation of an internal labour market is the product of workers' attempts to protect themselves from "direct competition by workers in the external labor market." They have also suggested that the "phenomenon of internal labor markets is closely akin to the problems other authors have identified as 'industrial feudalism,' 'the balkanization of labor markets,' and 'property rights' in a job."[23]

The fact that the existence of an internal labour market is conceptualized as a problem is particularly interesting in light of Edwards's acccount of its development. The internal labour market, according to Edwards, is designed by management to increase worker commitment to a firm-specific career. This, in turn, supposedly increases worker commitment to organizational objectives. It is here that the analytical inconsistency of the concept becomes evident. On the one hand, it is presented as a problem, criticized by management for producing rigidities which hinder organizational efficiency.[24] On the other hand, it is presented as a management strategy designed to increase employee commitment to organizational goals, including profitability. The fact that this inconsistency is not commented upon by the internal labour market theorists points to the analytical weakness of the concept.

As has been suggested above, the dialectical method of conceptualization, combined with the concepts of the social relations and forces of production, allows us to understand this apparent inconsistency as a manifestation of the contradictory nature of the employment relation.

Conceptualized dialectically, the employment relation is seen as having a built-in dynamism. This dynamism is derived from the various workplace practices and struggles engaged in by both employers-managers and employees as they attempt to achieve their structurally generated objectives. As has been suggested, employees have an interest in job security, and in certain circumstances management may have an interest in creating stable conditions of employment. Whether the establishment of workforce stability and job security is the product of management-worker cooperation or conflict, however, cannot be known *a priori*, as is claimed by the internal labour market theorists.

Although the concept of the internal labour market has little explanatory power, it can serve a useful descriptive function, much like the concept of bureaucracy to which it is closely related.[25] It is used in this study to describe the various mechanisms and processes involved in the creation of stability and predictability and security within the employment relation.

*Intramanagement Relations*

Although employer-employee relations are the central element of the social relations of production, other important relationships are also encompassed by the SRP. Management, for example, cannot properly be viewed as a unified entity. Different levels of management exist, and it cannot properly be assumed that persons differentially located within the management structure are characterized by an isomorphism of interests, except in the most general sense. This tends to be a particular problem for much Marxist analysis, which confuses occupational and management distinctions by the exclusive, and often inappropriate, use of the concept of class. Braverman, for example, has been criticized not only for assuming management to be a monolith, but also for reducing all management strategies and tactics to the principles of scientific management.[26] Wood and Kelly have criticized Braverman for assuming managerial homogeneity. They have gone even further to suggest it is inappropriate to assume the existence of a conscious and coherent management strategy. Thus they have argued that the existence and operation of a management strategy is a question which must be empirically answered.[27] In addition, even if it can be empirically demonstrated that a management strategy exists, the realization of that strategy through effective tactics must also be considered to be problematic. That is, the various workplace practices and struggles characteristic of an historically situated labour process are likely to result in a transmutation[28] of even the most clearsighted formulation of means and ends. This bit of common sense is often lost to the 'Bravermaniacs.'[29]

Thus, part of the reason that the formulation and implementation of management strategies are problematic is the segmented nature of management structure. In the case under investigation there are at least three levels of management: (1) the elected and appointed officials in the Department of Public Health;[30] (2) employees of the Psychiatric Services Branch of the Department of Public Health, charged with the general management of the province's psychiatric facilities; and (3) regional and unit managers responsible for specific psychiatric facilities. Although these three strata of management are all more or less directly concerned with securing control of the psychiatric labour process, they do not necessarily agree as to what that means in concrete situations. Nor do they necessarily agree about how best to achieve it even if there is a consensus regarding what it means. It would be expected that the nature and organization of psychiatric work would be significantly influenced by various intramanagement struggles which develop around these issues.

*Interoccupational Relations*

Relations between nonmanagement workers are also conceptualized in terms of a unity of the opposites, cooperation and conflict. These interoccupational relations are shifting and diffuse, with alliances forming and dissolving with respect to different issues and employee objectives. The psychiatric occupations examined in this study are medically trained psychiatrists, psychiatric nurses, psychiatric social workers and psychologists. These are the major occupational groups within the Saskatchewan psychiatric division of labour, especially as it has developed since World War II. Therefore, an understanding of the transformation of the nature and organization of psychiatric work necessitates an understanding of the relationships between these four occupations. It is important to note that Arnhoff et al., in their discussion of psychiatric manpower growth and development in postwar America, identified these same occupational groups as "the four major mental health disciplines." They added that

> The growth of the mental health movement, particularly post-World War II, has been intimately linked with the development of these four disciplines.[31]

This indicates that the transformation of psychiatric work associated with the development of community psychiatry in Saskatchewan is part of a more general process. Although the specifics of the historical development of community psychiatry as examined here are unique to Saskatchewan, it is likely that the major tendencies discerned can be generalized.

With four occupational groups, the possibility for complex combinations and permutations of interoccupational relationships and alliances is evident. This picture is further complicated because, until recently, medically trained psychiatrists occupied all management positions within PSB. The struggles leading to the break with this tradition in the mid-1970s form a significant aspect of what appears to be an incipient de-medicalization of public sector psychiatric work.

### *Intraoccupational Relations*

As Goldie has clearly demonstrated, there also exist intraoccupational relations based on both cooperation and conflict.[32] One cannot correctly assume all members of an occupation will share a common ideology or be characterized by common interests. This is especially true when the members of a given occupation are employed within different labour processes. This is the case with psychiatric nurses who are employed within the SRP of the mental hospital psychiatric labour process and the SRP of the community psychiatric labour process. All the occupational groups, of course, are characterized by this lack of unity, and the objectives and nature of their workplace practices and struggles are influenced by it.

## The Forces of Production

The forces of production (FP) are conceptualized as consisting of the means of production and the technical relations in production. The concept of means of production refers to the nonsocial elements of a labour process. In Marx's analysis of the nineteenth-century industrial labour process it was argued that the most important aspect of the means of production was technology, especially in the form of machinery. Marx maintained that machinery was "the material foundation of the capitalist mode of production."[33] The means of production, however, cannot properly be reduced to machinery. Included are all the material elements used in a labour process, such as raw materials and equipment, as well as the actual physical setting within which work is performed.[34]

The means of production are considered to be the proximate determinant of the technical relations in production. This refers to the specific way in which the material foundation of a labour process influences the specific organization of work. A very strong statement of this relationship is found in the following excerpt from a letter to P.V. Annenkov written by Marx in 1846:

> When new productive forces are won men change their method of production and with the method of production all the economic relations which are merely the necessary conditions of this particular method of production.[35]

The occupational division of labour referred to by Marx as cooperation, however, is also considered to be part of the FP: "When numerous workers work together side by side in accordance with a plan, whether in the same process, or in different but connected processes, this form of labour is called co-operation. . . . Not only do we have an increase in the productive power of the individual . . . *but the creation of a new productive power*."[36] [emphasis added] Thus, the FP are conceptualized as having a material and a social dimension, the material dimension being the means of production, and the social dimension the technical relations in production.

### *The Means of Production*

As suggested above, the means of production include *all* the nonsocial elements used in a given labour process. This includes raw materials, plant and equipment. With regard to the psychiatric labour process, raw materials are not significant, since no material object is produced.

With regard to plant and equipment, the asylum/mental hospital has, for the past 150 years, been the psychiatric "factory." As David Rothman has shown, the nineteenth-century proponents of the asylum system claimed incarceration in the asylum was itself the cure for insanity:

> Psychiatrists and their lay supporters insisted that insanity was curable, more curable than most other ailments. Spokesmen explained that their understanding of the causes of insanity equipped them to combat it, and the asylum was a first resort, the most important and effective weapon in their arsenal.[37]

Indeed, so convinced were these early proponents of the therapeutic efficacy of the asylum that they "confidently and aggressively asserted that properly organized institutions could cure almost every instance of the disease."[38] Thus, as originally conceived, the asylum itself was the treatment of choice; the principal element in the asylum physician's treatment regime. The fact that it was an ineffective technology for curing insanity is undoubtedly part of the reason that asylums became psychiatric warehouses.

Following the demise of the cult of curability, the asylum remained an integral element of the psychiatric labour process. The principal function was no longer to cure, however, but simply to control those persons who were problematical in the community and/or other institutional settings.[39] Regardless of whether the asylum was a technology of cure or control, as Scull has shown, control of the asylum was significant for the attainment of occupational dominance. Indeed, Freidson has argued, with regard to medicine in general, that the development of a secure and practical work technology was a precondition for a professional monopoly.[40]

Treacher and Baruch have maintained that, for psychiatry, this generalization cannot be substantiated, since the passage of the 1858 Medical Registration Act, which gave an effective monopoly of psychiatric work to British physicians, apparently predated "any major discoveries which could provide medicine with a valid technology."[41] Rothman has shown, however, that the asylum itself was the technological discovery which medical superintendents monopolized and upon which they established their domination of the psychiatric division of labour. Scull also made this point,[42] thus making it difficult to understand Treacher and Baruch's dismissal of its significance, especially given their heavy reliance on his analysis. Their subsequent suggestion that the achievement of a medical monopoly of psychiatric work in the nineteenth century must be understood "far more in ideological and class terms"[43] is somewhat trite due to their failure to give it any historical substance.

Scull placed great emphasis on the fact that medical control of the asylum constituted the material base from which the medical domination of the asylum-based division of labour arose. However, his assumption that the medical domination of the mental hospital labour process is *ipso facto* evidence of the medicalization of mental hospital work is questionable.

The thesis here is that the complete medicalization of psychiatric work did not occur until the introduction of a new technology, in the form of the psychotropic drugs, revolutionized the mental hospital labour process in 1954. It is suggested that the introduction of this medically monopolized pharmacological technology rendered the asylum technologically obsolete in the manufacture of manageable patients. This is not to say that these drugs are necessarily effective in producing symptom-free behaviour; often they are not, but they generally do produce manageable patients. As Clark has noted concerning the use of psychotropic drugs in the treatment of psychotic patients:

> It is well-known that patients can remain grossly psychotic and yet become passively co-operative, less overactive and destructive, or more docile. Such improvement may be more important to the custodian than the patient.[44]

Docile and passively cooperative patients do not need to be segregated in large mental hospitals. Nor do they need to be restrained by some of the more macabre paraphernalia associated with traditional psychiatric treatment. As Baumler and others have reported, the use of psychotropic drugs in mental hospitals has corresponded to a reduction in the use of shock therapy, cold water baths and other traditional methods of treatment.[45] Thus, the use of psychotropic drugs has not only rendered the asylums technologically obsolete, their use has rendered most of the other technologies of psychiatric control obsolete as well. Again, this is not necessarily because the drugs are more effective, or even more humane, than other forms of control. In fact, mounting evidence regarding the toxicity and side effects which result from the use of the psychotropic drugs stands as an indictment of their indiscriminate use. Crane, discussing the parkinsonism often caused by the use of these drugs, has stated that

> Often associated with parkinsonism is akinesia, which, in severe cases, is characterized by physical immobility as well as emotional indifference. The syndrome is poorly understood and often mistaken for psychomotor retardation. Some clinicians may even consider it a desirable effect because it helps control unruly behavior. In the early days of psychopharmacology, psychiatrists were accused of replacing a mechanical straight jacket with a chemical one, a criticism that is still justified when excessive doses of neuroleptics produce severe reduction of motor activity and a general loss of spontaneity.[46]

The rapid expansion in the use of these drugs must be ascribed not simply to technological efficiency nor humanitarian concern, but rather to the fact that their use is less expensive than asylum-based treatment, and the fact that they are the only psychiatric technology which is legislatively monopolized by those with medical training. Thus asylum physicians have used their position of dominance within the mental hospital to ensure the complete medicalization of that labour process. This was achieved by replacing the predrug forms of psychiatric treatment, which did not legally require medical participation, with chemotherapy, which did. It is further suggested that the complete medicalization of psychiatric work occurred in the middle of the twentieth century, not the end of the nineteenth century, as claimed by Scull.

The chemical production of manageable patients was also a precondition for the depopulation of the mental hospitals and the development of various community-based alternatives to them, such as hostels, day homes, halfway houses, group homes and so on. It would be wrong to argue that these developments followed directly from the introduction of the psychotropic drugs. Within the context of extreme overcrowding and rapidly escalating costs, however, the drug-generated possibility of developing alternatives to the mental hospitals was extremely attractive to legislators of all political persuasions. Community psychiatry thus received almost unanimous political support, both in North America and the United Kingdom.[47]

*The Technical Relations in Production*

The concept of technical relations in production, the social dimension of the FP, refers to the specific occupational division of labour which develops upon a specific material (technological) base of production. If one conceptualizes the asylum as part of the material foundation of the physician-dominated mental hospital labour process, it follows that the demise of the asylum, or the erosion of that material base, will correspond to a transformation of the technical relations in production, and consequently to a new interoccupational balance of power. If this change did not occur, it would be necessary to demonstrate the social and material conditions which sustained a given division of labour and balance of power. That is, it would be necessary to demonstrate how the medical domination of the community psychiatric labour process was sustained.

There is little doubt that community psychiatry is predominantly a medical labour process. It has a dual foundation which is based on the medical monopoly of drug prescription, and medical control of admissions and discharges to general hospitals where, since the early 1960s, most psychiatric patients requiring hospitalization have been treated. Thus community psychiatry corresponds to medical domination of the psychiatric division of labour and monopoly of the principal forces of psychiatric production, that is, to the medicalization of psychiatric work.

The psychotropic drugs, however, also formed the basis of an incipient de-medicalization of community psychiatric work. To the extent that they were effective in producing manageable patients, they facilitated the depopulation of the mental hospitals and the development of various community-based alternatives, as well as opening up "new possibilities for psychotherapy and psychagogy."[48]

Psychotherapy, however, is not monopolized by physicians. The nonmedical occupations, particularly social work and psychology, have attempted to secure autonomy from medical domination and control of their own work. This has taken the form of various attempts to develop alternative technologies and techniques for use in the production of community psychiatric services, including various psychotherapeutic procedures for helping clients cope with their problems with living. It is often argued by the nonmedical occupations that many of their clients do not require medical intervention, since their problems cannot be solved through drug therapy. This establishes the basis for interoccupational conflicts.

Another strategy for securing autonomy and control has been to develop new markets, examples of which are child-youth services, marriage counselling services, and other activities claimed to be preventive in orientation and nonmedical in nature. Thus, the nonmedical community psychiatric occupations have adapted the old public health ideology to meet their own ends. Rather than arguing for early medical intervention, however, they claim appropriate psycho-social intervention at an early stage can prevent a problem from worsening to the point where it requires more extensive and expensive intervention.

This promise is popular with legislators and the tax-paying public. The popular support constitutes a social base for the extension of the nonmedical aspects of public sector community psychiatric services and the bifurcation of psychiatric services in general. This draws attention to the fact that no labour process occurs in a vacuum. There are a myriad of social, political and economic forces which, although external to, are influential in the development of any given labour process. It is to these forces that attention is now turned.

## External Factors Influencing the Psychiatric Labour Process

The most significant external factor influencing the transformation of psychiatric work and the development of community psychiatry is the increase in demand for these services. It is estimated that one in six Canadians can expect to be hospitalized for a mental illness at least once during his/her lifetime. It is also estimated that between 10 and 30 percent of the population suffer from some sort of mental illness.[49] Most of these voluntarily seek treatment. In Saskatchewan approximately 90 percent of the people now consuming psychiatric services do so voluntarily. This is a dramatic reversal of the situation which existed in 1948, when less than 10 percent of all admissions to mental hospitals in the province were voluntary.

Although it is beyond the scope of the present study to explain why there has been an increase in the demand for psychiatric services, it is possible to make a few observations. Specifically, it seems theoretically fruitful to attempt to link the increased demand for psychiatric services to the processes of capital accumulation.

### *Capital Accumulation and the Creation of Needs*

Capital accumulation refers to much more than the accumulation of money and other forms of wealth.[50] It refers to the reproduction of the capital relationship itself, one aspect of which is the reproduction and incorporation of labour power into the wage (employment) relation. Marx stated in his discussion of the general law of capital accumulation:

> The reproduction of labour power which must incessantly be reincorporated into capital as its means of valorization, which cannot get free of capital, and whose enslavement to capital is only concealed by the variety of individual capitalists to whom it sells itself,

> forms, in fact, a major factor in the reproduction of capital itself. Accumulation of capital is therefore multiplication of the proletariat.[51]

Multiplication of the proletariat, or the incorporation of ever-increasing numbers of people into the wage relation transforms the conditions of peoples' lives. The conditions of existence give rise to social and individual needs and the means of satisfying those needs.

Within the context of the capitalist mode of production, social and individual needs increasingly come to be satisfied by the consumption of goods and services (use values) produced within the context of the capitalist labour process.[52]

Following this line of reasoning, it could presumably be argued that the transformation of the conditions of life brought about by the historical process of capital accumulation has produced a number of new needs, one of which is the need for psychiatric services. Psychiatric services can be argued to help people cope with their conditions of existence by removing, or at least making manageable, problematic (symptomatic) behaviour. The fact that the conditions of life have changed for a significant proportion of the population of Saskatchewan can be seen from Table 13. Although an analysis of the reasons for this dramatic shift of population from rural and farm to urban living is beyond the scope of the present study, a number of interesting studies linking it to the capitalization of agricultural production are available.[53]

One could presumably elaborate this 'new needs' thesis in terms of the forces generally operating within the capitalist mode of production. However, increased demand is here taken as a given, and a conjunctural analysis of what might be considered to be the proximate causes of the rise and development of community psychiatry has been undertaken. It is suggested that a conjunctural analysis is the only way to give historical specificity to an investigation. Analyses at the conceptual level of capital accumulation and the mode of production remain theoretical.[54]

**Table 13**
**Population: Saskatchewan Urban, Rural, and Farm, 1901-1981**

| | | | Rural | | |
|---|---|---|---|---|---|
| As at June 1 | Total | Urban | Total | Farm | Non-Farm |
| 1901 | 91,279 | 14,266 | 77,013 | | |
| 1911 | 492,432 | 131,395 | 361,037 | | |
| 1921 | 757,510 | 218,958 | 538,552 | | |
| 1931 | 921,785 | 187,121 | 734,664 | 561,407 | 173,257 |
| 1941 | 895,992 | 192,282 | 703,710 | 411,269 | 192,441 |
| 1951 | 931,729 | 252,470 | 579,258 | 398,279 | 180,979 |
| 1961 | 925,181 | 398,091 | 527,090 | 304,672 | 222,418 |
| 1971 | 926,245 | 490,635 | 435,610 | 233,335 | 202,275 |
| 1981 | 968,313 | 563,166 | 405,147 | 180,255 | 244,892 |

*Source:* Statistics Canada, Census of Canada.

*Conjunctural Forces Influential of Community Psychiatry in Saskatchewan*

A number of conjunctural forces are examined in this study of the transformation of the nature and organization of psychiatric work in Saskatchewan. These include: the activities of various lobby and special interest groups; the tenor of public opinion, and its manifestation in the form of support for and/or opposition to changes to the provincial psychiatric services system; the nature of the labour markets for various categories of psychiatric workers; and provincial government attempts to establish the principle of federal government cost-sharing in the provision of psychiatric services.

Other factors and forces identified as influencing the development of community psychiatry are also introduced at relevant points in the text.

For the purposes of this study the rise and development of community psychiatry is conceptualized in terms of the transformation of the nature and organization of psychiatric work. In order to undertake an analysis of this transformation, the concepts and analytical methods of a theory of the labour process are used. This theory conceptualizes a labour process as the purposive activity which occurs at the interface of the social relations and forces of production. It is argued that various workplace practices and struggles undertaken, as the several parties to the labour process attempt to achieve their objectives and realize their interests, result in a transformation of both the SRP and FP. In addition to these internal forces, a number of forces external to, but influential in determining the form and control of the relations and forces of the psychiatric labour process are examined. The elaboration of these relations forms the basis of a description of the development of community psychiatry in the province of Saskatchewan.

Within the historical materialist tradition, description is an integral element of explanation. The realist ontology of this tradition posits that phenomenal forms are caused by underlying invisible, but real, causal mechanisms. For this study, the phenomenal forms to be explained are the community psychiatric division of labour and the various technologies, techniques and facilities associated with the performance of psychiatric work. The underlying causal mechanisms are inferred from the various practices and struggles engaged in by interested groups, as they attempt to achieve structurally generated objectives. These social practices give the social relations and forces of psychiatric production their specific institutional form. Thus, working within this tradition, the explanation of the rise and development of community psychiatry entails a description of what entities were involved in the transformation of psychiatric work and how their interrelationships resulted in a specific institutional form.[55] This study is a contribution to a realist explanation of the rise of community psychiatry in Saskatchewan.

# Notes

## Chapter One

1. Leonard Schatzman and Anselm Strauss, "A Sociology of Psychiatry: A Perspective and Some Organizing Foci," in Eliot Freidson and Judith Lorber, eds., *Medical Men and Their Work* (Chicago and New York: Aldine-Atherton, 1972), 129.
2. Alex Robertson, "Sociology and the Study of Psychiatric Disorder," *The Sociological Review* 17 (1969): 378.
3. A representative list of such writings might include the following publications: Ivan Belknap, *Human Problems of a State Mental Hospital* (New York: McGraw-Hill, 1956); John A. Clausen, *Sociology and the Field of Mental Health* (New York: Russell Sage Foundation, 1956); Elaine and John Cumming, *Closed Ranks* (Cambridge: Harvard University Press, 1957); H. Warren Dunham and S. Kirson Weinberg, *The Culture of the State Mental Hospital* (Detroit: Wayne State University Press, 1960); H. Warren Dunham, *Sociological Theory and Mental Disorder* (Detroit: Wayne State University Press, 1959); Joseph W. Eaton and Robert J. Weil, *Culture and Mental Disorders* (New York: The Free Press, 1955); Robert F.L. Faris and H. Warren Dunham, *Mental Disorders in Urban Areas* (Chicago: University of Chicago Press, 1939); Erving Goffman, *Asylums* (Garden City, N.Y.: Doubleday, 1961); Herbert Goldhamer and Andrew Marshall, *Psychosis and Civilization* (New York: The Free Press, 1953); August B. Hollingshead and Frederick C. Redlich, *Social Class and Mental Illness* (New York: John Wiley, 1958); E. Gartley Jaco, "Social Factors in Mental Disorders in Texas," *Social Problems* 4 (April, 1957): 322-28; Henry L. Lennard and Arnold Bernstein, *The Anatomy of Psychotherapy* (New York: Columbia University Press, 1960); J. Myers and B. Roberts, *Family and Class Dynamics in*

*Mental Illness* (New York: John Wiley, 1959); Arnold M. Rose, ed., *Mental Health and Mental Disorder* (New York: W.W. Norton, 1957); Leo Srole et al., *Mental Health in the Metropolis* (New York: McGraw-Hill, 1962); Alfred H. Stanton and Morris S. Schwartz, *The Mental Hospital* (New York: Basic Books, 1954); Mervyn Susser, *Community Psychiatry: Epidemiologic and Social Themes* (New York: Random House, 1968); Gregory Bateson et al., "Toward a Theory of Schizophrenia," *Behavioral Science* 1 (1956): 251-64; Gregory Bateson, *Steps Toward an Ecology of Mind* (London: Granada Publishing, 1973); Jay Haley, "The Family of the Schizophrenic: A Model System," *Journal of Nervous and Mental Disease* 129 (1959): 357-74; Ronald D. Laing, *The Politics of the Family and Other Essays* (Harmondsworth: Penguin Books, 1976); Ronald D. Laing and A. Esterson, *Sanity, Madness and the Family, Volume I: Families of Schizophrenics* (London: Tavistock Publications Ltd., 1964); Theodore Lidz, *The Origin and the Treatment of Schizophrenic Disorders* (London: Hutchinson and Co. Ltd., 1975); Harry S. Sullivan, *Schizophrenia as a Human Process* (New York: W.W. Norton and Company, 1974).

4. Alfred J. Kahn, "Planning and Practice Perspectives on the Boundaries of Community Psychiatry," in Leigh M. Roberts, Seymour L. Halleck and Martin V. Loeb, eds., *Community Psychiatry* (Madison: University of Wisconsin Press, 1966), 171.
5. Rue Bucher and Joan Stelling, "Characteristics of Professional Organizations," *Journal of Health and Social Behavior* 10 (1969): 4.
6. Marie R. Haug, "Deprofessionalization: An Alternate Hypothesis for the Future," in Paul Halmos, ed., *Professionalization and Social Change* (Keele, Staffordshire: The University of Keele, 1973), 195-212; Martin Oppenheimer, "The Proletarianization of the Professional," in Halmos, *Professionalization and Social Change*, 213-28.
7. Eliot Freidson, "The Futures of Professionalisation," in Margaret Stacey et al., eds., *Health and the Division of Labour* (London: Croom Helm, 1977), 14.
8. Ibid.
9. Ibid., 14-15.
10. Karl Marx, *Capital, A Critique of Political Economy Volume 1* (Harmondsworth, Middlesex: Penguin Books Ltd., 1976), 764.

11. Harold L. Wilensky, "The Professionalization of Everyone?" *The American Journal of Sociology* 70 (September 1964): 137-58.
12. Robert W. Habenstein, "Critique of 'Profession' as a Sociological Category," *The Sociological Quarterly* 4 (Autumn 1963): 296.
13. Freidson, "The Futures of Professionalisation," 22.
14. Bucher and Stelling, "Characteristics of Professional Organizations," 4.
15. Freidson, "The Futures of Professionalisation," 22.
16. Bucher and Stelling, "Characteristics of Professional Organizations," 4.
17. Leonard Schatzman and Rue Bucher, "Negotiating a Division of Labor Among Professionals in the State Mental Hospital," *Psychiatry* 27 (1964): 277.
18. Ibid.
19. Freidson, "The Futures of Professionalisation," 22; for a similar approach see Philip Elliot, *The Sociology of the Professions* (London: Macmillan, 1972); and M.S. Larson, *The Rise of Professionalism: A Sociological Analysis* (Berkeley: University of California Press, 1977).
20. Freidson, "The Futures of Professionalisation," 22.
21. M.S. Larson, *The Rise of Professionalism*; Wilensky, "The Professionalization of Everyone?"
22. Freidson, "The Futures of Professionalisation," 35.
23. Ibid.
24. Good examples of these approaches can be found in R. Hunter and I.M. McAlpine, *Three Hundred Years of Psychiatry, 1535-1860* (New York: Oxford University Press, 1963); and F.G. Alexander and S.T. Seleznick, *The History of Psychiatry: An Evaluation of Psychiatric Thought and Practice from Pre-Historic Times to the Present* (New York: Harper and Row, 1966).
25. For a collection of descriptions of various medical treatments of the mentally ill in nineteenth-century England see Vieda Skultans, *English Madness: Ideas on Insanity, 1580-1890* (London: Routledge and Kegan Paul, 1979).
26. Andrew T. Scull, *Museums of Madness: The Social Organization of Insanity in Nineteenth-Century England* (London: Allen Lane, Penguin Books, 1979), 15.
27. Thomas S. Szasz, *The Manufacture of Madness: A Comparative Study of the Inquisition and the Mental Health Movement* (Frogmore, St. Albans, Herts.: Paladin, 1973).

28. Scull, *Museums of Madness*, 258.
29. Ibid.
30. Ibid.
31. Ibid.
32. Ibid., 259.
33. Ibid.
34. Sigmund Freud, "Psychoanalysis and Psychiatry," in James Strachey and Angela Richards, eds., *Introductory Lectures on Psychoanalysis, Vol. 1* (Harmondsworth: Penguin Books, 1973), 294.
35. Laurence J. Ray, "Models of Madness in Victorian Asylum Practice," *Archives of European Sociology* 22 (1981): 229-64.
36. Scull, *Museums of Madness*, 259.
37. I.K. Zola, "Medicine as an Institution of Social Control," *The Sociological Review* 20 (1972): 487.
38. Scull, *Museums of Madness*, 265-66. Within this quotation Scull has himself quoted and cited Szasz, *Manufacture of Madness*; N. Kittrie, *The Right to be Different* (Baltimore: Johns Hopkins University Press, 1971); Zola, "Medicine as an Institution of Social Control"; Eliot Freidson, *Profession of Medicine* (New York: Dodd, Mead and Co., 1970).
39. Andrew T. Scull, *Decarceration, Community Treatment and the Deviant* (Englewood Cliffs, N.J.: Prentice Hall, 1977), 3.
40. For a criticism of Scull on this point see Roger Matthews, "'Decarceration' and the Fiscal Crisis," in Bob Fine et al., eds., *Capitalism and the Rule of Law* (London: Hutchinson and Co., 1979), 102-4.
41. Scull, *Decarceration*, 11.
42. Ian Gough, "State Expenditures in Advanced Capitalism," *New Left Review* 92 (July-August 1975): 76, quoted in Scull, *Decarceration*, 138.
43. Scull, *Decarceration*, 140.
44. Ibid., 143.
45. Ibid., 152.
46. Ibid., 153.
47. Ibid., 73.
48. See Skultans, *English Madness*, 11, for a similar critique.
49. Scull, *Decarceration*, 140-41.
50. Kathleen Jones, *A History of the Mental Health Service* (London: Routledge and Kegan Paul, 1972).
51. Skultans, *English Madness*, 99.
52. Ibid.

53. See for example Matthews, "'Decarceration' and the Fiscal Crisis," 100-17.
54. Andrew T. Scull, "Community Corrections: Panacea, Progress or Pretence," in David Garland and Peter Young, eds., *The Power to Punish: Contemporary Penal and Social Analysis* (London: HEB, 1983), 160.
55. Diana Ralph, *Work and Madness: The Rise of Community Psychiatry* (Montreal: Black Rose Books, 1982), 42.
56. Scull, *Decarceration*, 134.
57. Diana Ralph, "Work and Madness: The Labour Theory of Community Psychiatry" (Ph.D. dissertation, University of Regina, 1980), 67.
58. Stanley F. Yolles, "The Future of Community Psychiatry," in W.E. Barton and C.J. Sanborn, eds., *An Assessment of the Community Mental Health Movement* (Lexington, Mass.: Lexington Books, 1977), 173. Also see Susser, *Community Psychiatry*, 71, 103, 243-46; Donald G. Langsley, "Community Mental Health: A Review of the Literature," in Barton and Sanborn, *Assessment of the Community Mental Health Movement*, 38; David F. Musto, "The Community Mental Health Center Movement in Historical Perspective," in Barton and Sanborn, *Assessment of the Community Mental Health Movement*, 8; Robert Shaplen, *Towards the Wellbeing of Mankind: Fifty Years of the Rockefeller Foundation* (London: Hutchinson, 1964); Raymond B. Fosdick, *The Story of the Rockefeller Foundation* (New York: Harper and Row Publishers, Inc., 1952); W.S. Maclay, "Experiments in Mental Hospital Organization," *The Canadian Medical Association Journal* 78 (15 June 1958): 9; and George Rosen, *Madness in Society: Chapters in the Historical Sociology of Mental Illness* (Chicago: University of Chicago Press, 1968), especially Chapter 10, 263-328.
59. Ralph, *Work and Madness*, 11.

## Chapter Two

1. Reported in Maurice Demay, "The Beginnings of Psychiatry in Saskatchewan," *Canada's Mental Health* 21 (January-February 1973): 19.
2. Ibid.
3. Ibid.
4. Ibid., 20.
5. Ibid., 20-21.
6. Ibid., 21.

7. Report, submitted to his Honour the Lieutenant Governor in Council, Regina, Saskatchewan, by David Low, M.D., 1 May 1907, pp. 2-3, (hereafter cited as the Low Report), Saskatchewan Archives Board (hereafter SAB), R-33.5, III, 127.(14-8). Douglas Papers: Mental Institutions.
8. Architects, 2 Leader Lane, Toronto, Ontario, to Deputy Commissioner, Public Works, Regina, Saskatchewan, 9 May 1908, SAB, R-33.5, III, 127.(14-8). Douglas Papers.
9. Saskatchewan, Haultain Royal Commission. SAB, R-195.4, Box 6.
10. Brief, submitted to the Premier, and Members of the Executive Council, Province of Saskatchewan, recommending the location of the proposed mental asylum at Battleford, 1910, SAB, R-33.5, III, 127.(14-8). Douglas Papers.
11. "Low Report," p. 1, SAB, R-33.5, III, 127.(14-8). Douglas Papers.
12. "Mental Hygiene Survey of Saskatchewan, 1920," *Sessional Paper No. 5*, Session 1921-22, p. 43.
13. "Low Report," p. 2, SAB, R-33.5, III, 127.(14-8). Douglas Papers.
14. J.W. MacNeill, "Why Was I Admitted to a Saskatchewan Hospital: Questions and Answers," n.d. I am indebted to the staff of SAB (Saskatoon) for bringing this uncatalogued pamphlet to my attention.
15. For a discussion of the use of patient labour power in the British mental hospital system see J.A.R. Bickford, "Economic Value of the Psychiatric Inpatient," *The Lancet* 1 (30 March 1963): 714-15.
16. Medical Superintendent, Saskatchewan Hospital Battleford, to Deputy Minister of Public Works, Province of Saskatchewan, 3 August 1932, SAB, PW, 195-2, 132.P. Public Works Department: Deputy Minister's Personal File, North Battleford Mental Hospital, 1910-1935.
17. Matthews, "'Decarceration' and the Fiscal Crisis," 113.
18. Ibid., 114.
19. Civil Service Commissioner, Province of Saskatchewan, to Joint Secretaries, Quebec Civil Service Commission, 24 September 1923, SAB, PS, G61. Public Service Commission: Information Regarding Operation of Civil Service Act, 1913-1928.
20. Ibid.
21. Ibid.

22. Civil Service Commissioner, Province of Saskatchewan, to Joint Secretaries, Quebec Civil Service Commission, 24 April 1923, SAB, PS, G61. Public Service Commission.
23. "Statement Regarding the Operation of the Civil Service Act, December 19, 1917," SAB, PS, G61. Public Service Commission.
24. Ibid.
25. Ibid.
26. Ibid.
27. Ibid.
28. Reported in Robin F. Badgley and Samuel Wolfe, *Doctors' Strike: Medical Care and Conflict in Saskatchewan* (Toronto: Macmillan, 1967), 26.
29. Report, "Facts and Observations Pertaining to the Mental Hygiene Situation in Saskatchewan," presented by Dr. C.M. Hincks to the Saskatchewan Cabinet in the Prime Minister's Office, 26 February 1937, SAB, R-97, 7. Uhrich Papers: New Mental Hospital.
30. Civil Service Commissioner, Province of British Columbia, to Civil Service Commissioner, Province of Saskatchewan, 18 October 1918, SAB, PS, G61. Public Service Commission.
31. Ibid.
32. "Account of the Tenth Annual Meeting of the National Committee for Mental Hygiene of the United States, held in New York, February 6, 1918," SAB, M4, I.153. Martin Papers: Social Welfare: Mental Defectives, 1917-1921, p. 40750.
33. "Account of the Proceedings of the Organizational Meeting of the Canadian National Committee for Mental Hygiene, held in Chateau Laurier, Ottawa, April 26, 1918," SAB, M4, I.153. Martin Papers, p. 40760.
34. "Provisional Constitution and By-Laws of the Canadian National Committee for Mental Hygiene, Adopted at the Organizational Meeting held at Chateau Laurier, Ottawa, April 26, 1918," SAB, M4,I.153. Martin Papers, p. 40764.
35. Associate Medical Director and Secretary, Canadian National Committee for Mental Hygiene, to Premier, Province of Saskatchewan, 20 March 1919, SAB, M4, I.153. Martin Papers, p. 40804.
36. It was also decided at the 1919 Annual Meeting of the United States National Committee for Mental Hygiene that an International Committee for Mental Hygiene would be organized using a donation from Mrs. Elizabeth Milbank Anderson. This

gift was to be used to enable the Medical Directors and Secretaries of the American and Canadian National Committees (this would have included Hincks in his role as Secretary) to go to England, and possibly France and Italy, to organize national committees in those countries. SAB, M4, I.153. Martin Papers, p. 40889.

37. Associate Medical Director and Secretary, Canadian National Committee for Mental Hygiene, to Premier, Province of Saskatchewan, 6 July 1920, SAB, M4, I.153. Martin Papers, p. 40927.
38. "Mental Hygiene Survey of Saskatchewan, 1920," *Sessional Paper No. 5*, Session 1921-22, pp. 121-22.
39. "Official Report of Conference held at Legislative Buildings, June 18, 1920," SAB, M6, X-16-2. Dunning Papers: Care of Mental Defectives, 1920, p. 25890.
40. F.S. Lawson, "Mental Hospitals: Their Size and Function," *Canadian Journal of Public Health* 49 (May 1958): passim.
41. "Official Report of the Conference held at Legislative Buildings, June 18, 1920," SAB, M6, X-16-2. Dunning Papers, p. 25871.
42. Saskatchewan Department of Public Works Annual Report 1921-22.
43. "Minutes of the Third Executive Committee Meeting of the Canadian National Committee for Mental Hygiene, held at 143 College St., Toronto, Wed. Feb. 12, 1919," SAB, M4, I.153. Martin Papers, p. 40882.
44. Superintendent, Saskatchewan Hospital Battleford, to Premier, Province of Saskatchewan, 30 November 1921, SAB, M4, I.154. Martin Papers: Social Welfare: Mental Hospitals, 1917-1921, p. 41125.
45. Ibid., pp. 41125-26.
46. Premier, Province of Saskatchewan, to Superintendent, Saskatchewan Hospital Battleford, 21 November 1921, SAB, M4, I.154. Martin Papers, p. 41124.
47. "Low Report," p. 2, SAB, R-33.5, III, 127.(14-8). Douglas Papers.
48. Superintendent, Saskatchewan Hospital Weyburn, to General Superintendent, Provincial Mental Hospital, British Columbia, 8 December 1936, SAB, PH.3, A13. Department of Public Health. Correspondence, A-X.
49. Superintendent, Saskatchewan Hospital Weyburn, to Superintendent, Regina General Hospital, Regina, Saskatchewan,

6 February 1936, SAB, PH.3, A13. Department of Public Health.

50. For an account of this strike see Donald Campbell Masters, *The Winnipeg General Strike* (Toronto: University of Toronto Press, 1950); David Jay Bercuson, *Confrontation at Winnipeg: Labour, Industrial Relations and the General Strike* (Montreal: McGill-Queen's University Press, 1974).
51. For a discussion of the little known Saskatoon support strike, see Glen Makahonuk, "Labour in the Prairie City: The Saskatoon Working Class Experience and Response to Capitalism, 1906-1919," in Harley D. Dickinson and Bob Russell, eds., *The Politics of Work in the West: Historical and Contemporary Perspectives* (Saskatoon: Social Research Unit, University of Saskatchewan, 1985), 5-69.
52. Superintendent, Saskatchewan Hospital Battleford, to Premier, Province of Saskatchewan, 6 December 1918, SAB, M4, I.154. Martin Papers, p. 41046.
53. Chief Engineer, Saskatchewan Hospital Battleford, to Superintendent, Saskatchewan Hospital Battleford, 28 June 1920, SAB, G132. Public Works Department: Saskatchewan Provincial Hospital, North Battleford; Cottages 1919-1944.
54. Superintendent, Saskatchewan Hospital Battleford, to Deputy Minister of Public Works, Province of Saskatchewan, 7 June 1919, SAB, PW, 195-2, 132.P. Public Works Department.
55. Medical Superintendent, The Ontario Hospital, London, Ontario, to Superintendent, Saskatchewan Hospital Battleford, 3 December 1923, SAB, PH.3, A13. Department of Public Health.
56. Superintendent, Saskatchewan Hospital Battleford, to Medical Superintendent, The Ontario Hospital, London, Ontario, 11 December 1923, SAB, PH.3, A13. Department of Public Health.
57. Acting Superintendent, Saskatchewan Hospital Battleford, to Director, Toronto Mental Hospital, Toronto, Ontario, 7 May 1945, SAB, R-33.5, 103.(13-4-3-1). Douglas Papers: Mental Hospital: North Battleford: Inquiry, Correspondence.
58. Ibid.
59. Ibid.
60. For a good example of this technique see the following letter: Superintendent, Saskatchewan Hospital Battleford, to Deputy Minister, Department of Public Works, Province of Saskatchewan, 27 December 1912, SAB, PW, 195-2, 132.P. Public Works Department.

61. Superintendent, Saskatchewan Hospital Battleford, to Deputy Minister of Public Health, Province of Saskatchewan, 21 November 1914, SAB, PW, 195-2, 132.P. Public Works Department.
62. Ibid.
63. J.W. MacNeill, *Rules and Regulations for Employees of Mental Hospitals* (Regina: Thomas McConnica, King's Printer, 1943).
64. Ibid.
65. "Regulations for Residents of Nurses' Home," SAB, PH.3, A13. Department of Public Health.
66. Superintendent, Saskatchewan Hospital Weyburn, to Employee, Saskatchewan Hospital Weyburn, 13 June 1922, SAB, PH.3, A13. Department of Public Health.
67. MacNeill, *Rules and Regulations.*
68. Civil Service Commissioner, Province of Saskatchewan, to Civil Service Commissioner, State of Wisconsin, U.S.A., 16 January 1918, SAB, PS, G61. Public Service Commission.
69. "Graduated Increases for Probationers as Adopted by Mental Hospitals," SAB, PS, A17. Public Service Commission: Mental Hospitals, Perquisites.
70. Superintendent, Saskatchewan Hospital Battleford, to Public Service Commissioner, Province of Saskatchewan, 22 December 1930, SAB, PS, A17. Public Service Commission.
71. Richard C. Edwards, *Contested Terrain: The Transformation of the Workplace in the Twentieth Century* (New York: Basic Books, 1979).
72. Superintendent, Saskatchewan Hospital Battleford, to Public Service Commission, Province of Saskatchewan, 22 December 1930, SAB, PS, A17. Public Service Commission.
73. "Notes on Visit of P.G. Ward, Deputy Chairman, and Mrs. V. Beilly, Commissioner, to Weyburn Mental Hospital, July 18, 1930," SAB, PS, A17. Public Service Commission.
74. Civil Service Commission, Province of Saskatchewan, to Superintendent, Saskatchewan Hospital Weyburn, 19 December 1930, SAB, PS, A17. Public Service Commission.
75. Memorandum, Superintendent, Saskatchewan Hospital Weyburn, to Married Women Employees, Saskatchewan Hospital Weyburn, 13 October 1930, SAB, PH.3, A13. Department of Public Health.
76. Ibid.
77. "Journals of the Legislative Assembly, April 4, 1930," SAB, R-594,46. Uhrich Papers: Sterilization of Insane, 1930-1946.

78. Memorandum, Director, Psychiatric Services Branch, Province of Saskatchewan, to Minister of Public Health, Province of Saskatchewan, SAB, R-11, 14-19. Bentley Papers: Saskatchewan Mental Institutions, 1944-52.
79. Commissioner of Mental Institutions and Director of Mental Health, Province of Alberta, to Superintendent, Saskatchewan Hospital Weyburn, 21 December 1932, SAB, PH.3, A13. Department of Public Health.
80. Superintendent, Saskatchewan Hospital Weyburn, to Commissioner of Mental Institutions and Director of Mental Health, Province of Alberta, 15 December 1932, SAB, PH.3, A13. Department of Public Health.
81. Commissioner of Mental Institutions and Director of Mental Health, Province of Alberta, to Superintendent, Saskatchewan Hospital Weyburn, 21 December 1932, SAB, PH.3, A13. Department of Public Health.
82. Superintendent, Saskatchewan Hospital Battleford, to Public Service Commission, Province of Saskatchewan, 22 December 1930, SAB, PS, A17. Public Service Commission.
83. Superintendent, Saskatchewan Hospital Battleford, to Deputy Minister of Public Health, Province of Saskatchewan, 3 August 1932, SAB, PW, 195-2, 132.P. Public Works Department.
84. For a fascinating exposé of this process of 'income supplementation' written by a former superintendent of an American mental hospital at the turn of the century, see S.V. Clevenger, "Treatment of the Insane," *Journal of the American Medical Association* 27 (October 1896): 894-901. Excerpts of this are reproduced in Thomas Szasz, ed., *The Age of Madness: History of Involuntary Mental Hospitalization Presented in Selected Texts* (London: Routledge and Kegan Paul, 1975), 84-88.
85. Superintendent, Saskatchewan Hospital Battleford, to Deputy Minister of Public Works, Province of Saskatchewan, 1 October 1915, SAB, PW, 195-2, 132.P. Public Works Department.
86. Superintendent, Saskatchewan Hospital Battleford, to Deputy Minister of Public Works, Province of Saskatchewan, 3 August 1932, SAB, PW, 195-2, 132.P. Public Works Department.
87. Ibid.
88. Ex-employee, Saskatchewan Hospital Battleford, to Premier, Province of Saskatchewan, 8 December 1948, SAB, R-33.5, 103. (13-4-3-1). Douglas Papers.

89. Minister of Public Health, Province of Saskatchewan, to Executive Director, Canadian National Committee for Mental Hygiene, 4 December 1940, SAB, R-97, 7. Uhrich Papers.
90. Report, "Facts and Observations Pertaining to the Mental Hygiene Situation in Saskatchewan," presented by Dr. C.M. Hincks to the Saskatchewan Cabinet in the Prime Minister's Office, 26 February 1937, SAB, R-97, 7. Uhrich Papers.
91. Minister of Public Health, Province of Saskatchewan, to Executive Director, Canadian National Committee for Mental Hygiene, 4 December 1940, SAB, R-97, 7. Uhrich Papers.
92. Report, "Facts and Observations Pertaining to the Mental Hygiene Situation in Saskatchewan," presented by Dr. C.M. Hincks to the Saskatchewan Cabinet in the Prime Minister's Office, 26 February 1937, SAB, R-97, 7. Uhrich Papers.
93. Ibid.
94. Ibid.
95. Ibid.
96. Ibid.
97. News Release, n.d. (c. September 1943), SAB, R-97, 7. Uhrich Papers.
98. Report, Chief Attendant, Saskatchewan Hospital Battleford, to Commissioner of Mental Services and Superintendent of Saskatchewan Hospital Battleford, 3 July 1944, SAB, R-11, 14-19. Bentley Papers.
99. Commissioner of Mental Services and Superintendent of Saskatchewan Hospital Battleford, to Deputy Minister of Public Health, Province of Saskatchewan, 5 July 1944, SAB, R-11, 14-19. Bentley Papers.
100. Report, Chief Attendant, Saskatchewan Hospital Battleford, to Commissioner of Mental Services and Superintendent of Saskatchewan Hospital Battleford, 3 July 1944, SAB, R-11, 14-19. Bentley Papers.
101. Joseph Smucker, *Industrialization in Canada* (Scarborough, Ontario: Prentice-Hall Inc., 1980), 193.

## Chapter Three

1. Seymour Martin Lipset, *Agrarian Socialism* (Berkeley: University of California Press, 1974).
2. John Richards and Larry Pratt, *Prairie Capitalism: Power and Influence in the New West* (Toronto: McClelland and Stewart, 1979).

3. "Regina Manifesto: Programme of the Cooperative Commonwealth Federation," in Walter D. Young, *The Anatomy of a Party: The National CCF, 1932-61* (Toronto: University of Toronto Press, 1969), 309.
4. Ibid.
5. Ibid., 313.
6. "Working Group on the Relationship between Government and Private Enterprise," Minutes of First Meeting, 27 March 1946, SAB, R-33.4. Douglas Papers: Committee on Labour Policy in Government Enterprises.
7. Richards and Pratt, *Prairie Capitalism.*
8. Interview with the Honourable T.C. Douglas, former premier and minister of public health of the province of Saskatchewan, Ottawa, Ontario, 17 December 1982 (hereafter cited as Douglas, interview).
9. Ibid.
10. Regional Director — United States, Canada and Mexico, International Health Division, Rockefeller Foundation, to Premier and Minister of Public Health, Province of Saskatchewan, 8 September 1944, SAB, R-33.5, 140.(14-35). Douglas Papers: The Rockefeller Foundation.
11. Fosdick, *Rockefeller Foundation,* 133-34.
12. Saskatchewan, Health Services Survey Commission (Sigerist): Dr. Sigerist and Members of the Commission. SAB, Collection 251, RC[M13], 12.
13. Clarence M. Hincks, *Mental Hygiene Survey of Saskatchewan* (Regina: Thomas A. McConnica, King's Printer, 1945), 8; Henry E. Sigerist, *Saskatchewan Health Services Survey Commission* (Regina: Thomas A. McConnica, King's Printer, 1944), 7.
14. Ibid.
15. Ibid.
16. Ray, "Models of Madness," passim.
17. Harley D. Dickinson and Glenn Andre, "Community Psychiatry: The Institutional Transformation of Psychiatric Work," in B. Singh Bolaria and Harley D. Dickinson, eds., *Sociology of Health Care in Canada* (Toronto: HBJ, 1988), 295-308.
18. Hincks, *Mental Hygiene Survey,* 6.
19. Ibid.
20. Ibid.
21. Sigerist, *Saskatchewan Health Services,* 7.
22. Hincks, *Mental Hygiene Survey,* 17.

23. John Urry, *Anatomy of Capitalist Societies: The Economy, Civil Society and the State* (London: Macmillan, 1981), 144.
24. Howard A. Scarrow, "The Civil Service Commissions in the Canadian Provinces," *Journal of Politics* 19 (1957).
25. Douglas, interview.
26. Member of the Legislative Assembly, Cooperative Commonwealth Federation (hereafter cited as MLA(CCF)), Battlefords, Province of Saskatchewan, to Premier, Province of Saskatchewan, 31 July 1944, SAB, R-11, 14-17. Bentley Papers: Saskatchewan Hospital North Battleford, 1944-1950.
27. Premier, Province of Saskatchewan, to MLA(CCF) Battlefords, Province of Saskatchewan, 23 July 1945, SAB, R-11, 14-17. Bentley Papers.
28. Ibid.
29. Fanny H. Kahan, *A Different Drummer: The History of the Saskatchewan Psychiatric Nurses Association, 1948-1973* (Regina: SPNA Pamphlet, 1973), 4.
30. Director, Research and Statistics Branch, Department of Labour, Government of Canada, to Premier's Office, Province of Saskatchewan, 29 August 1945, SAB, R-33.5, 98.(13-4-1-4). Douglas Papers: Mental Hospitals and the United Civil Servants of Canada.
31. "Agreement between the Government of Saskatchewan and the United Civil Servants of Canada, Numbers 2 and 3, being chartered local unions of the Canadian Congress of Labour," 21 March 1945, SAB, R-11, 14-38. Bentley Papers: Union Agreements and Staff of Mental Institutions, 1945-1947.
32. Ibid.
33. "Voluntary Statement Made Jointly and Severally, by Employees of the North Battleford Hospital, and Members of Local No. 3 of the Congress of Labour," 12 July 1945, SAB, R-11, 14-38. Bentley Papers.
34. Ibid.
35. Ibid.
36. "Full Investigation of North Battleford Mental Hospital Follows Thefts: Don Williams Appointed Administrator," Press Release, 8 January 1946, SAB, R-33.5, 103.(13-4-3-1). Douglas Papers.
37. Ibid.
38. Ibid.
39. William C. Menninger, "Lessons from Military Psychiatry for Civilian Psychiatry," reprinted in Nolan D.C. Lewis and Bernice Engle, eds., *Wartime Psychiatry: A Compendium of the*

*International Literature* (New York: Oxford University Press, 1954), 886.

40. Saskatchewan Department of Public Health Annual Report 1947, p. 80.
41. Deputy Minister of Public Health, Province of Saskatchewan, to Superintendents, Provincial Institutions, Province of Saskatchewan, 9 March 1949, SAB, R-11, 14-19. Bentley Papers.
42. Interview with Dr. Frank Coburn, psychiatrist, Saskatoon, Saskatchewan, 8 September 1982 (hereafter cited as Coburn, interview).
43. Ibid.
44. Ibid.
45. Memorandum, Public Service Commission, Province of Saskatchewan, to Premier, Province of Saskatchewan, 28 November 1950, SAB, R-33.5, III, 127.(14-8). Douglas Papers.
46. Memorandum, Deputy Minister of Public Works, Province of Saskatchewan, to Premier's Office, Province of Saskatchewan, 27 March 1946, SAB, R-33.5, 100.(13-4-2-1). Douglas Papers: Health, Mental Hospitals, North Battleford, Employees of.
47. Memorandum, Deputy Minister of Public Health, Province of Saskatchewan, to Minister of Public Health, Province of Saskatchewan, 6 July 1961, SAB, R-34, 110A. Erb Papers: Personnel Collective File.
48. Director, Psychiatric Services Branch, Province of Saskatchewan, to Minister of Public Health, Province of Saskatchewan, 18 October 1954, SAB, R-11, 14-18. Bentley Papers: Saskatchewan Hospital Weyburn, 1954.
49. Commissioner of Mental Services, Province of Saskatchewan, to Deputy Minister of Public Health, Province of Saskatchewan, 5 July 1944, SAB, R-11, 14-19. Bentley Papers.
50. Memorandum, Director, Psychiatric Services, Province of Saskatchewan, to Minister of Public Health, Province of Saskatchewan, 10 February 1951, SAB, R-11, 14-19. Bentley Papers.
51. "CMHA Brief to Cabinet, 1955," SAB, R-33.5, 135.(14-26). Douglas Papers: Canadian Mental Health Association.
52. "Brief on Professional Salaries," prepared by Saskatchewan Psychiatric Association, May 1956, SAB, R-34, 013T.(15). Erb Papers: Saskatchewan Psychiatric Association.
53. Larson, *The Rise of Professionalism*, xvi.
54. Noel Parry and José Parry, "Social Closure and Collective Social Mobility," in Richard Scase, ed., *Industrial Society: Class,*

*Cleavage and Control* (London: George Allen and Unwin, 1977), 112.

55. Freidson, "The Futures of Professionalisation," 27.
56. Larson, *The Rise of Professionalism*, xvii.
57. Freidson, "The Futures of Professionalisation."
58. Littler and Salaman discuss this point in their critique of Braverman (1974). It is suggested that a category of labour-power that has income options will be able to use this in an attempt to struggle against management initiatives that are deemed to be counter to worker interests.
59. Within the context of the wage-relation, professionalism as an occupational organizational strategy becomes less effective. In the face of managerial cost reduction/productivity enhancing strategies, occupations increasingly turn to other organizational strategies. Discussing this point, Parry and Parry conclude: "Consequently, it seems pertinent to suggest that professionalism is now less relevant than in the past as a strategy for collective mobility." Parry and Parry, "Social Closure," 121.
60. Memorandum, Deputy Minister of Public Health, Province of Saskatchewan, to Minister of Public Health, Province of Saskatchewan, 6 July 1961, SAB, R 33.1, XIV, 554.(14-8). Douglas Papers: Mental Institutions and Psychiatric Services.
61. Memorandum, Deputy Minister of Public Health, Province of Saskatchewan, to Minister of Public Health, Province of Saskatchewan, 6 July 1961, SAB, R-33.1, XIV, 554.(14-8). Douglas Papers.
62. For example see "Report on the Provincial Mental Hospitals of Saskatchewan," Central Inspection Board, American Psychiatric Association, September 1950, p. 18, and p. 54.
63. Employee, Saskatchewan Hospital North Battleford, Province of Saskatchewan, to Minister of Public Health, Province of Saskatchewan, 18 March 1959, SAB, R-34, 172D1. Erb Papers: Saskatchewan Hospital North Battleford.
64. President, Saskatchewan Psychiatric Association, to Premier, Province of Saskatchewan, 26 February 1959, SAB, R-34, 116A. Erb Papers.
65. Memorandum, Deputy Minister of Public Health, Province of Saskatchewan, to Minister of Public Health, Province of Saskatchewan, 6 July 1961, SAB, R-33.1, XIV, 554.(14-8). Douglas Papers.
66. Ibid.

67. Secretary-Treasurer, Saskatchewan Psychiatric Association, Province of Saskatchewan, to Premier, Province of Saskatchewan, 4 September, 1957, SAB, R-34, 013T.(15). Erb Papers.
68. Executive, Saskatchewan Psychiatric Association, to Premier, Province of Saskatchewan, 23 August 1957, SAB, R-34, 013T.(15). Erb Papers.
69. Premier, Province of Saskatchewan, to Secretary-Treasurer, Saskatchewan Psychiatric Association, 9 September 1957, SAB, R-34, 013T.(15). Erb Papers.
70. "Saskatchewan Hospital, North Battleford and Saskatchewan Hospital, Weyburn," n.d., circa 1951, SAB, R-11, 14-19. Bentley Papers.
71. Ibid.
72. Commissioner of Mental Services, Province of Saskatchewan, to Deputy Minister of Public Health, Province of Saskatchewan, 5 July 1944, SAB, R-11, 14-19. Bentley Papers.
73. Superintendent, Saskatchewan Hospital Weyburn, to Premier's Office, Province of Saskatchewan, 4 June 1945, SAB, R-33.5, 98.(13-4-1-4). Douglas Papers.
74. Premier's Office, Province of Saskatchewan, to Canadian Congress of Labour, SAB, R-33.5, 98.(13-4-1-4). Douglas Papers.
75. "Report of the Conciliation Board in the Dispute between United Civil Servants of Canada, Locals 2, 3 and 4, C.C.L. and the Government of the Province of Saskatchewan, Department of Public Health, 1953," SAB, R-33.5, III, 127.(14-8). Douglas Papers.
76. Ibid.
77. CCF party member to Premier's Office, Province of Saskatchewan, 1 April 1946, SAB, R-33.5, 98.(13-4-1-4). Douglas Papers.
78. Union Executive, Local No. 3, Saskatchewan Hospital North Battleford, to Deputy Minister of Public Health, Province of Saskatchewan, 12 June 1946, SAB, R-33.5, 100.(13-4-2-1). Douglas Papers.
79. Public Service Commission, Province of Saskatchewan, to Local No. 3 Union Executive, Saskatchewan Hospital North Battleford, 20 June 1946, SAB, R-33.5, 100.(13-4-2-1). Douglas Papers.
80. Secretary-Treasurer, Local No. 3, United Civil Servants of Canada, to Economic Advisor to the Premier, Premier's Office,

Province of Saskatchewan, 8 September 1945, SAB, R-33.5, 98.(13-4-1-4). Douglas Papers.

81. Memorandum, Acting Deputy Minister of Public Health, Province of Saskatchewan, to Premier, Province of Saskatchewan, 30 August 1948, SAB, R-11, 14-17. Bentley Papers.
82. Ibid.
83. Minister of Public Health, Province of Saskatchewan, to MLA (CCF) Battlefords, Province of Saskatchewan, 23 December 1954, SAB, R-11, 14-17. Bentley Papers.
84. Official, United Civil Servants of Canada, Local No. 3, to Premier's Office, Province of Saskatchewan, 2 May 1947, SAB, R-33.5, 98. (13-4-1-4). Douglas Papers.
85. Memorandum, for file Premier's Office, Province of Saskatchewan, 5 May 1947, SAB, R-33.5, 98.(13-4-1-4). Douglas Papers.
86. John Storey, *Managerial Prerogative and the Question of Control* (London: Routledge and Kegan Paul, 1983), 58.
87. Michael Mann, *Consciousness and Action Among the Western Working Class* (London: Macmillan; Atlantic Highlands, New Jersey: Humanities Press International, Inc., 1973), 21.
88. Storey, *Managerial Prerogative*, 59.
89. "Labour Policy for Government Enterprises," Minutes of Fourth Meeting of the sub-committee of the Economic Advisory and Planning Board, Meeting of 20 May 1946, SAB, R-33.4. Douglas Papers.
90. Kahan, *A Different Drummer*, 7.
91. Coburn, interview.
92. Ibid.
93. Memorandum, Director, Psychiatric Services, Province of Saskatchewan, to Minister of Public Health, Province of Saskatchewan, 10 February 1951, SAB, R-11, 14-19. Bentley Papers.
94. Report, "Background to Ward Staff Recruitment Program," from Commissioner of Mental Services, Province of Saskatchewan, to Executive-Secretary, Minnesota Mental Hygiene Society, Inc., n.d., circa March 1948, SAB, R-11, 14-37. Bentley Papers: Director of Psychiatric Services.
95. Executive of Local No. 3, North Battleford, Province of Saskatchewan, to Premier's Office, Province of Saskatchewan, 2 April 1947, SAB, R-33.5, 109.(13-5-2). Douglas Papers: Psychiatric Nurses.
96. Ibid.
97. Coburn, interview.

98. Memorandum, Premier's Office, Province of Saskatchewan, to Commissioner of Mental Services, Province of Saskatchewan, 13 February 1948, SAB, R-33.5, 100.(13-5-2). Douglas Papers: Health: Incorporation: Psychiatric Nurses Civil Servants Union of Canada, Local No. 3.
99. Premier's Office, Province of Saskatchewan, to Union Executive, Local No. 3, North Battleford, Province of Saskatchewan, 14 April 1947, SAB, R-33.5, 109.(13-5-2). Douglas Papers.
100. Memorandum, Premier's Office, Province of Saskatchewan, to Public Service Commission, Province of Saskatchewan, 23 March 1946, SAB, R-33.5, 100.(13-4-2-1). Douglas Papers.
101. Ibid.
102. Psychiatric Nurses Act, 1948.
103. Interview with Bill Ford, psychiatric nurse, Saskatoon, Saskatchewan, 2 May 1983 (hereafter cited as Ford, interview).
104. Memorandum, Premier, Province of Saskatchewan, to Acting Deputy Minister of Public Health, Province of Saskatchewan, 2 September 1949, SAB, R-11, 14-17. Bentley Papers.
105. CCF Advisor to Premier's Office, Province of Saskatchewan, 15 April 1946, SAB, R-33.5, 106.(13-4-4-1). Douglas Papers: Mental Hospital Weyburn.
106. Memorandum, Psychiatric Services Branch, Province of Saskatchewan, to Minister of Public Health, Province of Saskatchewan, 7 January 1958, SAB, R-33.5, III, 127.(14-8). Douglas Papers.
107. Doeringer and Piore, *Internal Labor Markets*, 6.
108. Edwards, "Social Relations of Production".
109. Premier, Province of Saskatchewan, to Minister of Public Health, Province of Saskatchewan, 6 May 1958, SAB, R-33.5, III, 127.(14-8). Douglas Papers.
110. Memorandum, MLA(CCF) Battlefords, Province of Saskatchewan, to Minister of Public Health, Province of Saskatchewan, 25 November 1958, SAB, R-33.1, XIV, 554.(14-8). Douglas Papers.
111. Ibid.
112. MLA(CCF) Battlefords, Province of Saskatchewan, to Premier, Province of Saskatchewan, 31 March 1959, SAB, R-33.1, XIV, 554.(14-8). Douglas Papers.
113. Memorandum, Premier, Province of Saskatchewan, to Minister of Public Health, Province of Saskatchewan, 10 February 1950, SAB, R-33.5, III, 127.(14-8). Douglas Papers.

114. "Business Managers, Mental Hospital," SAB, R-34, 172A1. Erb Papers: Collective File, 1957-1959.
115. Ibid.
116. Memorandum, Deputy Minister of Public Health, Province of Saskatchewan, to Minister of Public Health, Province of Saskatchewan, 25 March 1959, SAB, R-33.1, XIV, 554.(14-8). Douglas Papers.
117. Ibid.
118. Storey, *Managerial Prerogative*, 1.
119. Memorandum, Commissioner of Mental Services, Province of Saskatchewan, to Minister of Public Health, Province of Saskatchewan, 29 April 1952, SAB, R-11, 14-19. Bentley Papers.
120. "A Psychiatric Nurse Training Program — Progress Report 1950," SAB, R-11, 14-37. Bentley Papers.
121. "1955 Brief to the Cabinet: Re. Basement Wards," Saskatchewan Psychiatric Nurses' Association, Weyburn Branch, SAB, R-33.5, III, 127. (14-8). Douglas Papers.
122. Ibid.
123. See A. Kornhauser, *Mental Health of the Industrial Worker* (New York: John Wiley and Sons, 1965); and Charles Hampden-Turner, "The Factory as an Oppressive and Non-Emancipatory Environment," in G. Hunnius, G.D. Garson and John Case, eds., *Workers' Control: A Reader on Labor and Social Change* (New York: Vintage Books, 1973), 30-45.
124. Goffman, *Asylums.*
125. Ford, interview.
126. Ibid. As far as I am able to determine, the term pro-baths is simply a shortened version of prolonged baths.
127. Ibid
128. "Factors in Defining Psychiatric Nursing," *The Bulletin* 2 (November 1961). SAB, R-34, 172C1. Erb Papers: Saskatchewan Hospital Weyburn.
129. Ibid.
130. Ibid.
131. Ibid.
132. See H. Jamous and B. Peloille, "Professions or Self-Perpetuating Systems? Changes in the French University-Hospital System," in J.A. Jackson, ed., *Professions and Professionalization* (Cambridge: Cambridge University Press, 1970), 111-52.
133. Memorandum, Director, Psychiatric Services Branch, Province of Saskatchewan, to Minister of Public Health, Province of Saskatchewan, 3 October 1960, SAB, R-34, 172A1. Erb Papers.

134. "Saskatchewan Department of Public Health: Outline of Services," Regina: Division of Health Education, n.d., p. 40.
135. Scull, *Decarceration*, 79.
136. Peter Conrad and Joseph W. Schneider, *Deviance and Medicalization: From Badness to Sickness* (St. Louis: The Mosby Company, 1980), 52.
137. Kathleen Jones, *History of the Mental Health Service*; see also Henry M. Hurd, *The Institutional Care of the Insane in the United States and Canada*, 4 volumes (New York: Arno Press, 1973).
138. Conrad and Schneider, *Deviance and Medicalization*, 48.
139. Scull, *Decarceration*, 91.
140. For a discussion of this process as it occurred in Canada see David Coburn et al., "Medical Dominance in Canada in Historical Perspective: The Rise and Fall of Medicine?," *International Journal of Health Services* 13 (1983): 407-32.
141. Conrad and Schneider, *Deviance and Medicalization*, 44.
142. Marglin, "Origins and Functions of Hierarchy."
143. David J. Rothman, *The Discovery of the Asylum: Social Order and Disorder in the New Republic* (Boston: Little, Brown and Company, 1971).
144. L.D. Clark, "Evaluation of the Therapeutic Effects of Drugs in Psychiatric Patients," *Diseases of the Nervous System* 17 (1956): 283.
145. Ibid.

## Chapter Four

1. President, Canadian Mental Health Association, Saskatchewan Division, to Premier, Province of Saskatchewan, 9 February 1951, SAB, R-33.5, 135.(14-26). Douglas Papers.
2. Cumming and Cumming, *Closed Ranks*.
3. Ibid., foreword by John A. Clausen, xiv.
4. Memorandum, Director, Psychiatric Services, Province of Saskatchewan, to Minister of Public Health, Province of Saskatchewan, 25 September 1959, SAB, R-34, 172A1. Erb Papers.
5. Maxwell Shaw Jones, *Social Psychiatry in Practice: The Idea of the Therapeutic Community* (Harmondsworth, Middlesex: Penguin Books, 1968).
6. Stanley Cohen, *Folk Devils and Moral Panics* (New York: St. Martin's Press, 1972).

7. Memorandum, Director Psychiatric Services, Province of Saskatchewan, to Minister of Public Health, Province of Saskatchewan, 25 September 1959, SAB, R-34, 172A1. Erb Papers.
8. Superintendent, Saskatchewan Hospital Weyburn, to Premier, Province of Saskatchewan, 25 October 1959, SAB, R-33.5, III, 127.(14-8). Douglas Papers.
9. Canadian Mental Health Association, *This is Your Mental Health Association* (Regina: CMHA, 1975), 4.
10. Coburn, interview.
11. Ibid.
12. Minister of Public Health, Province of Saskatchewan, to Minister of Health and Public Welfare, Province of Manitoba, 23 June 1955, SAB, R-11, 14-84. Bentley Papers: Canadian Mental Health Association (Sask. Division).
13. Canadian Mental Health Association, *This is Your Mental Health Association*, 4.
14. Memorandum, Minister of Public Health, Province of Saskatchewan, to Deputy Minister of Public Health, Province of Saskatchewan, 3 May 1951, SAB, R-11, 14-84. Bentley Papers.
15. Memorandum, Premier, Province of Saskatchewan, to Minister of Public Health, Province of Saskatchewan, 31 January 1957, SAB, R-33.1, 572.(14-26). Douglas Papers: Canadian Mental Health Association Jan. 1957-Mar. 1961.
16. Minister of Public Health, Province of Saskatchewan, to Administrative Assistant to the Leader of the Opposition, Province of British Columbia, 13 February 1961, SAB, R-34, 172A1. Erb Papers.
17. Saskatchewan Department of Public Health Annual Report 1947, p. 47.
18. D.G. McKerracher, *Trends in Psychiatric Care*, Report of the Royal Commission on Health Services in Canada, 1964 (Ottawa: Queen's Printer, 1966), 109.
19. Private Psychiatrist, Saskatoon, Saskatchewan, to Minister of Public Health, Province of Saskatchewan, 29 December 1950, SAB, R-11, 14-19. Bentley Papers.
20. Saskatchewan Department of Public Health Annual Report 1952-53, p. 77.
21. Ibid.
22. Ibid.
23. Memorandum, Director, Psychiatric Services, Province of Saskatchewan, to Minister of Public Health, Province of

Saskatchewan, 10 February 1951, SAB, R-11, 14-19. Bentley Papers.

24. Meyer Harvey Brenner, *Mental Illness and the Economy* (Cambridge, Mass.: Harvard University Press, 1973).
25. Ford, interview.
26. "Mental Health Program," n.d., circa 1957, SAB, R-34, 172G. Erb Papers: Proposed Regional Mental Hospital.
27. F. Grunberg, "The Role and Function of a Community Mental Health Clinic in Relation to the Mental Hospital," n.d., circa 1959, p. 1, SAB, R-33.5, III, 127.(14-8). Douglas Papers.
28. Ibid., pp. 7-8.
29. Ibid., p. 10.
30. "Sask. Psychiatrists Welcome Health Scheme for Mentally Ill," *Saskatoon Star Phoenix*, 22 July 1958, SAB, R-34, 172A1. Erb Papers.
31. Coburn, interview.
32. "Surveys of Saskatchewan Hospital Weyburn," SAB, R-33.5, III, 127.(14-8). Douglas Papers.
33. Goffman, *Asylums*, 203.
34. Fanny H. Kahan, *Brains and Bricks: The History of the Yorkton Psychiatric Centre* (Regina: White Cross Publications, 1965), 82.
35. Lawson, "Mental Hospitals," p. 186.
36. J.D. McMillan, "Community Mental Hospital," *The Canadian Hospital* (May 1957): 41-42.
37. Scull, *Museums of Madness*, 103-4.
38. Ibid.
39. "Low Report," SAB, R-33.5, III, 127.(14-8). Douglas Papers.
40. For a complete elaboration of this design see McMillan, "Community Mental Hospital."
41. Kahan, *Brains and Bricks*, 84.
42. Professor of Psychiatry, University of Saskatchewan, to Minister of Public Health, Province of Saskatchewan, 17 April 1956, SAB, R-11, 14-84. Bentley Papers.
43. Quoted in Lawson, "Mental Hospitals," 188.
44. Coburn, interview.
45. Lawson, "Mental Hospitals," 188-89.
46. "Canadian Mental Health Association Submission to the Federal Minister of Health and Welfare, 1956," SAB, R-11, 14-84. Bentley Papers.
47. All figures taken from the following Psychiatric Services Branch submission to the Minister of Public Health, Province

of Saskatchewan: "A Plan to Given Adequate Care to Saskatchewan," SAB, R-34, 172G2. Erb Papers: Saskatchewan Plans.

48. Memorandum, Premier, Province of Saskatchewan, to Minister of Public Health, Province of Saskatchewan, 31 January 1957, SAB, R-34, 172A1. Erb Papers.
49. Ibid.
50. Premier, Province of Saskatchewan, to Mr. Bill Walker, 14 November 1955, SAB, R-33.5, III, 127.(14-8). Douglas Papers.
51. Douglas, interview.
52. Professor of Psychiatry, University of Saskatchewan, to Premier, Province of Saskatchewan, 10 October 1957, SAB, R-33.1, 572.(14-26). Douglas Papers.
53. Premier, Province of Saskatchewan, to President, Canadian Mental Health Association, Saskatchewan Division, 21 October 1957, SAB, R-33.1, 572.(14-26). Douglas Papers.
54. Ibid.
55. Professor of Psychiatry, University of Saskatchewan, to Premier, Province of Saskatchewan, 30 July 1958, SAB, R-34, 051A. Erb Papers: Hospital Insurance: General Correspondence.
56. Minister of Public Health, Province of Saskatchewn, to Federal Minister of Health and Welfare, 31 July 1958, SAB, R-34, 051A. Erb Papers.
57. Federal Minister of Health and Welfare, to Minister of Public Health, Province of Saskatchewan, 22 August 1958, SAB, R-34, 015A. Erb Papers.
58. Saskatchewan Department of Public Health Annual Report 1946, p. 71.
59. Memorandum, Director of Psychiatric Services, Province of Saskatchewan, to Minister of Public Health, Province of Saskatchewan, 10 February 1951, SAB, R-11, 14-19. Bentley Papers.
60. Professor of Psychiatry, University of Saskatchewan, to Premier, Province of Saskatchewan, 10 October 1957, SAB, R-33.1, 572.(14-26). Douglas Papers.
61. "Psychiatric Wards Rapped," *Saskatoon Star Phoenix*, 21 January 1958.
62. Professor of Psychiatry, University of Saskatchewan, to Premier, Province of Saskatchewan, 10 October 1957, SAB, R-33.1, 572.(14-26). Douglas Papers.
63. D.G. McKerracher, "Research at Saskatchewan," in Richard H. Williams and Lucy D. Ozarin, eds., *Community Mental Health:*

*An International Perspective* (San Francisco: Jossey-Bass, 1968), 370-81; W.J. McCorkell and D.G. McKerracher, "The Family Doctor and the Psychiatric Ward," *Mental Hospitals* 11 (1962): 300-302; D.G. McKerracher et al., "General Practice Psychiatry — An Account of Two Canadian Experiments," *Lancet* 2 (1965): 1005-7; C.M. Smith and D.G. McKerracher, "The Comprehensive Psychiatric Unit in the General Hospital," *American Journal of Psychiatry* 121 (1964): 52-57; C.M. Smith and D.G. McKerracher, "The Family Doctor in a Program of Comprehensive Psychiatric Care," in Hugh Freeman and James Farndale, eds., *New Aspects of the Mental Health Service* (Oxford: Pergammon Press, 1967).

64. Coburn, interview.
65. "Saskatchewan Psychiatric Nurses' Association, Weyburn Branch, Brief to Cabinet, 1955, re: Basement Wards," SAB, R-33.5, III, 127.(14-18). Douglas Papers.
66. Premier, Province of Saskatchewan, to Minister of Education, Province of Saskatchewan, 4 April 1961, SAB, R-12.3, IV, 9, (box 20). Blakeney Papers: New Party.
67. Badgley and Wolfe, *Doctors' Strike.*
68. Secretary-Treasurer, Saskatchewan Psychiatric Nurses' Association, to Minister of Public Health, Province of Saskatchewan, 1 March 1960, SAB, R-34, 172G3. Erb Papers: Yorton Community Mental Hospital.
69. "Duties," attachment to Letter, Secretary-Treasurer, Saskatchewan Psychiatric Nurses' Association, to Minister of Public Health, Province of Saskatchewan, 24 September 1960, SAB, R-34, 172A1. Erb Papers.
70. Chairman and Secretary-Treasurer, Saskatchewan Psychiatric Nurses' Association, to Minister of Public Health, Province of Saskatchewan, 16 March 1962, SAB, R-30.3, 15A, D289. Davies Papers: Saskatchewan Psychiatric Nurses' Association.
71. "Psychiatrist Hits Govt. Indifference," *Regina Leader-Post*, 21 October 1961, SAB, R-34, 110A. Erb Papers.
72. Memorandum, Minister of Public Health, Province of Saskatchewan, to Premier, Province of Saskatchewan, 25 October 1961, SAB, R-34, 110A. Erb Papers.
73. Professor of Psychiatry, University of Saskatchewan, to Minister of Public Health, Province of Saskatchewan, 7 February 1961, SAB, R-34, 172A. Erb Papers: Psychiatric Services.

74. Memorandum, Minister of Public Health, Province of Saskatchewan, to Premier, Province of Saskatchewan, 25 October 1961, SAB, R-34, 110A. Erb Papers.
75. Crane, "Clinical Psychopharmacology," 126; Dr. Douglas Bennett, a leading figure in British community psychiatry, told me in a personal interview that the developments in Saskatchewan had some influence on the programs he developed out of Maudsley Hospital. Interview with Dr. Douglas Bennett, psychiatrist, Maudsley Hospital, London, England.
76. Director, Psychiatric Research, Psychiatric Services Branch, Province of Saskatchewan, to Premier, Province of Saskatchewan, 15 October 1957, SAB, R-33.5, III, 127.(14-8). Douglas Papers.
77. Professor of Psychiatry, University of Saskatchewan, to Minister of Public Health, Province of Saskatchewan, 7 February 1961, SAB, R-34, 172A. Erb Papers.
78. Memorandum, Minister of Public Health, Province of Saskatchewan, to Premier, Province of Saskatchewan, 25 October 1961, SAB, R-34, 110A. Erb Papers.

## Chapter Five

1. F. Grunberg et al., "Reducing the Population of a Mental Hospital," n.d., p. 30, SAB, R-94, 120.(9-1). Steuart Papers: Psychiatric Services, December 1963-December 1964.
2. For a brief discussion of the basic changes to the Saskatchewan Mental Health Act, 1961, see "New Mental Health Act for Saskatchewan," *Canada's Mental Health* 9 (1961): 4-6.
3. D.G. McKerracher, *Trends*, 115.
4. Memorandum, Deputy Minister of Public Health, Province of Saskatchewan, to Minister of Public Health, Province of Saskatchewan, 25 September 1967, SAB, R-45, 78a.(9-3). Grant Papers: Psychiatric Services Division: Committees and Reports (various).
5. Richards and Pratt, *Prairie Capitalism*, 201.
6. Ibid., 199.
7. David Smith, *Prairie Liberalism: The Liberal Party in Saskatchewan, 1905-71* (Toronto: University of Toronto Press, 1975), Chapter 8, passim.
8. Richards and Pratt, *Prairie Capitalism*, 200.
9. Saskatchewan, Royal Commission on Government Administration (Regina: Queen's Printer, 1965), 12.
10. Ibid.

11. Ibid., 399.
12. Figures taken from the 1964 Saskatchewan Department of Public Health Annual Report, and the 1965 Royal Commission on Government Administration, p. 452.
13. Saskatchewan, Royal Commission on Government Administration (Regina: Queen's Printer, 1965), p. 409.
14. Howard A. Scarrow, "Employer-Employee Relationships in the Civil Services of the Canadian Provinces," *Public Administration* 398 (Spring 1957).
15. Saskatchewan, Royal Commission on Government Administration (Regina: Queen's Printer, 1965), p. 410.
16. Ibid.
17. Ibid., 427.
18. Ibid., 426.
19. Ibid., 408.
20. Smith, *Prairie Liberalism*, 310. This refers to the application in 1966 of the Essential Services Emergency Act, which in effect denied government workers designated as being employed in the essential services the right to strike.
21. Editorial, "A Return to the Dark Ages," *The Dome: Official Publication of the Saskatchewan Government Employees Association* 43 (June 1969): 94.
22. Ibid.
23. Ibid., 94-95.
24. Saskatchewan, Royal Commission on Government Administration (Regina: Queen's Printer, 1965).
25. "The Treatment of the Mentally Ill in Saskatchewan: The 'Saskatchewan Plan' and the Future of the Mental Hospitals in the Province by 1970," p. 4, undated Department of Public Health Report, filed 8 August 1966, SAB, R-45, 75.(9-1). Grant Papers.
26. Ibid., p. 12.
27. Memorandum, Deputy Minister of Public Health, Province of Saskatchewan, to Secretary, Treasury Board, Province of Saskatchewan, 13 March 1969, SAB, R-45, 102.(9-19). Grant Papers: Psychiatric Services: Half-Way House, Swift Current.
28. The membership of the Ad Hoc Committee on the Resettlement of Mental Hospital Patients was as follows: Mr. Sam Murray, Weyburn, Chairman; Miss Isabel Butters, Weyburn; Rev. Ross Mc Murtry, Weyburn; Mr. Ernie Neufeld, Weyburn; Dr. John P. Falkingham, Swift Current; Mrs. William Fyles,

Regina; Dr. Colin Smith, Saskatoon; and Mr. Ken Torrance, Regina.

29. Memorandum, Minister of Public Health, Province of Saskatchewan, to Minister of Industry and Commerce, Province of Saskatchewan, 17 February 1966, SAB, R-45, 97.(1-16). Grant Papers.
30. "The Report of the Ad Hoc Committee on the Resettlement of Mental Hospital Patients," submitted to the Minister of Public Health, Province of Saskatchewan, 27 June 1966, p. 1.
31. Ibid., p. 10.
32. Submission to Premier, Province of Saskatchewan, and Minister of Public Health, Province of Saskatchewan, from President, Weyburn Chamber of Commerce and Secretary Manager, Weyburn Chamber of Commerce, concerning the resettlement and care of mental patients, n.d., circa February-March 1966, SAB, R-45, 97.(9-16). Grant Papers: Committee on Resettlement of Mental Hospital Patients.
33. "The Report of the Ad Hoc Committee on the Resettlement of Mental Hospital Patients," submitted to the Minister of Public Health, Province of Saskatchewan, 27 June 1966, p. 11.
34. "The Treatment of the Mentally Ill in Saskatchewan," p. 2.
35. Ford, interview.
36. "The Treatment of the Mentally Ill in Saskatchewan," p. 4.
37. Memorandum, Director, Psychiatric Services Branch, Province of Saskatchewan, to Deputy Minister of Public Health, Province of Saskatchewan, 15 June 1966, SAB, R-45, 97.(9-16). Grant Papers.
38. Shervert H. Frazier and Alex D. Pokorny, "Report of a Consultation to the Minister of Public Health on the Psychiatric Services of Saskatchewan," p. 28 (hereafter cited as the Frazier Report), n.d., circa January 1968.
39. "The Treatment of the Mentally Ill in Saskatchewan," pp. 3-4.
40. Ibid., pp. 5-6.
41. Ibid., p. 6.
42. Dennis Guest, *The Emergence of Social Security in Canada* (Vancouver: University of British Columbia Press, 1980), 155.
43. Coburn, interview.
44. President, Sherbrooke Nursing Home Ltd., Saskatoon, Saskatchewan, to Minister of Public Health, Province of Saskatchewan, 23 March 1966, SAB, R-45, 97.(9-16). Grant Papers.
45. "The Treatment of the Mentally Ill in Saskatchewan," pp. 5-6.
46. Ibid., p. 6.

47. Ibid., p. 3.
48. Ibid., p. 4.
49. Frazier Report, 35-37.
50. "The Report of the Ad Hoc Committee on the Resettlement of Mental Hospital Patients," p. 14.
51. Ibid.
52. Canadian Mental Health Association, Saskatchewan Division, to Minister of Public Health, Province of Saskatchewan, 3 January 1966, SAB, R-45, 97.(9-16). Grant Papers.
53. P. Allderidge, "Hospitals, Madhouses and Asylums: Cycles in the Care of the Insane," *British Journal of Psychiatry* 134 (1979): 330. Also see W.L. Parry-Jones, *The Trade in Lunacy* (London: Routledge and Kegan Paul, 1972); and Andrew Scull, "Community Care of the Mentally Ill: Current Realities in the Context of Past Developments," in A. Johnson, O. Grusky and B. Raven, eds., *Contemporary Health Services: Social Science Perspectives* (Boston, Mass.: Auburn House, 1982), 237-49.
54. The Saskatchewan Assistance Plan (SAP) is the provincial counterpart to the CAP established in 1966.
55. Saskatchewan Department of Public Health Annual Report 1972-73, p. 78.
56. Scull, "Community Corrections."
57. According to the Mental Health Act, 1961, p. 2, facility refers to institution, psychiatric center, psychiatric ward, mental health clinic or any other building or portion thereof set aside for the care, treatment or training of mentally disordered persons.
58. Helen K. Mussallem, *Nursing Education in Canada*, Report of the Royal Commission on Health Services in Canada, 1964 (Ottawa: Queen's Printer, 1966), 108.
59. Ibid.
60. "Report of the Ad Hoc Committee on Nursing Education, Province of Saskatchewan" (Regina: Queen's Printer, 1966), 32.
61. Mussallem, *Nursing Education*, 107.
62. "Report of the Ad Hoc Committee on Nursing Education, Province of Saskatchewan," p. 32.
63. *Saskatchewan Psychiatric Nurse Newsletter* 2 (March 1964): 2.
64. Quoted in Kahan, *A Different Drummer*, 45.
65. Ibid., 45-46.
66. Ibid, 46.
67. Ibid.

68. "Weyburn Staffing Establishment 8 May 1969," SAB, R-45, 98b.(9-16). Grant Papers: Psychiatric Services: Weyburn Mental Hospital 1967-1969.
69. Mussallem, *Nursing Education*, 135.
70. "Report of the Ad Hoc Committee on Nursing Education, Province of Saskatchewan," p. 144.
71. Ibid., 145.
72. Ibid., 1.
73. Ibid., 147.
74. "Presentation to the Minister of Public Health by the SPNA," n.d., circa 1967, SAB, R-45, 85.(9-7). Grant Papers: Psychiatric Services; North Battleford Mental Hospital.
75. Ibid.
76. "Weyburn Staffing Establishment 8 May 1969," SAB, R-45, 98b.(9-16). Grant Papers.
77. "Submission to Minister of Public Health, Province of Saskatchewan, by the Saskatchewan Psychiatric Nurses' Association," circa June 1969, SAB, R-45, 85.(9-7). Grant Papers.
78. Ibid.
79. Ibid.
80. "Criteria for Conducting a Psychiatric Affiliation Program," submission of the SRNA to Minister of Public Health, Province of Saskatchewan, 10 April 1967, SAB, R-45, 85.(9-7). Grant Papers.
81. Interview with Glenn Rutherford, Director of Social Work, Saskatoon Mental Health Clinic, Saskatoon, Saskatchewan, 10 May 1983 (hereafter cited as Rutherford, interview).
82. Ibid.
83. W. Rempel, "A Reappraisal of the Role of Social Worker in a Mental Health Clinic," Personal Files: Glenn Rutherford.
84. Bernard Vandermeer, "Program Priorities," 10 January 1970, p. 3, prepared for Chief Social Workers Meeting held 28-29 January 1970, Personal Files: Glenn Rutherford.
85. For an interesting discussion of the non-confrontational deskilling of work in an historical context see Craig Littler, "De-Skilling and Changing Structures of Control," in Stephen Wood, ed., *The Degradation of Work? Skill, De-Skilling and the Labour Process* (London: Hutchinson, 1983), 125-45.
86. Bernard Vandermeer, "Program Priorities," 10 January 1970, p. 2.
87. Ibid. This same general strategy was subsequently proposed to the DPH by PSB management as one of a number of possible

solutions to the chronic shortage of trained psychiatrists — it was in fact this solution which was finally adopted.

88. Ibid., 3.
89. Ibid., 2.
90. Ibid.
91. Ibid., 4.
92. Ibid.
93. Memorandum, Deputy Minister of Public Health, Province of Saskatchewan, to Minister of Public Health, Province of Saskatchewan, 25 September 1967, SAB, R-45, 78a.(9-3). Grant Papers.
94. Memorandum, Minister of Public Health, Province of Saskatchewan, to Premier, Province of Saskatchewan, 17 November 1967, SAB, R-45, 87a. Grant Papers: Psychiatric Services Division, Staff, 1967.
95. Dr. A. Spellman, "State of Psychiatry in Saskatchewan," n.d., circa 1967, SAB, R-45, 84.(9-6). Grant Papers: Psychiatric Services: North Battleford Mental Hospital.
96. Memorandum, Director, Psychiatric Services Branch, Province of Saskatchewan, to Deputy Minister of Public Health, Province of Saskatchewan, 24 October 1967, SAB, R-45, 87a. Grant Papers.
97. The MCIC was the culmination of a long series of bitter struggles undertaken by the CCF in their attempt to establish a complete system of socialized medicine promised in their 1944 election campaign. By 1962, however, the plan for socialized medicine had been transmuted into a state-run insurance scheme which provided for guaranteed payment to physicians on a fee-for-service basis. This included payment for both specialist and GP-provided psychotherapeutic services. It was on the basis of this that private sector psychiatry developed. It must be recognized that private sector medical practice in Saskatchewan after 1963 and indeed throughout all of Canada after 1968 was, and is, largely financed from state revenues, and in this sense might more accurately be called semi-private or quasi-public sector psychiatry. For the sake of simplicity and clarity, however, I shall refer to the PSB-managed psychiatric services as public and MCIC-financed psychiatric services as private. For a discussion of the various struggles leading to, and surrounding, the creation of MCIC see Badgley and Wolfe, *Doctors' Strike,* and Edwin A. Tollefson, "The Medicare Dispute," in Norman Ward and Duff Spafford, eds., *Politics in*

*Saskatchewan* (Don Mills, Ontario: Longmans Canada Ltd., 1968), 238-79.

98. Frazier Report, 14.
99. Registrar, Saskatchewan College of Physicians and Surgeons, to Minister of Public Health, Province of Saskatchewan, 21 September 1966, SAB, R-45, 97.(9-16). Grant Papers.
100. Minister of Public Health, Province of Saskatchewan, to Registrar, Saskatchewan College of Physicians and Surgeons, 28 September 1966, SAB, R-45, 97.(9-16). Grant Papers.
101. "Working Paper: Private Practice Outside Hours for Full Time Psychiatrists," p. 1, 3 December 1969, SAB, R-45, 101.(9-18). Grant Papers: Steering Committee Agenda and Minutes.
102. Ibid.
103. Ibid.
104. Ibid., p. 3
105. "Survey of Provinces Regarding Part-time Private Practice, 1969," SAB, R-45, 101.(9-18). Grant Papers.
106. Wood and Kelly, "Taylorism," 77-89.
107. "Department of Public Health, PSB, Psychiatrist Staffing, Exhibit F," n.d., circa 1970, presentation to the Budget Bureau, SAB, R-82, 549, 1-19(n). Smishek Papers: Staff 1970-71.
108. "And Don't Blame the CCF," *Weyburn Review*, no date, SAB, R-45, 75.(9-1). Grant Papers.
109. Ibid.
110. Ibid.
111. Frazier Report, 7.
112. Ibid., 26-27.
113. Memorandum, Deputy Minister of Public Health, Province of Saskatchewan, to Minister of Public Health, Province of Saskatchewan, 14 December 1967, SAB, R-45, 88.(9-9). Grant Papers.
114. Ibid., p. 38.
115. Ibid., p. 29.
116. Frazier Report, 35.
117. Memorandum, Deputy Minister of Public Health, Province of Saskatchewan, to Minister of Public Health, Province of Saskatchewan, 14 December 1967, SAB, R-45, 88.(9-9). Grant Papers.
118. Memorandum, Director, Psychiatric Services Branch, Province of Saskatchewan, to Minister of Public Health, Province of Saskatchewan, 23 February 1968, SAB, R-45, 88.(9-9). Grant Papers.

119. For an account of the historical struggles leading to the creation of federal health care policy see Donald Swartz, "The Politics of Reform: Conflict and Accommodation in Canadian Health Policy," in Leo Panitch, ed., *The Canadian State: Political Economy and Political Power* (Toronto: University of Toronto Press, 1977), 311-43; also see Vivienne Walters, "State, Capital and Labour: The Introduction of Federal-Provincial Insurance for Physician Care in Canada," *The Canadian Review of Sociology and Anthropology* 19 (May 1982): 157-72.
120. Memorandum, Deputy Minister of Public Health, Province of Saskatchewan, to Minister of Public Health, Province of Saskatchewan, 14 December 1967, SAB, R-45, 88.(9-9). Grant Papers.
121. Memorandum, Deputy Minister of Public Health, Province of Saskatchewan, to Minister of Public Health, Province of Saskatchewan, 29 March 1968, SAB, R-45, 203b.(24-C-4). Grant Papers.
122. Memorandum, Deputy Minister of Public Health, Province of Saskatchewan, to Minister of Public Health, Province of Saskatchewan, 8 March 1968, SAB, R-45, 203b.(24-C-4). Grant Papers: Canadian Mental Health Association.
123. Memorandum, Deputy Minister of Public Health, Province of Saskatchewan, to Minister of Public Health, Province of Saskatchewan, 4 July 1968, SAB, R-45, 203b.(24-C-4). Grant Papers.
124. Ex-executive Director, Canadian Mental Health Association, Saskatchewan Division, to Director, Psychiatric Services Branch, Province of Saskatchewan, 2 July 1968, SAB, R-45, 203b.(24-C-4). Grant Papers.
125. Ibid.
126. Ibid.
127. Memorandum, Deputy Minister of Public Health, Province of Saskatchewan, to Minister of Public Health, Province of Saskatchewan, 4 July 1968, SAB, R-45, 203b.(24-C-4). Grant Papers.
128. MDT Associates, Winnipeg, Manitoba, to Deputy Minister of Public Health, Province of Saskatchewan, 24 February 1968, SAB, R-45, 90.(9-10). Grant Papers: Psychiatric Services Division Study — Prefontaine (MDT).
129. Memorandum, Director, Psychiatric Services Branch, Province of Saskatchewan, to Minister of Public Health, Province of

Saskatchewan, 23 February 1968, SAB, R-45, 88.(9-9). Grant Papers: Psychiatric Services, Frazier Report.

130. Saskatchewan Department of Public Health Annual Report 1968, p. 69.
131. The figure for SHW was reported as $21.20 and for SHNB $10.52 in September 1968. Memorandum, Director, Psychiatric Services Branch, Province of Saskatchewan, to Deputy Minister of Public Health, Province of Saskatchewan, 19 September 1968, SAB, R-45, 90.(9-10). Grant Papers.
132. Ibid.
133. Memorandum, MDT Associates, Winnipeg, Manitoba, to Minister of Public Health, Province of Saskatchewan, 26 June 1968, SAB, R-45, 90.(9-10). Grant Papers.
134. Ibid.
135. Ibid.
136. Ibid.
137. "An outline of Psychiatric Services in Saskatchewan," p. 10. A talk given at the Minister's Meeting of Chairmen and Administrators, Saskatchewan Hospitals, Saskatoon, 27 June 1968, by Colin M. Smith, Director, Psychiatric Services Branch, SAB, R-45, 84.(9-6). Grant Papers.
138. Ibid., p. 3.
139. Colin M. Smith, "Crisis and Aftermath: Community Psychiatry in Saskatchewan, 1963-69," *Canadian Psychiatric Association Journal* 16 (1971): 70.
140. The number of deaths in the institutions declined from a high of 405 in 1963 to 14 in 1981. Saskatchewan Department of Public Health Annual Reports.

## Chapter Six

1. Interview with Peter Griffiths, Social Worker, Prince Albert Psychiatric Center, Prince Albert, Saskatchewan, 5 May 1983.
2. "Confidential Report to Walter E. Smishek, Minister of Public Health," 30 December 1971, pp. 2-3, SAB, R-82, 549, 9-14. Smishek Papers: Hospital North Battleford.
3. Ibid., p. 9.
4. Memorandum, Legislative Secretary, Province of Saskatchewan, to Minister of Public Health, Province of Saskatchewan, 13 October 1971, SAB, R-82, 549, 9-14. Smishek Papers.
5. Carl D'Arcy, Janet A. Schmitz and Guin Bold, "Patterns in the Delivery of Psychiatric Care in Saskatchewan 1969-1974: Service Interface Study (SIS) Final Report" (Regina: Psychiatric

Services Branch, Department of Health, Province of Saskatchewan, 1979), 173.

6. Ibid.
7. Ibid., 172.
8. Ibid.
9. Saskatchewan MCIC Annual Report 1975, p. 30.
10. D'Arcy, Schmitz and Bold, "Service Interface Study," xiii.
11. Ibid., xv.
12. Ibid., xiv.
13. For a discussion of the expected impact of this on the demand for psychiatric services see Kent Silzer, "Saskatchewan's Population — 1976 to 2001: An Examination of Anticipated Changes with Particular Reference to the Demand for Mental Health Services" (Regina: Department of Public Health, Psychiatric Services Branch, 1981).
14. D'Arcy, Schmitz and Bold, "Service Interface Study," xiv.
15. For an account of the development of medical insurance in Canada see Malcolm G. Taylor, *Health Insurance and Canadian Public Policy: The Seven Decisions that Created the Canadian Health Insurance System* (Montreal: McGill-Queen's University Press, 1978).
16. For a brief history of the Saskatoon Community Clinic to 1972 see Dennis Gruending, *The First Ten Years* (Saskatoon: Community Clinic, 1974).
17. Ibid.
18. "The Community Health Centre in Canada: Report of the Community Health Centre Project to the Conference of Health Ministers," 21 July 1972, Foreword, p.v. (hereafter cited as Hastings Report).
19. T. Kue Young, "Lay-Professional Conflict in a Canadian Community Health Centre: A Case Report," *Medical Care* (1974): 898.
20. Hastings Report, p. 35.
21. For an excellent account of this event see T.K. Young, "Lay-Professional Conflict."
22. Wayne B. Fritz, "A Critical Assessment of Proposals for a Compulsory Mental Health Care Act," Applied Research Unit, Psychiatric Research Division, Saskatchewan, 1982. (Mimeographed.)
23. John Weingust, "When Therapy Becomes Assault," *Toronto Globe and Mail*, 26 April 1984, p. 7.

24. *Report of the Thrust Working Party: Community Based Alternatives for Mental Health Care* (Regina: Policy Research and Management Services Branch, Saskatchewan Health, 1980), 52.
25. Ibid.
26. Saskatchewan Health Annual Report 1980-81, p. 91.
27. "The Neufeldt Report," p. 72, January 1969, SAB, R-45, 103.(9-20). Grant Papers: Study-Dr. Aldred Neufeldt.
28. "The Neufeldt Report: Position of the Department of Public Health," 2 July 1969, SAB, R-45, 103.(9-20). Grant Papers.
29. John E. Gray, "Role Conflicts Within a Provincial Community Mental Health Program," *The Saskatchewan Psychologist: Bulletin of the Psychological Society of Saskatchewan* 72 (November 1972): 41.
30. Saskatchewan Department of Public Health Annual Report 1976-77, p. 65.
31. Marc Lalonde, *A New Perspective on the Health of Canadians* (Ottawa: Information Canada, 1974), 26.
32. B. Singh Bolaria, "Self-Care and Lifestyles: Ideological and Policy Implications," in John A. Fry, ed., *Economy, Class and Social Reality* (Toronto: Butterworths, 1979), 359.
33. This ideology is disseminated in many different forms. For example, the 21 March 1984 edition of the *Globe and Mail* included a twenty-four-page "advertising special report" entitled "Close-up on Health." This "advertising special report" was "produced in collaboration with Health and Welfare Canada" and covered a broad range of "lifestyles and self-care" topics ranging from alcohol, drug use and how to avoid herpes, to diets, exercise, menopause and more. One article entitled "Accepting Situation a Way Out of Stress" suggests the best way to cope with "negative stress" linked to things like "unemployment, marriage problems, death of a spouse, money worries, poor housing or concerns about children" is by "accepting it and adjusting to it." It is particularly interesting to note that the advertising special report was partly financed by approximately sixty-five different companies selling 'healthy lifestyles,' or the accoutrements of such. The ideological emphasis on lifestyles and self-care is also accompanied by the commodification of health, and the lifestyles ideology is thereby disseminated not only by the state, but by private businesses attempting to sell their health products. This

includes everything from exercise classes to yoga to running shoes.

34. D'Arcy, Schmitz and Bold, "Service Interface Study," xiv.
35. Interview with Mary Jane Katz, Executive Director, Saskatchewan Psychiatric Nurses Association, Regina, Saskatchewan, 20 March 1983 (hereafter cited as Katz, interview).
36. St. Paul's Hospital, the other large general hospital in Saskatoon, was/is privately owned and operated by the Grey Nuns religious order. They had made it clear they had no intention of ever opening a psychiatric service in their hospital, although they would allow the occasional emergency psychiatric admission to medical beds. Section of Psychiatry, Department of Medicine, Saskatoon City Hospital, Saskatoon, Saskatchewan, to Minister of Public Health, Province of Saskatchewan, 5 September 1972, SAB, R-82, 549, 9-4. Smishek Papers: Correspondence-Psych. Services.
37. Ibid.
38. Memorandum, Director, Psychiatric Services Branch, Province of Saskatchewan, to Minister of Public Health, Province of Saskatchewan, 11 September 1972, SAB, R-82, 549, 9-4. Smishek Papers.
39. Ibid.
40. Memorandum, Director, Psychiatric Services Branch, Province of Saskatchewan, to Minister and Deputy Minister of Public Health, Province of Saskatchewan, 24 November 1972, SAB, R-82, 549, 3-15(b). Smishek Papers: Psychiatric Bed Needs, 1972-1975.
41. Memorandum, Director, Psychiatric Services Branch, Province of Saskatchewan, to Associate Deputy Minister of Public Health, Province of Saskatchewan, 26 May 1972, SAB, R-82, 549, 3-15(b). Smishek Papers.
42. "Psychiatrist Slams Mental Health Plans," *Regina Leader-Post*, 2 March 1972.
43. Private Psychiatrist, Saskatoon, Saskatchewan, to Minister of Public Health, Province of Saskatchewan, 18 May 1972, SAB, R-82, 549, 9-4. Smishek Papers.
44. It should be noted that in a 1976 amendment to the Mental Health Act provision was made for the contracting out of psychiatric services to "any hospital or association or corporation whose objectives include the preservation or restoration of health." This appears to clear the way for the creation and

operation of private hospitals or other psychiatric facilities. Previous to this amendment contractors could only operate "in conjunction" with DPH.

45. Memorandum, Director, Psychiatric Services Branch, Province of Saskatchewan, to Minister of Public Health, Province of Saskatchewan, 19 July 1971, SAB, R-82, 549, 9-8. Smishek Papers: Staff, 1970.
46. Tollefson, "The Medicare Dispute," 244.
47. The threat to unilaterally change the medical licensing procedures in part prompted the SCPS to request the establishment of a Minister's Advisory Committee on Medical Licensure. This nine-member committee, chaired by Dr. R.G. Murray, Dean of Medicine, University of Saskatchewan, submitted a report in 1974, wherein fourteen recommendations were made for changing medical licensing procedures. The first recommendation, however, was that "The College of Physicians and Surgeons of Saskatchewan should be maintained as an independent licensing and regulatory body." "Report of the Advisory Committee on Medical Licensure," (Regina: Department of Public Health, 1974), 13.
48. "Care of Chronic Psychotics," *British Medical Journal* (15 May 1971): 351-52.
49. Psychiatrists, Department of Public Health, Prince Albert Psychiatric Centre, Prince Albert, Saskatchewan, to Editor, British Medical Journal, Re: "Care of Chronic Psychotics," *British Medical Journal* (18 September 1971): 703.
50. Private Psychiatrists, Province of Saskatchewan, to Editor, British Medical Journal, Re: "Care of Chronic Psychotics," *British Medical Journal* (20 November 1971): 489.
51. Memorandum, Director, Psychiatric Services Branch, Province of Saskatchewan, to Minister of Public Health, Province of Saskatchewan, 11 January 1972, SAB, R-82, 549, 9-4. Smishek Papers.
52. Director, Psychiatric Services Branch, Province of Saskatchewan, to Minister of Public Health, Province of Saskatchewan, 13 January 1972, SAB, R-82, 549, 9-4. Smishek Papers.
53. Saskatchewan Department of Public Health Annual Reports.
54. Saskatchewan Department of Public Health Annual Report 1976-77, p. 84.
55. Notice, "Saskatchewan Hospital North Battleford, Social Service Department," 18 January 1972, agreed to and signed by an MD

and two MSW social workers, SAB, R-82, 549, 9-14. Smishek Papers.

56. Memorandum, Director, Psychiatric Services Branch, Province of Saskatchewan, to Minister of Public Health, Province of Saskatchewan, 10 February 1972, SAB, R-82, 549, 9-12. Smishek Papers: Mental Health Clinics, 1970-71.
57. Memorandum, Director, Psychiatric Services Branch, Province of Saskatchewan, to Minister of Public Health, Province of Saskatchewan, 26 June 1972, SAB, R-82, 549, 9-14. Smishek Papers.
58. Memorandum, Minister of Public Health, Province of Saskatchewan, to Minister of Industry and Commerce, Province of Saskatchewan, 17 October 1966, SAB, R-45, 339. Grant Papers: Information for Mr. Grant.
59. The relationships between psychiatrists, social workers and community psychiatric nurses in the Weyburn region were not much better. In one anonymous letter forwarded to the premier in late 1971 they were described as having "regressed into a state of confusion and indecision." It was added that "the present state of interdiscipline warfare must be terminated to preserve some sense of balance. A Personnel Director who can take charge of personnel is an immediate necessity to prevent further spreading of inter-discipline jealousies." SAB, R-565, 335a.8. Blakeney Papers: Psychiatric Services, 1971-72.
60. Provincial Councillor, Saskatoon Mayfair NDP, to Minister of Public Health, Province of Saskatchewan, 28 June 1972, SAB, R-82, 549, 9-14. Smishek Papers.
61. Administrative Supervisor, Social Work Department, Saskatchewan Hospital North Battleford, to Director, Psychiatric Services Branch, Province of Saskatchewan, 12 May 1972, SAB, R-82, 549, 9-14. Smishek Papers.
62. Provincial Councillor, Saskatoon Mayfair NDP, to Minister of Public Health, Province of Saskatchewan, 28 June 1972, SAB, R-82, 549, 9-14. Smishek Papers.
63. Memorandum, Executive Director, Saskatchewan Hospital North Battleford, to All Medical Staff and All Social Service Staff, 26 June 1972. SAB, R-82, 549, 9-14. Smishek Papers.
64. Social Worker, Saskatchewan Hospital North Battleford, to Minister of Public Health, Province of Saskatchewan, 15 June 1972, SAB, R-82, 549, 9-14. Smishek Papers.
65. Memorandum, Executive Director, Psychiatric Services Branch, Province of Saskatchewan, to Minister of Public Health,

Province of Saskatchewan, 26 June 1972, SAB, R-82, 549, 9-14. Smishek Papers.

66. Chairman, Psychological Society of Saskatchewan Annual Institute, to Minister of Public Health, Province of Saskatchewan, 2 June 1972, SAB, R-82, 549, 9-4. Smishek Papers.
67. Ibid.
68. Memorandum, Associate Director, Psychiatric Services Branch, Province of Saskatchewan, to Executive Officer to the Minister of Public Health, Province of Saskatchewan, 8 June 1972, SAB, R-82, 549, 9-4. Smishek Papers.
69. Ibid.
70. "Saskatchewan Psychological Association, Summary of SPA Ad Hoc Committee Meetings to Investigate Possible Alterations to the Registered Psychologists Act," n.d., circa December 1971, SAB, R-82, 549, 9-4. Smishek Papers.
71. Social Worker, Saskatchewan Hospital North Battleford, to Minister of Public Health, Province of Saskatchewan, n.d., received Minister's Office 26 June 1972, SAB, R-82, 549, 9-14. Smishek Papers.
72. Memorandum, Executive Officer to the Minister of Public Health, Province of Saskatchewan, to Minister of Public Health, Province of Saskatchewan, 12 July 1972, SAB, R-82, 549, 9-14. Smishek Papers.
73. Ibid.
74. Ibid.
75. Executive Director, Saskatchewan Hospital North Battleford, to Minister of Public Health, Province of Saskatchewan, 18 July 1972, SAB, R-82, 549, 9-14. Smishek Papers.
76. Ibid.
77. Memorandum, Deputy Minister of Public Health, Province of Saskatchewan, to Minister of Public Health, Province of Saskatchewan, 8 August 1972, SAB, R-82, 549, 9-14. Smishek Papers.
78. Memorandum, Minister of Public Health, Province of Saskatchewan, to Premier, Province of Saskatchewan, 8 August 1972, SAB, R-565, 335a.8. Blakeney Papers.
79. Memorandum, Premier, Province of Saskatchewan, to Minister of Public Health, Province of Saskatchewan, 11 August 1972, SAB, R-565, 335a.8. Blakeney Papers.
80. Memorandum, Minister of Public Health, Province of Saskatchewan, to Premier, Province of Saskatchewan, 8 August 1972, SAB, R-565, 335a.8. Blakeney Papers.

81. Memorandum, Executive Director, Saskatchewan Hospital North Battleford, to Director, Psychiatric Services Branch, Province of Saskatchewan, 15 August 1972, SAB, R-82, 549, 9-14. Smishek Papers.
82. Ibid.
83. Memorandum, Director, Psychiatric Services Branch, Province of Saskatchewan, to All Unit Heads, PSB Facilities, 14 August 1972, SAB, R-82, 549, 9-4. Smishek Papers.
84. Memorandum, Director of Social Work, Psychiatric Services Branch, Province of Saskatchewan, to Director, Psychiatric Services Branch, Province of Saskatchewan, 25 August 1972, SAB, R-82, 549, 9-4. Smishek Papers.
85. Memorandum, Director, Psychiatric Services Branch, Province of Saskatchewan, to Minister of Public Health and Executive Assistant, Department of Public Health, Province of Saskatchewan, 28 August 1972, SAB, R-82, 549, 9-4. Smishek Papers.
86. Ibid.
87. News Release, "New Executive Director," n.d., circa October 1972, SAB, R-82, 549, 9-14. Smishek Papers.
88. Gray, "Role Conflicts," 40.
89. Saskatchewan Health Annual Report 1975-76, p. 90.
90. Griffiths, interview.
91. "Report of the Ad Hoc Committee on Psychiatric Team Structure," May 1973, p. 1. Personal Files: Glenn Rutherford.
92. Ibid., p. 15.
93. "A Position Paper by Psychiatrists Employed by the Psychiatric Services Branch on the Ad Hoc Committee Report on Psychiatric Team Structure," submitted to Director, Psychiatric Services Branch, Province of Saskatchewan, by two Psychiatrists, Psychiatric Services Branch, 26 September 1973, p. 1. Personal Files: Glenn Rutherford.
94. Ibid.
95. Ibid.
96. Ibid.
97. Ibid.
98. Ibid.
99. "Proposed Guidelines on Interrelationships Amongst Mental Health Professionals," p. 1. Personal Files: Glenn Rutherford.
100. Ibid., p. 2.
101. Ibid., p. 3.
102. Memorandum, Director of Social Work, Saskatoon Mental Health Clinic, Saskatoon, Saskatchewan, to Director, Psychi-

atric Services Branch, Province of Saskatchewan, 29 August 1973. Personal Files: Glenn Rutherford.

103. Director, Psychiatric Services Branch, Province of Saskatchewan, to Director of Social Work, Saskatoon Mental Health Clinic, Saskatoon, Saskatchewan, 4 September 1973. Personal Files: Glenn Rutherford.
104. Regional Director, Saskatoon Mental Health Clinic, Saskatoon, Saskatchewan, to Chairman, Ad Hoc Committee on Psychiatric Team Structure, 28 March 1983. Personal Files: Glenn Rutherford.
105. Ibid.
106. Memorandum, Director, Munroe Youth Services, Regina, Saskatchewan, to Ad Hoc Committee on Psychiatric Team Structure, 26 March 1973. Personal Files: Glenn Rutherford.
107. Ibid.
108. "Statement Regarding Resignation of Yorkton Psychiatrists," 5 March 1973, SAB, R-565, 335b. Blakeney Papers: Psychiatric Services; 1973.
109. "Inpatient Nursing Reaction to the Report of the Ad Hoc Committee on Team Structure and Psychiatric Services Proposed Guidelines," n.d., circa September 1973, p. 2. Personal Files: Glenn Rutherford.
110. Memorandum, Home Care Department, Munroe Wing and Clinic, Regina, Saskatchewan, to Chairman and Committee Members, Ad Hoc Committee on Psychiatric Team Structure, n.d., circa March 1973, p. 10. Personal Files: Glenn Rutherford.
111. "Inpatient Nursing Reaction to the Report of the Ad Hoc Committee on Team Structure and Psychiatric Services Proposed Guidelines," n.d., circa September, 1973, p. 2. Personal Files: Glenn Rutherford.
112. Dr. C.F. Lipscomb, "An Organization for Psychiatric Services," January 1973, p. 1. Personal Files: Glenn Rutherford.
113. "Taking a Look at Team Structure," submitted by Community Psychiatric Nurses, Weyburn Psychiatric Center, to Ad Hoc Committee on Psychiatric Team Structure, n.d., circa February 1973, pp. 3-4. Personal Files: Glenn Rutherford.
114. Memorandum, Home Care Department, Munroe Wing and Clinic, Regina, to Chairman and Committee Members, Ad Hoc Committee on Psychiatric Team Structure, n.d., circa March 1973, p. 11. Personal Files: Glenn Rutherford.
115. Ibid.

116. Alan McKinnon, "Role Conflict in Saskatchewan Psychiatric Services," *The Saskatchewan Psychologist* 73 (November 1973): 26.
117. President, Psychological Society of Saskatchewan, to Federal Minister of Health and Welfare, Ottawa, 14 December 1982. Reprinted in *The Saskatchewan Psychologist* 83 (February 1983): 58.
118. Ibid., 59.
119. Ibid.
120. Ibid.
121. For an interesting discussion of the development and organization of psychiatry for profit in the United States see Theodore L. Gessner and Delores S. Morrisseau, "Under the Golden Psi: The Franchising of Mental Health," *Psychiatry* 43 (1980).
122. The privatization of medical care is already underway in Canada, primarily in the province of Ontario. For a brief discussion of this see "Private Health Care Creeps into Canada," *Commonwealth* 43 (9 March 1983): 7.
123. Moshe H. Spero, "Thoughts on Computerized Psychotherapy," *Psychiatry* 41 (1978): 280. Also see M. Fink, "Computers and Psychiatry," in A. Freedman and H. Kaplan, eds., *Comprehensive Textbook of Psychiatry* (Baltimore: Williams and Wilkins, 1967), 232-37; B. Glueck and C. Stroebel, "Computers and Clinical Psychiatry," in A. Freedman, H. Kaplan and B. Sadock, eds., *Comprehensive Textbook of Psychiatry*, 2d ed. (Baltimore: Williams and Wilkins, 1975), 413-27; M. Klein, et.al., "Computers and Psychiatry," *Archives of General Psychiatry* 32 (1975): 837-46; H. Rome et al., "Symposium in Automatic Techniques in Personality Assessment," *Mayo Clinical Proceedings* 37 (1962): 61-79; R. Spitzer and J. Endicott, "DIAGNO: A Computer Program for Psychiatric Diagnosis Utilizing Differential Diagnostic Procedure," *Archives of General Psychiatry* 18 (1968): 746-56; R. Spitzer and J. Endicott, "Computer Applications in Psychiatry," in S. Arieti, ed., *American Handbook of Psychiatry*, 2d ed. (New York: Basic Books, 1975); J. Weizenbaum, "ELIZA — A Computer Program for the Study of Natural Language Between Man and Machine," *Communication Association of Computing Machines* 9 (1966): 36-45; K. Colby et al., "A Computer Method of Psychotherapy: Preliminary Communication," *Journal of Nervous and Mental Disease* 142 (1966): 148-52.

124. Ibid.
125. Interview with Tim Greenough, Director, Psychological Services, North Battleford Psychiatric Centre, North Battleford, Saskatchewan, 2 March 1983 (hereafter cited as Greenough, interview).
126. Saskatchewan Department of Public Health Annual Report 1964-65, p. 92.
127. Greenough, interview.
128. "Report of the Thrust Working Party: Community Based Alternatives for Mental Health Care" (Regina: Policy Research and Management Services Branch, Saskatchewan Health, August 1980), 26. The Thrust Committee was a central planning committee of the Saskatchewan Department of Health. The goal of the committee was "to develop a health programming strategy for the 1980s." Although recommendations of the committee do not constitute government policy, they do indicate the dominant line of thought.
129. Ibid.

## Chapter Seven

1. Michel Foucault, *Madness and Civilization: A History of Insanity in the Age of Reason* (New York: Vintage Books, 1973).
2. Scull, *Museums of Madness.*

## Appendix

1. Karl Marx, *Capital, A Critique of Political Economy Volume 1* (Harmondsworth, Middlesex: Penguin Books Ltd., 1976), 1045.
2. Quoted in Harry Braverman, *Labour and Monopoly Capital: The Degradation of Work in the Twentieth Century* (New York: Monthly Review Press, 1974), 79-80.
3. Ibid., 83.
4. Vincente Navarro, "The Labor Process and Health: A Historical Materialist Interpretation," *International Journal of Health Services* 12 (1982): 23.
5. Marx, *Capital, Volume 1*, p. 284; Ali Rattansi, *Marx and the Division of Labour* (London: Macillan, 1982), 126; Christian Palloix, "The Labour Process: From Fordism to Neo-Fordism," in *CSE Pamphlet No. 1* (London: CSE Books, 1976), 46; Storey, *Managerial Prerogative.*

6. George E. Crane, "Clinical Psychopharmacology in its 20th Year: Late, Unanticipated Effects of Neuroleptics May Limit Their Use in Psychiatry," *Science* 181 (13 July 1973): 125; also see Scull, *Decarceration*, especially footnote 28, pp. 90-91; and Ernst Baumler, *In Search of the Magic Bullet: Great Adventures in Modern Drug Research* (London: Thames and Hudson, 1965).
7. Andrew Scull, "Mad-doctors and Magistrates: English Psychiatry's Struggle for Professional Autonomy in the Nineteenth Century," *Archives of European Sociology* 17 (1976): 279-305.
8. Gelvin Stevenson, "Social Relations of Production and Consumption in the Human Service Occupations," *Monthly Review* 28 (July-August 1973): 78.
9. Karl Marx, *Grundrisse: Foundations of the Critique of Political Economy* (New York: Vintage Books, a division of Random House, Inc., 1973), 94.
10. Ibid.
11. Ibid., p. 92.
12. Eliot Freidson, *Professional Dominance: The Social Structure of Medical Care* (New York: Atherton Press, 1970), 156.
13. Batya Weinbaum and Amy Bridges, "The Other Side of the Paycheck: Monopoly Capital and the Structure of Consumption," *Monthly Review* 28 (July-August 1976): 94.
14. Jones, *Social Psychiatry in Practice.*
15. David Robinson and Yvonne Robinson, *A Guide to Self-Help Groups, From Self-Help to Health* (London: Concord Books, 1979); Donald M. Vickery et al., *Take Care of Yourself* (London: George Allen and Unwin, 1979), especially Chapter 22.
16. See Gerald A. Cohen, "On Some Criticisms of Historical Materialism," *Supplementary Proceedings of the Aristotlean Society* 44 (1970): 121-41; and Russel Keat and John Urry, *Social Theory as Science* (London: Routledge and Kegan Paul, 1982), 101.
17. For example see Eric Olin Wright, "Class Boundaries in Advanced Capitalist Societies," *New Left Review* 98 (1976): 3-43; Eric Olin Wright, *Class, Crisis and the State* (London: NLB, 1978); Guglielmo Carchedi, *On the Economic Identification of Classes* (London: RKP, 1977).
18. Freidson, "The Futures of Professionalisation," 22.
19. Ibid.
20. Robert Blauner, *Alienation and Freedom: The Factory Worker and His Industry* (Chicago: The University of Chicago Press, 1964), 19, see also footnote 19.

21. For example see P. Doeringer and M. Piore, *Internal Labor Markets and Manpower Analysis* (Lexington, Mass.: Lexington Books, 1971); Richard C. Edwards, "The Social Relations of Production in the Firm and Labor Market Structure," in Richard C. Edwards, Michael Reich and David M. Gordon, eds., *Labor Market Segmentation* (Lexington, Mass.: D.C. Heath, 1973), 3-26.
22. Edwards, "Social Relations of Production," 5.
23. Doeringer and Piore, *Internal Labor Markets*, 2.
24. Ibid., 6.
25. For a discussion of this relationship see Craig R. Littler, *The Development of the Labour Process in Capitalist Societies: A Comparative Study of the Transformation of Work Organization in Britain, Japan and the USA* (London: Heineman Educational Books, 1982), 15-17; also see Peter Burke, *Sociology and History* (London: George Allen and Unwin, 1980), 70-72, for an interesting discussion of the concept of bureaucracy and its use in historical analyses.
26. See for example A. Friedman, "Responsible Autonomy versus Direct Control over the Labor Process," *Capital and Class* 1 (1977): 43-57; and Edwards, *Contested Terrain.*
27. Stephen Wood and John Kelly, "Taylorism, Responsible Autonomy and Management Strategy," in Stephen Wood, ed., *The Degradation of Work? Skill, De-skilling and the Labour Process* (London: Hutchinson, 1983), 89.
28. Urry, *The Anatomy of Capitalist Societies.*
29. Craig R. Littler and Graeme Salaman, "Bravermania and Beyond: Recent Theories of the Labour Process," *Sociology* 16 (1982): 251-69.
30. In fiscal year 1973-74 the Department of Public Health became Saskatchewan Health. For simplicity's sake, I have referred to it as DPH throughout.
31. Franklyn N. Arnhoff et al., "The Mental Health Fields: An Overview of Manpower Growth and Development," in Franklyn N. Arnhoff, Eli A. Rubinstein and Joseph C. Speisman, eds., *Manpower for Mental Health* (Chicago: Aldine Publishing Co., 1969), 1.
32. Nigel Goldie, "The Division of Labour Among the Mental Health Professionals — a Negotiated or an Imposed Order?," in Margaret Stacey et al., eds., *Health and the Division of Labour* (London: Croom Helm, 1977), 141-64.
33. Marx, *Capital, Volume 1*, 554.

34. For an interesting discussion of the factory as part of the means of production see Stephen Marglin, "The Origins and Functions of Hierarchy in Capitalist Production," in Theo Nichols, ed., *Capital and Labour: A Marxist Primer* (Glasgow: Fontana Paperbacks, 1980), 237-54.
35. Marx to Annenkov, P.V., Brussels, 28 December 1846, in *Karl Marx and Friedrich Engels, Correspondence 1846-1895: A Selection with Commentary and Notes* (London: Martin Lawrence Ltd., 1934), 8.
36. Marx, *Capital, Volume 1*, 441.
37. David J. Rothman, *The Discovery of the Asylum.*
38. Ibid.
39. Scull, *Museums of Madness*, 41-43.
40. Quoted in Andy Treacher and Geoff Baruch, "Towards a Critical History of the Psychiatric Profession," in David Ingleby, ed., *Critical Psychiatry: The Politics of Mental Health* (Harmondsworth: Penguin Books, 1981), 130.
41. Ibid., 131.
42. Scull, "Mad-doctors and Magistrates," quoted in Treacher and Baruch, "Towards a Critical History of the Psychiatric Profession," 130; see also Scull, *Museums of Madness.*
43. Treacher and Baruch, "Towards a Critical History of the Psychiatric Profession," 131.
44. Clark, "Therapeutic Effects of Drugs," 283.
45. Baumler, *In Search of the Magic Bullet*, 155.
46. Crane "Clinical Psychopharmacology in Its 20th Year," 126.
47. Susser, *Community Psychiatry*, 4.
48. Baumler, *In Search of the Magic Bullet*, 154.
49. "One of Eight: Mental Illness in Canada," Statistics Canada, 1981.
50. This probably finds its clearest expression in Karl Marx, *Capital, A Critique of Political Economy Volume III* (Moscow: Progress Publishers, 1959), 814-15.
51. Marx, *Capital, Volume 1*, 763-64.
52. Ibid., 1041-42.
53. See for example Gucharan Basran, "The Rural De-population of the Prairies," in John Allan Fry, ed., *Economy, Class and Social Reality* (Toronto: Butterworths, 1979), 391-410; Theodore P. Lianos, "Concentration and Centralization of Capital in Agriculture," *Studies in Political Economy: A Socialist Review* 14 (Summer 1984): 99-116.

54. Probably the best known conjunctural analysis done by Marx is *The Eighteenth Brumaire of Louis Bonaparte*, vol. 1 of *Karl Marx and Frederick Engels, Selected Works in Two Volumes* (Moscow: Foreign Languages Press, 1962), 247-344.
55. Keat and Urry, *Social Theory as Science*, 31.

# Selected Bibliography


## 1. Archival Materials — Restricted

Saskatchewan Archives Board

Bentley Papers; Blakeney Papers; Davies Papers; Erb Papers; Grant Papers; Smishek Papers; Steuart Papers.

## 2. Archival Materials — Unrestricted

Saskatchewan Archives Board

Douglas Papers; Dunning Papers; Martin Papers; Uhrich Papers.

Department of Public Health: Correspondence, A-X. Saskatchewan Archives Board (hereafter SAB), PH.3, A13.

MacNeill, J.W. "Why Was I Admitted to a Saskatchewan Hospital: Questions and Answers." n.d.

Public Service Commission: Mental Hospitals, Perquisites. SAB, P5, A17.

________: Information Regarding Operation of Civil Service Act, 1913- 1928. PS, G61.

Public Works Department: Saskatchewan Provincial Hospital, North Battleford; Cottages 1919-1944. SAB, G132.

________: Deputy Minister's Personal File, North Battleford Mental Hospital, 1910-1935. SAB, PW, 195-2, 132.P.

Saskatchewan. Haultain Royal Commission. SAB, R-195.4, Box 6.

Saskatchewan. Health Services Survey Commission (Sigerist): Dr. Sigerist and Members of the Commission. SAB, Collection 251, RC[M13], 12.

## 3. Published Material

Alexander, F.G., and Seleznick, S.T. *The History of Psychiatry: An Evaluation of Psychiatric Thought and Practice from Pre-*

*Historic Times to the Present.* New York: Harper and Row, 1966.

Allderidge, P. "Hospitals, Madhouses and Asylums: Cycles in the Care of the Insane." *British Journal of Psychiatry* 134(1979): 321-34.

Arnhoff, Franklyn N.; Rubinstein, E.A.; Shriver, B.M.; and Jones D.R. "The Mental Health Fields: An Overview of Manpower Growth and Development." In *Manpower for Mental Health,* edited by Franklyn N. Arnhoff, Eli A. Rubinstein and Joseph C. Speisman, 1-37. Chicago: Aldine Publishing Co., 1969.

Badgley, Robin F., and Wolfe, Samuel. *Doctors' Strike: Medical Care and Conflict in Saskatchewan.* Toronto: Macmillan, 1967.

Basran, Gucharan. "The Rural De-population of the Prairies." In *Economy, Class and Social Reality,* edited by John A. Fry, 391-410. Toronto: Butterworths, 1979.

Bateson, Gregory. *Steps Toward an Ecology of Mind.* London: Granada Publishing, 1973.

Bateson, Gregory; Jackson, Donald; Haley, Jay; and Weakland, J. "Toward a Theory of Schizophrenia." *Behavioral Science* 1 (1956): 251-64.

Baumler, Ernst. *In Search of the Magic Bullet: Great Adventures in Modern Drug Research.* London: Thames and Hudson, 1965.

Belknap, Ivan. *Human Problems of a State Mental Hospital.* New York: McGraw-Hill, 1956.

Bercuson, David Jay. *Confrontation at Winnipeg: Labour, Industrial Relations and the General Strike.* Montreal: McGill-Queen's University Press, 1974.

Bickford, J.A.R. "Economic Value of the Psychiatric Inpatient." *The Lancet* 1 (30 March 1963): 714-15.

Blauner, Robert. *Alienation and Freedom: The Factory Worker and His Industry.* Chicago: The University of Chicago Press, 1964.

Bolaria, B. Singh. "Self-Care and Lifestyles: Ideological and Policy Implications." In *Economy, Class and Social Reality,* edited by John A. Fry, 350-64. Toronto: Butterworths, 1979.

Braverman, Harry. *Labour and Monopoly Capital: The Degradation of Work in the Twentieth Century.* New York: Monthly Review Press, 1974.

Brenner, Meyer Harvey. *Mental Illness and the Economy.* Cambridge, Mass.: Harvard University Press, 1973.

*British Medical Journal* (15 May 1971): 351-52; (18 September 1971): 703; (20 November 1971): 489.

Bucher, Rue, and Stelling, Joan. "Characteristics of Professional Organizations." *Journal of Health and Social Behavior* 10 (1969): 3-15.

Burke, Peter. *Sociology and History.* London: George Allen and Unwin, 1980.

Canadian Mental Health Association. *This is Your Mental Health Association.* Regina: CMHA, 1975.

Carchedi, Guglielmo. *On the Economic Identification of Classes.* London: Routledge and Kegan Paul, 1977.

Clark, L.D. "Evaluation of the Therapeutic Effects of Drugs in Patients." *Diseases of the Nervous System* 17 (1956): 282-86.

Clausen, John A. *Sociology and the Field of Mental Health.* New York: Russel Sage Foundation, 1956.

Clevenger, S.V. "Treatment of the Insane." *Journal of the American Medical Association* 27 (October 1896): 894-901.

Cohen, Gerald A. "On Some Criticisms of Historical Materialism." *Supplementary Proceedings of the Aristotlean Society* 44 (1970): 121-41.

Cohen, Stanley. *Folk Devils and Moral Panics.* New York: St. Martin's Press, 1972.

Colby, K.; Watt, J.; and Gilbert, J. "A Computer Method of Psychotherapy: Preliminary Communication." *Journal of Nervous and Mental Disease* 142 (1966): 148-52.

"The Community Health Centre in Canada: Report of the Community Health Centre Project to the Conference of Health Ministers." 21 July 1972, Foreword, v.

Conrad, Peter, and Schneider, Joseph W. *Deviance and Medicalization: From Badness to Sickness.* St. Louis: The Mosby Company, 1980. © 1985 Merrill Pub. Co., Columbus, OH.

Crane, George E. "Clinical Psychopharmacology in its 20th year: Late, Unanticipated Effects of Neuroleptics May Limit Their Use in Psychiatry." *Science* 181 (13 July 1973): 124-28. © 1973 by the AAAS.

Cumming, Elaine, and Cumming, John. *Closed Ranks: An Experiment in Mental Health Education.* Cambridge: Harvard University Press, 1957.

D'Arcy, Carl; Schmitz, Janet A; and Bold, Guin. "Patterns in the Delivery of Psychiatric Care in Saskatchewan 1969-1974: Service Interface Study (SIS) Final Report." Regina: Psychiatric Services Branch, Department of Health, Province of Saskatchewan, 1979.

Demay, Maurice. "The Beginnings of Psychiatry in Saskatchewan." *Canada's Mental Health* 21 (January-February 1973): 18-24.

Dickinson, Harley D., and Andre, Glenn. "Community Psychiatry: The Institutional Transformation of Psychiatric Work." In *Sociology of Health Care in Canada*, edited by B. Singh Bolaria and Harley D. Dickinson, 295-308. Toronto: HBJ-Holt, 1988.

Doeringer, P., and Piore, M. *Internal Labour Markets and Manpower Analysis*. Lexington, Mass.: Lexington Books, 1971.

Dunham, H. Warren. *Sociological Theory and Mental Disorder*. Detroit: Wayne State University Press, 1959.

Dunham, H. Warren, and Weinberg, S.K. *The Culture of the State Mental Hospital*. Detroit: Wayne State University Press, 1960.

Eaton, Joseph W., and Weil, Robert J. *Culture and Mental Disorders*. New York: The Free Press, 1955.

Edwards, Richard C. "The Social Relations of Production in the Firm and Labor Market Structure." In *Labor Market Segmentation*, edited by Richard Edwards, Michael Reich and David M. Gordon, 3-26. Lexington, Mass.: D.C. Heath, 1973.

________. *Contested Terrain: The Transformation of the Workplace in the Twentieth Century*. New York: Basic Books, 1979.

Elliot, Philip. *The Sociology of the Professions*. London: Macmillan, 1972.

Faris, Robert L., and Dunham, H. Warren. *Mental Disorders in Urban Areas*. Chicago: University of Chicago Press, 1939.

Fink, M. "Computers and Psychiatry." In *Comprehensive Textbook of Psychiatry*, edited by A. Freedman, H. Kaplan, and B. Sadock, 232-37. Baltimore: Williams and Wilkins, 1967.

Fosdick, Raymond B. *The Story of the Rockefeller Foundation*. New York: Harper and Row, Publishers Inc., 1952.

Foucault, Michel. *Madness and Civilization: A History of Insanity in the Age of Reason*. New York: Vintage Books, 1973.

Frazier, Shervert H., and Pokorny, Alex D. "Report of a Consultation to the Minister of Public Health on the Psychiatric Services of Saskatchewan." Circa January 1968.

Freidson, Eliot. *Profession of Medicine*. New York: Dodd, Mead and Co., 1970.

________. *Professional Dominance: The Social Structure of Medical Care*. New York: Atherton Press, 1970.

________. "The Futures of Professionalisation." In *Health and the Division of Labour*, edited by Margaret Stacey, Margaret Reid, Christian Heath and Robert Dingwall, 14-38. London: Croom Helm, 1977.

Freud, Sigmund. "Psychoanalysis and Psychiatry." In *Introductory Lectures on Psychoanalysis*, edited by James Strachey and Angela Richards, translated by James Strachey, 281-95. Harmondsworth: Penguin Books, 1973.

Friedman, A. "Responsible Autonomy versus Direct Control over the Labor Process." *Capital and Class* 1 (1977): 43-57.

Fritz, Wayne B. "A Critical Assessment of Proposals for a Compulsory Mental Health Care Act." Applied Research Unit, Psychiatric Research Division, Saskatoon, Saskatchewan, 1982.

Gessner, Theodore L., and Morrisseau, Delores S. "Under the Golden Psi: The Franchising of Mental Health." *Psychiatry* 43 (1980): 294-302.

Glueck, B., and Stroebel, C. "Computers and Clinical Psychiatry." In *Comprehensive Textbook of Psychiatry*. 2d ed., vol. I, edited by A. Freedman, H. Kaplan and B. Sadock, 413-27. Baltimore: Williams and Wilkins, 1975.

Goffman, Erving. *Asylums: Essays on the Social Situation of Mental Patients and Other Inmates*. New York: Doubleday and Company, 1961.

Goldhamer, Herbert, and Marshall, Andrew. *Psychosis and Civilization*. New York: The Free Press, 1953.

Goldie, Nigel. "The Division of Labour Among the Mental Health Professionals — a Negotiated or an Imposed Order?" In *Health and the Division of Labour*, edited by Margaret Stacey, Margaret Reid, Christian Heath and Robert Dingwall, 141-64. London: Croom Helm, 1977.

Gough, Ian. "State Expenditures in Advanced Capitalism." *New Left Review* 92 (July-August 1975): 53-92.

Gray, John E. "Role Conflicts Within a Provincial Community Mental Health Program." *The Saskatchewan Psychologist* 72 (November 1972): 41.

Gruending, Dennis. *The First Ten Years*. Saskatoon: Community Clinic, 1974.

Guest, Dennis. *The Emergence of Social Security in Canada*. Vancouver: University of British Columbia Press, 1980.

Habenstein, Robert W. "Critique of 'Profession' as a Sociological Category." *The Sociological Quarterly* 4 (Autumn 1963): 291-300.

Haley, Jay. "The Family of the Schizophrenic: A Model System." *Journal of Nervous and Mental Disease* 129 (1959): 357-74.

Hampden-Turner, Charles. "The Factory as an Oppressive and Non-Emancipatory Environment." In *Workers' Control: A Reader on*

*Labor and Social Change*, edited by G. Hunnius, G.D. Garson and John Case, 30-45. New York: Vintage Books, 1973.

Haug, Marie R. "Deprofessionalization: An Alternate Hypothesis for the Future." In *Professionalization and Social Change*, edited by Paul Halmos, 195-212. Keele, Staffordshire: The University of Keele, 1973.

Hincks, Clarence M. *Mental Hygiene Survey of Saskatchewan.* Regina: King's Printer, 1945.

Hollingshead, August B., and Redlich, Frederick C. *Social Class and Mental Illness.* New York: John Wiley, 1958.

Hunter, R., and McAlpine, I.M. *Three Hundred Years of Psychiatry, 1535-1860.* New York: Oxford University Press, 1963.

Hurd, Henry M. *The Institutional Care of the Insane in the United States and Canada.* 4 vols. New York: Arno Press, 1973.

Jaco, E. Gartley. "Social Factors in Mental Disorders in Texas," *Social Problems* 4 (April 1957): 322-28.

Jamous, H., and Peloille, B. "Professions or Self-Perpetuating Systems? Changes in the French University-Hospital System." In *Professions and Professionalization*, edited by J.A. Jackson, 111-52. Cambridge: Cambridge University Press, 1970.

Jones, Kathleen. *A History of the Mental Health Service.* London: Routledge and Kegan Paul, 1972.

Jones, Maxwell Shaw. *Social Psychiatry in Practice: The Idea of the Therapeutic Community.* Harmondsworth: Penguin Books, 1968.

Kahan, Fanny H. *Brains and Bricks: The History of the Yorkton Psychiatric Centre.* Regina: White Cross Publications, 1965.

________. *A Different Drummer: The History of the Saskatchewan Psychiatric Nurses Association, 1948-1973.* Regina: SPNA Pamphlet, 1973.

Kahn, Alfred J. "Planning and Practice Perspectives on the Boundaries of Community Psychiatry." In *Community Psychiatry*, edited by Leigh M. Roberts, Seymour L. Halleck and Martin B. Loeb, 165-82. Madison: University of Wisconsin Press, 1966.

Keat, Russel and Urry, John. *Social Theory as Science.* 2d ed. London: Routledge and Kegan Paul, 1982.

Kittrie, N. *The Right to be Different.* Baltimore: Johns Hopkins University Press, 1971.

Klein, M.; Greist, J.; and Van Cura, J. "Computers and Psychiatry." *Archives of General Psychiatry* 32 (1975): 837-46.

Kornhauser, A. *Mental Health of the Industrial Worker.* New York: John Wiley and Sons, 1965.

Laing, Ronald D. *The Politics of the Family and Other Essays.* Harmondsworth: Penguin Books, 1976.

Laing, Ronald D., and Esterson, A. *Sanity, Madness and the Family.* Vol. 2, *Families of Schizophrenics.* London: Tavistock Publications Ltd., 1964.

Lalonde, Marc. *A New Perspective on the Health of Canadians.* Ottawa: Information Canada, 1974.

Langsley, Donald G. "Community Mental Health: A Review of the Literature." In *An Assessment of the Community Mental Health Movement,* edited by W.E. Barton and C.J. Sanborn, 35-64. Lexington, Mass.: Lexington Books, 1977.

Larson, M.S. *The Rise of Professionalism: A Sociological Analysis.* Berkeley: University of California Press, 1977.

Lawson, F.S. "Mental Hospitals: Their Size and Function." *Canadian Journal of Public Health* 49 (May 1958): 186-95.

Lennard, Henry L., and Bernstein, Arnold. *The Anatomy of Psychotherapy.* New York: Columbia University Press, 1960.

Lianos, Theodore P. "Concentration and Centralization of Capital in Agriculture." *Studies in Political Economy: A Socialist Review.* 14 (Summer 1984): 99-116.

Lidz, Theodore. *The Origin and the Treatment of Schizophrenic Disorders.* London: Hutchinson and Co. Ltd., 1975.

Lipset, Seymour Martin. *Agrarian Socialism.* Berkeley: University of California Press, 1974.

Littler, Craig R. *The Development of the Labour Process in Capitalist Societies: A Comparative Study of the Transformation of Work Organization in Britain, Japan and the USA.* London: Heineman Educational Books, 1982

________. "De-Skilling and Changing Structures of Control." In *The Degradation of Work? Skill, De-Skilling and the Labour Process,* edited by Stephen Wood, 122-45. London: Hutchinson, 1983.

Littler, Craig R., and Salaman, Graeme. "Bravermania and Beyond: Recent Theories of the Labour Process." *Sociology* 16 (1982): 251-69.

Maclay, W.S. "Experiments in Mental Hospital Organization." *The Canadian Medical Association Journal* 78 (15 June 1958): 909-16.

MacNeil, J.W. *Rules and Regulations for Hospital Employees.* Regina: King's Printer, 1943.

Makahonuk, G. "Labour in the Prairie City: The Saskatoon Working Class Experience and Response to Capitalism, 1906-1919." In *The Politics of Work in the West: Historical and Contemporary*

*Perspectives*, edited by Harley D. Dickinson and Bob Russell, 5-69. Saskatoon: Social Research Unit, Dept. of Sociology, University of Saskatchewan, 1985.

Mann, Michael. *Consciousness and Action Among the Western Working Class.* London and Atlantic Highlands, New Jersey: Macmillan and Humanities Press International, Inc., 1973.

Marglin, Stephen. "The Origins and Functions of Hierarchy in Capitalist Production." In *Capital and Labour: A Marxist Primer*, edited by Theo Nichols, 237-54. Glasgow: Fontana Paperbacks, 1980.

Marx to Annenkov, P.V., Brussels, 28 December 1846. In *Karl Marx and Friedrich Engels, Correspondence 1846-1895: A Selection with Commentary and Notes*, pp. 5-18. London: Martin Lawrence Ltd., 1934.

Marx, Karl. "The Eighteenth Brumaire of Louis Bonaparte." In *Karl Marx and Frederick Engels, Selected Works in Two Volumes.* Vol. 1. Moscow: Foreign Languages Press, 1962.

________. *Capital, A Critique of Political Economy Volume III.* Moscow: Progress Publishers, 1959.

________. *Capital, A Critique of Political Economy Volume I.* Harmondsworth: Penguin Books Ltd., 1976.

________. *Grundrisse: Foundations of the Critique of Political Economy*, translated with a Foreword by Martin Nicolaus. New York: Vintage Books, a division of Random House, Inc., 1973.

Masters, Donald Campbell. *The Winnipeg General Strike.* Toronto: University of Toronto Press, 1950.

Matthews, Roger. "'Decarceration' and the Fiscal Crisis." In *Capitalism and the Rule of Law*, edited by Bob Fine, Richard Kinsey, John Lea, Sol Picciotto and Jock Young, 100-117. London: Hutchinson and Co., 1979.

McCorkell, W.J., and McKerracher, D.G. "The Family Doctor and the Psychiatric Ward." *Mental Hospitals* 11 (1962): 300-302.

McKerracher, D.G. *Trends in Psychiatric Care.* Report of the Royal Commission on Health Services in Canada, 1964. Ottawa: Queen's Printer, 1966.

________. "Research at Saskatchewan." In *Community Mental Health: An International Perspective*, edited by Richard H. Williams and Lucy D. Ozarin, 370-81. San Francisco: Jossey-Bass, 1968.

McKerracher, D.G.; Smith, C.M.; Coburn, F.E.; and McDonald, I.M. "General Practice Psychiatry — An Account of Two Canadian Experiments." *Lancet* 2 (1965): 1005-1007.

McKinnon, Alan. "Role Conflict in Saskatchewan Psychiatric Services." *The Saskatchewan Psychologist* 73 (November 1973): 25-30.

McMillan, J.D. "Community Mental Hospital." *The Canadian Hospital* (May 1957): 40-46.

Menninger, William C. "Lessons from Military Psychiatry for Civilian Psychiatry." Reprinted in *Wartime Psychiatry: A Compendium of the International Literature*, edited by Nolan D.C. Lewis and Bernice Engle. New York: Oxford University Press, 1954.

Mussallem, Helen K. *Nursing Education in Canada.* Report of the Royal Commission on Health Services in Canada, 1964. Ottawa: Queen's Printer, 1966.

Musto, David F. "The Community Mental Health Center Movement in Historical Perspective." In *An Assessment of the Community Mental Health Movement*, edited by W.E. Barton and C.J. Sanborn, 1-11. Lexington, Mass.: Lexington Books, 1977.

Myers, J., and Roberts, B. *Family and Class Dynamics in Mental Illness.* New York: John Wiley, 1959.

Navarro, Vincente. "The Labour Process and Health: A Historical Materialist Interpretation." *International Journal of Health Services* 12 (1982): 15-29.

"New Mental Health Act for Saskatchewan." *Canada's Mental Health* 9 (1961): 4-6.

Oppenheimer, Martin. "The Proletarianization of the Profession." In *Professionalization and Social Change*, edited by Paul Halmos, 213-28. Keele, Staffordshire: The University of Keele, 1973.

Palloix, Christian. "The Labour Process: From Fordism to Neo-Fordism." In *CSE Pamphlet No. 1*, 46-47. London: CSE Books, 1976.

Parry, Noel, and Parry, José. "Social Closure and Collective Social Mobility." In *Industrial Society: Class, Cleavage and Control*, edited by Richard Scase, 111-21. London: George Allen and Unwin, 1977.

Parry-Jones, W.L. *The Trade in Lunacy.* London: Routledge and Kegan Paul, 1972.

"Private Health Care Creeps into Canada." *Commonwealth* 43, no. 9 (March 1983): 7.

Ralph, Diana. "Work and Madness: The Labour Theory of Community Psychiatry." Ph.D. diss., University of Regina, 1980.

________. *Work and Madness: The Rise of Community Psychiatry.* Montreal: Black Rose Books, 1983.

Rattansi, Ali. *Marx and the Division of Labour.* London: Macmillan, 1982.

Ray, Laurence J. "Priests of the Body." Ph.D. diss., University of Sussex, 1981.

________. "Models of Madness in Victorian Asylum Practice." *Archives of European Sociology* 22 (1981): 229-64.

*Regina Leader-Post.* "Psychiatrist Slams Mental Health Plans," 2 March 1972.

"Report of the Ad Hoc Committee on Nursing Education, Province of Saskatchewan." Regina: Queen's Printer, 1966.

"Report of the Advisory Committee on Medical Licensure." Regina: Department of Public Health, 1974.

"Report of the Thrust Working Party: Community Based Alternatives for Mental Health Care." Regina: Policy Research and Management Services Branch, Saskatchewan Health, August 1980.

"A Return to the Dark Ages." *The Dome: Official Publication of the Saskatchewan Government Employees Association* 43 (1969): 94.

Richards, John, and Pratt, Larry. *Prairie Capitalism: Power and Influence in the New West.* Toronto: McClelland and Stewart, 1979.

Robertson, Alex. "Sociology and the Study of Psychiatric Disorder." *The Sociological Review* 17 (1969): 377-97.

Robinson, David, and Robinson Yvonne. *A Guide to Self-Help Groups, From Self-Help to Health.* London: Concord Books, 1979.

Rome, H.; Swenson, W.; Mataya P.; McCarthy, C.; Pearson J.; Keating, F.; and Hathaway, S. "Symposium in Automatic Techniques in Personality Assessment." *Mayo Clinic Proceedings* 37 (1962): 61-79.

Rose, Arnold M., ed. *Mental Health and Mental Disorder.* New York: W.W. Norton, 1957.

Rosen, George. *Madness in Society: Chapters in the Historical Sociology of Mental Illness.* Chicago: University of Chicago Press, 1968.

Rothman, David J. *The Discovery of the Asylum: Social Order and Disorder in the New Republic.* Boston: Little, Brown and Company, 1971.

Saskatchewan Department of Public Health. Annual Reports 1914-1981.

"Saskatchewan Department of Public Health: Outline of Services." Regina: Division of Health Education, n.d.

Saskatchewan Department of Public Works. Annual Report 1921-22.

Saskatchewan Economic Review, 1982.

Saskatchewan Health. Annual Reports 1963-1981.

Saskatchewan Hospital Services Plan. Annual Reports 1944-1981.

Saskatchewan Medical Care Insurance Commission. Annual Reports 1963-1981.

*Saskatchewan Psychiatric Nurse Newsletter* 2 (March 1964): 2.

*The Saskatchewan Psychologist* 83 (February 1983): 58. Letter, President, Psychological Society of Saskatchewan, to Federal Minister of Health and Welfare, Ottawa, 14 December 1982.

Saskatchewan Public Accounts Committee. Annual Reports 1944-1981.

Saskatchewan. Royal Commission on Government Administration. Regina: Queen's Printer, 1965.

*Saskatoon Star-Phoenix.* "Psychiatric Wards Rapped," 21 January 1958.

Scarrow, Howard A. "The Civil Service Commissions in the Canadian Provinces." *Journal of Politics* 19 (1957).

________. "Employer-Employee Relationships in the Civil Services of the Canadian Provinces." *Public Administration* (Spring 1957).

Schatzman, Leonard, and Bucher, Rue. "Negotiating a Division of Labor Among Professionals in the State Mental Hospital." *Psychiatry* 27 (1964): 266-77.

Schatzman, Leonard, and Strauss, Anselm. "A Sociology of Psychiatry: A Perspective and Some Organizing Foci." In *Medical Men and Their Work*, edited by Eliot Freidson and Judith Lorber, 128-44. Chicago and New York: Aldine Atherton, 1972.

Scull, Andrew. "Mad-doctors and Magistrates: English Psychiatry's Struggle for Professional Autonomy in the Nineteenth Century." *Archives of European Sociology* 17 (1976): 279-305.

________. *Decarceration, Community Treatment and the Deviant*. Englewood Cliffs, N.J.: Prentice Hall, 1977.

________. *Museums of Madness: The Social Organization of Insanity in Nineteenth-Century England.* London: Allen Lane, Penguin Books, 1979.

________. "Community Care of the Mentally Ill: Current Realities in the Context of Past Developments." In *Contemporary Health Services: Social Science Perspectives*, edited by A. Johnson,

O. Grusky and B. Raven, 237-49. Boston, Mass.: Auburn House, 1982.

________. "Community Corrections: Panacea, Progress or Pretence." In *The Power to Punish: Contemporary Penal and Social Analysis*, edited by David Garland and Peter Young, 146-65. London: HEB, 1983.

Shaplen, Robert. *Towards the Wellbeing of Mankind: Fifty Years of the Rockefeller Foundation*. London: Hutchinson, 1964.

Sigerist, Henry E. *Saskatchewan Health Services Survey Commission*. Regina: King's Printer, 1944.

Silzer, Kent. "Saskatchewan's Population — 1976 to 2001: An Examination of Anticipated Changes with Particular Reference to the Demand for Mental Health Services." Regina: Department of Public Health, Psychiatric Services Branch, 1981.

Skultans, Vieda. *English Madness: Ideas on Insanity, 1580-1890*. London: Routledge and Kegan Paul, 1979.

Smith, Colin M. "Crisis and Aftermath: Community Psychiatry in Saskatchewan, 1963-69." *Canadian Psychiatric Association Journal* 16 (1971): 65-76.

Smith, C.M., and McKerracher, D.G. "The Comprehensive Psychiatric Unit in the General Hospital." *American Journal of Psychiatry* 121 (1964): 52-57.

________. "The Family Doctor in a Program of Comprehensive Psychiatric Care." In *New Aspects of the Mental Health Service*, edited by Hugh Lionel Freeman and James Farndale, 237-45. Oxford: Pergammon Press, 1967.

Smith, David. *Prairie Liberalism: The Liberal Party in Saskatchewan 1905-7*. Toronto: University of Toronto Press, 1975.

Smucker, Joseph. *Industrialization in Canada*. Scarborough, Ontario: Prentice-Hall, Inc., 1980.

Spero, Moshe H. "Thoughts on Computerized Psychotherapy." *Psychiatry* 41 (1978): 279-88.

Spitzer, R., and Endicott, J. "DIAGNO: A Computer Program for Psychiatric Diagnosis Utilizing Differential Diagnostic Procedure." *Archives of General Psychiatry* 18 (1968): 746-56.

________. "Computer Applications in Psychiatry." In *American Handbook of Psychiatry*. 2d ed., vol. 6, edited by S. Arieti. New York: Basic Books, 1975.

Srole, Leo; Langner, Thomas S.; Michael, Stanley T.; Kirkpatrick, Price; Opler, Marvin K.; Rennie, Thomas A.C. *Mental Health in the Metropolis*. New York: McGraw-Hill, 1962.

Stanton, Alfred H., and Schwartz, Morris S. *The Mental Hospital.* New York: Basic Books, 1954.
Statistics Canada. Census of Canada.
Statistics Canada. Consumer Price Index Cat. No.: 62-001.
Statistics Canada. Mental Health Statistics, Vol. I. Cat. No.: 83-204.
Statistics Canada. National Income and Expenditure Accounts 1926-1981.
Statistics Canada. "One of Eight: Mental Illness in Canada." 1981.
Stevenson, Gelvin. "Social Relations of Production and Consumption in the Human Service Occupations." *Monthly Review* 28 (July-August 1973): 78-87.
Storey, John. *Managerial Prerogative and the Question of Control.* London: Routledge and Kegan Paul, 1983.
Sullivan, Harry S. *Schizophrenia as a Human Process.* New York: W.W. Norton and Company, 1974.
Susser, Mervyn. *Community Psychiatry: Epidemiologic and Social Themes.* New York: Random House, 1968.
Swartz, Donald. "The Politics of Reform: Conflict and Accommodation in Canadian Health Policy." In *The Canadian State: Political Economy and Political Power,* edited by Leo Panitch, 311-43. Toronto: University of Toronto Press, 1977.
Szasz, Thomas S. *The Manufacture of Madness: A Comparative Study of the Inquisition and the Mental Health Movement.* Frogmore, St. Albans, Herts.: Paladin, 1973.
________., ed. *The Age of Madness: History of Involuntary Mental Hospitalization Presented in Selected Texts.* London: Routledge and Kegan Paul, 1975.
Taylor, Malcolm G. *Health Insurance and Canadian Public Policy: The Seven Decisions that Created the Canadian Health Insurance System.* Montreal: McGill-Queen's University Press, 1978.
Tollefson, Edwin A. "The Medicare Dispute." In *Politics in Saskatchewan,* edited by Norman Ward and Duff Spafford, 238-79. Don Mills, Ontario: Longman's Canada Ltd., 1968.
*Toronto Globe and Mail.* "Close-up on Health," 21 March 1984.
Treacher, Andy, and Baruch, Geoff. "Towards a Critical History of the Psychiatric Profession." In *Critical Psychiatry: The Politics of Mental Health,* edited by David Ingleby, 120-49. Harmondsworth: Penguin Books, 1981.
Urry, John. *The Anatomy of Capitalist Societies: The Economy, Civil Society and the State.* London: Macmillan, 1981.

Vickery, Donald M.; Fries, J.F.; Muir Gray, J.A.; and Smail, S.A. *Take Care of Yourself.* London: George Allen and Unwin, 1979.

Walters, Vivienne. "State Capital and Labour: The Introduction of Federal Provincial Insurance for Physician Care." *The Canadian Review of Sociology and Anthropology* 19 (May 1982): 157-72.

Weinbaum, Batya, and Bridges, Amy. "The Other Side of the Paycheck: Monopoly Capital and the Structure of Consumption." *Monthly Review* 28 (July-August 1976): 88-103.

Weingust, John. "When Therapy Becomes Assult." *Toronto Globe and Mail,* 26 April 1984.

Weizenbaum, J. "ELIZA — A Computer Program for the Study of Natural Language Between Man and Machine." *Communication Association of Computing Machines* 9 (1966): 36-45.

Wilensky, Harold L. "The Professionalization of Everyone?" *The American Journal of Sociology* 70 (September 1964): 137-58.

Wood, Stephen, and Kelly, John. "Taylorism, Responsible Autonomy and Management Strategy." In *The Degradation of Work? Skill, De-skilling and the Labour Process,* edited by Stephen Wood, 74-89. London: Hutchinson, 1983.

Wright, Eric Olin. "Class Boundaries in Advanced Capitalist Societies." *New Left Review* 98 (1976): 3-43.

________. *Class, Crisis and the State.* London: NLB, 1978.

Yolles, Stanley F. "The Future of Community Psychiatry." In *An Assessment of the Community Mental Health Movement,* edited by W.E. Barton and C.J. Sanborn, 169-85. Lexington, Mass.: Lexington Books, 1977.

Young, T. Kue. "Lay-Professional Conflict in a Canadian Community Health Centre: A Case Report." *Medical Care* (1975): 889-905.

Young, Walter D. *The Anatomy of a Party: The National CCF, 1932-61.* Toronto: University of Toronto Press, 1969.

Zola, I.K. "Medicine as an Institution of Social Control." *The Sociological Review* 20 (1972): 487-504.

## 4. Interviews

Bennett, Douglas. Psychiatrist, Maudsley Hospital, London, England. Interview, 21 June 1982.

Coburn, Frank. Psychiatrist, Saskatoon, Saskatchewan. Interview, 8 September 1982.

Douglas, T.C. Former Premier and Minister of Public Health, Province of Saskatchewan. Interview, 17 December 1982.

Ford, Bill. Psychiatric Nurse, Saskatoon, Saskatchewan. Interview, 2 May 1983.

Greenough, Tim. Director, Psychological Services, North Battleford Psychiatric Centre, North Battleford, Saskatchewan. Interview, 2 March 1983.

Griffiths, Peter. Social Worker, Prince Albert Psychiatric Center, Prince Albert, Saskatchewan. Interview, 5 May 1983.

Katz, Mary Jane. Executive Director, Psychiatric Nurses' Association, Regina, Saskatchewan. Interview, 20 March 1983.

Rutherford, Glenn. Director of Social Work, Saskatoon Mental Health Clinic, Saskatoon, Saskatchewan. Interview, 10 May 1983.

## 5. Unpublished Material

Adults Working Paper: Task Force on Mental Health in Saskatchewan. Circa 1980.

Coburn, David. "Mental vs. Class Domination: Implications for Canada." Paper presented at the annual meeting of the Canadian Sociology and Anthropology Association, Vancouver, B.C., June 1983.

Coburn, David; Torrance, George M.; and Kaufert, Joseph M. "Medical Dominance in Canada in Historical Perspective: The Rise and Fall of Medicine?" Revised version of paper presented at the annual meeting of the Canadian Sociology and Anthropology Association, Halifax, N.S., May 1981.

Commission into Affairs and Administration of Saskatchewan Hospital North Battleford. Minutes of Evidence and Proceedings, 17 and 18 January 1946.

"Mental Hygiene Survey of Saskatchewan, 1920." *Sessional Paper No. 5*, Session 1921-22.

"The Report of the Ad Hoc Committee on the Resettlement of Mental Hospital Patients." Submitted to the Minister of Public Health, Province of Saskatchewan, 27 June 1966.

"Report on the Provincial Mental Hospitals of Saskatchewan." Central Inspection Board, American Psychiatric Association, September 1950.

Rutherford, Glenn. Saskatoon, Saskatchewan. Personal Files.

# Proper Name Index